# Notable Medical Books

## From the Lilly Library Indiana University

The Lilly Research Laboratories
Indianapolis, Indiana

Prepared by

**William R. LeFanu**
Emeritus Librarian, Royal College of Surgeons
of England, London

Edited by

**S. O. Waife, M.D., F.A.C.P.**
Director, Medical Services Division

**Elizabeth McCain and Ruth Weber**
Medical Science Writers, Medical Services Division

**Charles E. Hammond**
Senior Art Director

Published by

The Lilly Research Laboratories
Indianapolis, Indiana

# Contents

# Notable Medical Collections

The collecting of books is nearly as ancient a pursuit as the writing of them. The great manuscript libraries of the Greco-Roman world at Alexandria, Pergamum, and Rome (300 B.C.-A.D. 600) held many medical books, and their tradition continued at Byzantium for nearly a thousand years. At the height of Arabic culture (A.D. 800-1200), Greek medical texts were gathered and translated for the libraries of Baghdad and Bukhara in the East and Córdoba in Spain. A few places in Europe, such as Salerno in southern Italy and Chartres in northern France, were centers of medical learning in the Middle Ages, and surviving catalogues and books show that other monastic libraries possessed many medical texts, including translations from the Greek and Arabic physicians.

Books were gathered by the medical faculties of the new universities in Italy and in Paris before the end of the fourteenth century; with the spread of printing a hundred years later, it became possible for private individuals at last to possess more than a few books. There are records of physicians in the sixteenth century who owned two or three hundred volumes. Many such private collections are known only from their catalogues; others passed intact into college or university libraries. Sir Hans Sloane (1660-1753), a London physician and an insatiable collector, amassed a splendid medical library, which he made freely available to his colleagues; his collection and library were the nucleus of the British Museum. The comparable holdings of Dr. Richard Mead (1673-1754) were scattered through an unparalleled sale that lasted for twenty-eight days. Dr. William Hunter (1718-1783), the great anatomist and obstetrician, bequeathed his library to the University of Glasgow; it includes a wide-ranging collection of rare medical editions. This pattern of dispersal and preservation was repeated in other countries. In Italy, the famous physician Giovanni Maria Lancisi (1654-1720) dedicated his library to the use of the public, as he recorded on the title page of his edition of Eustachius's *Tabulae Anatomicae* in 1714; this collection is still intact at the San Spirito Hospital in Rome. In Germany, the University of Erlangen owns the huge library of the eminent physician and botanist, C. J. Trew (1695-1769). In our own time, Dr. Erik Waller (1875-1955), a Swedish surgeon, presented his large collection, notable for its rarities, to the University of Uppsala.

The library of Dr. J. F. Payne (1840-1910), a London physician and scholar, was bought by Henry Wellcome, developer of a prominent pharmaceutical firm and an obsessive collector, who left his wealth and multiple collections to found the Wellcome Institute of the History of Medicine in London. Sir William Osler (1849-1919), perhaps the most famous physician of his time and equally at home in Canada, the United States, and England, bequeathed his library of some seven thousand titles to McGill University in Montreal. Osler was the first to set apart a special collection within his library of "the essential medical literature grouped about the men of the first rank, whether a great Aldine edition of Aristotle or a pamphlet of Roentgen." Inspired by Osler, three outstanding medical collectors—Arnold Klebs (1870-1943), Harvey Cushing (1869-1939), and John Fulton (1899-1960)—concentrated their collecting, each in a different period, and joined in presenting their magnificent libraries to Yale to form the Medical Historical Library.

Many other American medical libraries owe not a little of their rare book collections to individual physicians. The library of the Warren family, eminent in Boston medicine through four generations, is at Harvard, and Oliver Wendell Holmes's books passed to the Boston Medical, now the Countway, Library. The fine historical medical books gathered by Dr. LeRoy Crummer (1872-1934) were divided among the universities of Michigan and Nebraska and various other libraries. Dr. Logan Clendening (1884-1945) bequeathed his collection to the University of Kansas Medical Center, and Dr. Josiah C. Trent (1914-1948) left his rare books to form the medical library at Duke University.

Great collections have been amassed by institutions and are housed in the large and small libraries of the world, and private holdings are often enhanced by fortuitous single-volume acquisitions. The National Library of Medicine in Washington, D. C., possesses the most nearly complete collection in the world of incunabula, manuscripts, books, and journals past and current. The Countway Library, formed by the fusion of the Boston Medical and Harvard Medical School libraries, is considered the second largest in the United States and serves the medical historian, the student, and the practitioner. Impressive collections exist in the British Museum, the Vatican, the Bibliothèque de la Faculté de Médecine in Paris, and Uppsala University in Sweden. Many other notable libraries are too numerous to list.

The Lilly Library at Indiana University holds some of the most important of these historical medical books—those of the late J. K. Lilly, Jr. His collection, small in size and yet highly selective, is particularly notable for its remarkable range of the most influential early editions from the classical period to modern times.

*William R. LeFanu*

# The Lilly Library

## THE RARE BOOK COLLECTION AT INDIANA UNIVERSITY

Josiah Kirby Lilly, Jr., a grandson of the founder of Eli Lilly and Company and former president and chairman of the board of that company, was a most unusual and versatile collector. He was so shy and retiring in his hobbies that none but a few friends were aware of the wide range of his interests and expertise. His collection of American gold coins, for example, was the most complete in the world and after his death in 1966 was acquired by the Smithsonian Institution. Equally outstanding were his collections of stamps and miniature soldiers.

To this very private person, however, his first collecting love was books. He assembled some 20,000 items (books, manuscripts, and documents) of English, American, and Continental literature, history, and science; Greek and Latin classics; Americana; and, most notably, rare treasures recording the history of medicine. When, in 1956, Mr. Lilly made his varied collections available to scholars and historians by presenting them to Indiana University, rare book experts assessed them as one of the largest and most valuable gifts of that kind ever made to an American university. This was the genesis of the distinguished Lilly Library of rare books at Indiana University. Named, at Mr. Lilly's request, not for him but for his family, the library was dedicated and opened to the public in 1960.

The Lilly rarities attracted others, including the medical collection of Dr. Edgar F. Kiser, of Indianapolis. Even with the addition of Dr. Kiser's books, however, the medical collection at the Lilly Library, consisting of some fifteen hundred volumes, remains only a small portion of the library's more than 300,000 printed works and more than 3,000,000 manuscripts. It will probably remain a highly selective group of representative works in the history of medicine, in the tradition of Mr. Lilly's discriminating method of collecting. Like many of the other small and distinguished collections housed at the Lilly Library, it has an unusually large proportion of pieces of great rarity and value.

Other historic holdings acquired by the Lilly Library include the Bernardo Mendel collection of Latin Americana, detailing the discovery, exploration, and colonization of the western world; the C. L. Ricketts collection of medieval manuscripts, from the seventh century onward; the Poole collection of early printing; the Ellison collection of Western Americana, containing overland narratives and other materials pertaining to the great westward movement from the Mississippi to the Pacific; the Oakleaf collection of Abraham Lincoln; the Watkins Wordsworth Library; and the War of 1812 collection. Among the twentieth-century materials are the papers and libraries of Upton Sinclair, Max Eastman, and Louis Untermeyer.

Mr. Lilly's manner of collecting was methodical and challenging. He preferred to seek out items from a selective list rather than randomly acquire whatever became available. Before World War II, his collecting interests were primarily literary. He purchased little during the war, and when he resumed in 1945, his interests had broadened. Desiring to specialize only in books that had had an important influence on the progress of mankind, he turned naturally to the field of medicine, the profession his family had served since 1876, when his grandfather, Colonel Eli Lilly, started the pharmaceutical firm.

Since no suitable list of medical books existed, he characteristically set about having one created. Past experience had taught him that there could be pitfalls in such a method. He had once asked a well-known bookdealer to prepare for him a list of significant works on a specific subject, only to learn subsequently that most of the editions recommended already reposed on the dealer's shelves.

After much consideration, William R. LeFanu, librarian of the Royal College of Surgeons of England and distinguished medical historian, was asked to draw up the list.

LeFanu's list of *Two Hundred Key Books in the History of Medicine and Surgery,* compiled with consideration only for the historical importance of the items and not for their availability, contained many of such legendary rarity that to complete the collection would be impossible. Mr. Lilly used the list simply as a guide. If a desired volume was unobtainable, he sought another that was representative of the author's achievements. This policy has been continued by the library since Mr. Lilly's death, and many books on Mr. LeFanu's list as well as others have been added.

No account of the Lilly Library and the collection of J. K. Lilly, Jr., would be complete without a tribute to the late David A. Randall, librarian of the Lilly Library from its inception until his death in May, 1975. Before coming to Indiana University as rare books librarian in 1956, he had for twenty years been manager of the rare books department of Charles Scribner's Sons, New York, where he first became an adviser to Mr. Lilly and assisted him in acquiring books. An internationally recognized authority on literary rarities, Randall had an intimate knowledge of books and history that is exquisitely preserved for us in the quality and scholarliness of Mr. Lilly's own collections and those of the Lilly Library.

*William R. Cagle*
Acting Librarian

*Josiah Q. Bennett*
Senior Cataloger

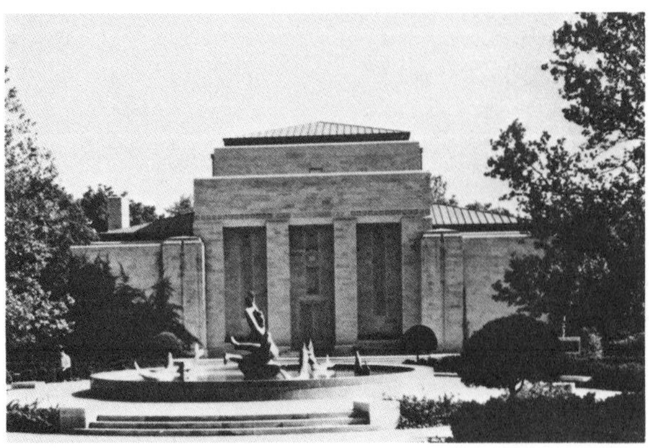

The Lilly Library at Indiana University
Bloomington, Indiana

# Introduction

One hundred and thirty medical books from the collection of J. K. Lilly, Jr., are described and illustrated in this volume; each one, when it was new, made some striking contribution to the increase of knowledge or the advance of medical care. Most of the books are first editions, often in superb condition.

This volume, then, is only a partial record of special treasures in the Lilly Library at Indiana University. It does not aim to be a full survey of medical literature, still less a history of medicine. It samples great discoveries as recorded by those who made them. The history of medicine is preserved in the written word, but books are not mere impersonal accounts. They carry the mark of their authors' character and personality. Therefore, an attempt has been made to include here a brief account of each author's life and his other work and to provide a historical framework for the contribution he made to medical knowledge.

The age of an author when he wrote his influential work is often noted, for it is remarkable how many noteworthy scientific contributions were made by men in their twenties and thirties. Laënnec was thirty-three when he introduced the stethoscope in his masterly study of thoracic disease and Vesalius only twenty-eight when he published his monumental *De Humani Corporis Fabrica,* and they were not exceptional. On the other hand, Morgagni waited until he was seventy-nine to publish his encyclopedic collection of pathologic reports.

The illustrations that occupy one-half of this volume lend an element of personality and humanity to the stark records of fact. They are man-made creations endowed, as Milton said, "with a life beyond life"; often they are beautiful products of the engraver's and printer's art. Most of the illustrations are taken directly from the book described. In some instances, when the book contains no artwork or the illustrations lack graphic interest if lifted out of context, appropriate illustrations have been selected from other sources.

*Notable Medical Books* is a tribute to the scholarship and generosity of J. K. Lilly, Jr., who was personally responsible for collecting works of primary significance for the story of medicine and who presented his acquisitions to Indiana University to attract others—as he had been attracted—to study and appreciation of the past.

Special thanks must be extended to James G. Armstrong, M.D., for research and editorial assistance in the preparation of this book and to Dean Timmerman for photographing many of the illustrations. The enthusiasm and helpfulness of Josiah Q. Bennett, senior cataloger of the Lilly Library, are greatly appreciated and gratefully acknowledged.

*S. O. Waife, M.D.*

For out of olde feldes, as men ſayth
Cōmeth al this newe corne fro yere to yere
And out of olde bokes, in good fayth
Cōmeth all this newe ſcience that men lere

Facsimile of lines from *The Workes of Geffray Chaucer Newlye Printed* (London, 1542) in the Lilly Library collection of rare books.

# Notable Medical Books

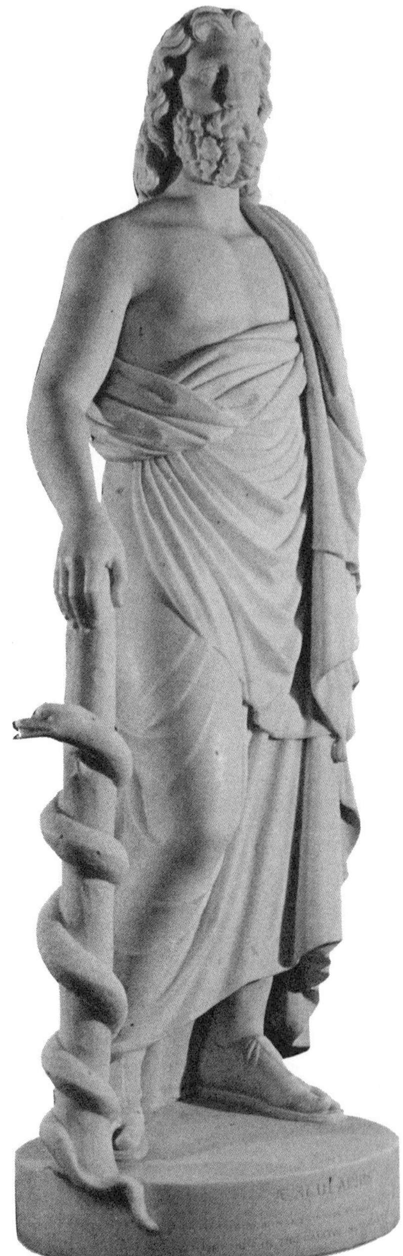

# Hippocrates

## APHORISMS

Hippocrates (460-375 B.C.) was born on the Greek island of Cos, site of a temple of Aesculapius (Asklepios), the Greek god of medicine. According to the ancient biographers, his father, a teacher of medicine, provided him with his first training in the healing arts. Later, Hippocrates studied in Athens and then gained wide experience from practicing in cities throughout Macedonia, Thessaly, and Thrace. The writings attributed to him (though undoubtedly composed by many authors over a long period of time) were assembled two hundred years after his death.

Long before the day of Hippocrates, followers of Aesculapius (mortal, god, and myth all in one) had taken the practice of medicine into the temples. Disease and its cure were associated with the wrath of the gods, divine miracles, and the interpretation and control of dreams. Hippocrates taught that disease is a physical disturbance attributable to or resulting in disorders in the body fluids. To detect these changes, Hippocrates and his followers recommended a careful history and a complete physical examination, with study of the patient by all the physician's senses.

Although Hippocrates paid homage to the past (the Hippocratic oath invokes Apollo, Aesculapius, Panacea, and "all the gods and goddesses"), it is to him that medicine owes the beginning of clinical observation and rational study of the body.

Whereas other physicians concealed their errors, Hippocrates advocated learning from one's mistakes by frankly examining them and seeking their causes. His honesty, high ideals, and deep respect for his patients set Hippocrates apart from all earlier physicians. He has rightly come to be regarded as the "Father of Medicine," largely because he established the first rational school of medicine.

The "Aphorisms" are the best known of the Hippocratic writings. The first aphorism has become a universal proverb: *Vita brevis: ars longo: occasio praeceps: experimentum fallax: iudicium difficile est* (life is short, art long, opportunity fleeting, experiment dangerous, decision difficult). The rest of the aphorisms are more technical and record precise clinical observations only occasionally modified by traditional beliefs.

In this book published in Florence in 1494, the aphorisms have accompanying notes by the translator, Lorenzo Lorenzini, and then follows Galen's commentary, similarly translated from Greek into Latin. The handsome volume in beautiful Florentine type, now a treasured rarity, thus includes the two most famous names in Greco-Roman medicine: Hippocrates, the earliest truly scientific physician, and Galen, the Greek from Pergamum, who practiced in Rome around A.D. 160 to 190, nearly six centuries after Hippocrates. Galen was considered the absolute master of medical knowledge for fifteen hundred years.

Hippocrates of Cos. *Hippocratis Medici Sententiarum Particula Prima Interprete Laurentio Laurentiano Florentino* [*Aphorismoi*]. Florence, 16 Oct., 1494.

This statue of Aesculapius, a copy of one found in Nero's palace at Antium, was commissioned by J. K. Lilly, Sr., in 1911. Carved of Carrara marble in the Gazzeri studios of Rome, it graces the research headquarters of Eli Lilly and Company in Indianapolis. The original is in the Capitoline Museum in Rome.

anguſtam intelligenciam legis acceperat &
ꝑ anguſtam voluntatem ꝑdicacionis omnia
īfirmiter ꝑdicauit. ſi aūt terrena ſapienter
ac dilig̃eter reſpiciam⁹ ſpiritaliter ac miſti
ce intelligenda ſūt. Item alio modo chor⁹ cō
cordia eſt caritatis. vbi & ſupra. laudate eū
in timpano & choro: & in aliā partem. vt in
hieremia. verſus eſt in luctū chorus noſter:
& alibi & organum meum in vocem flenciū
Cymbalum acitabula quedā ſūt que ꝑcuſſa
inuicem ſe tangunt. & faciunt ſonum. dicta
autem cymbala quia cum ballemacia ſimꝉ ꝑ
cuciunt̄ cū enī greci dicūt cībala ballemacia
de q̄ ī pſalmo ſcriptū eſt. laudate eū ī cimba
lis bene ſonantibus. Cymbala bene ſonancia
labia noſtra debemus accipere. que non ī me
merito inter muſica inſtrumenta poſita ſūt.
quia & ſimilitudo quedā eſt cymbalorū. &
per ea voces humane armoniam reddere ſu-
auiſſimā comprobantur. Armonia eſt enim
diuerſarū rerum ī vnam conueniēciā redac
ta copulacio. qđ & ī voce humana cōſtat ac
cidere. quando & tempora ipſa & ſillabe in
vnam vocis concordiā perducūtur. ſiſtrū ab
inuentrice vocatum: yſis enim regina egyp
ciorum id genus inueniſſe probatur. Iuue-
nalis yſis & irato feriat mea lumina ſiſtro.
inde & hoc mulieres percuciunt eo quod in
uentrix huius generis mulier fuit. vnde &
apud amazonas ſiſtro ad bellum feminarum
exercitus vocabatur. Tintinnabulū de ſono
vocis nomen habet. ſicut & plauſus manuū.
ſtridor valuarū. Simphonia vulgo appellat̄
lignum cauū ex vtraq; parte pelle extenta
quā virgulis hinc & inde muſici feriunt. fit
q; ī ea ex concordia grauis & acuti ſuauiſſi-
mus cantus.

¶ De medicina. v.

Medicina eſt que corporis vel tuetur.
vel reſtaurat ſalutem. cuius materia
verſatur in morbis vel vulneribus.
Ad hanc itaq; pertinēt non ea tantū que ars
eorum exhibet. qui proprie medici nominan
tur: ſed eciam cibus & potus tegmen & te-
gumen: defenſio deniq; omnis atq; municō q̄
ſanum corp⁹ aduerſus externos ictus. caſ⁹q;
ſeruatur. Nomen aūt medicine a modo id ē
temperamento īpoſitū eſtimatur. Nam ī ea
multū contriſtatur natura mediocriter aūt
gaudet: vnde & qui pigmenta & antidota
ſatis vel aſſidue biberint vexantur. Immode
ratio enim omnis non ſalutem ſed periculum
affert. Medicine aūt artis auctor ac reptor
apud grecos perhibetur apollo: hanc filius
eius aſcolapius laude vel opere ampliauit. ſ
poſtq; fulminis ictu aſcolapius interiit. īter
dicta fertur medendi cura. & ars ſimul cum
auctore defecit. latuitq; per annos pene quī
gentos vſq; ad tempus artarxerſis regii per
ſarum. tunc eam reuocauit in lucem ypo-
cras a ſclepio patre geīt⁹ ī inſula choo. Sani
tas eſt integritas corporis & temperācia. ex
calido & humido quod eſt ſanguis. vnde &
ſanitas dicta eſt quaſi ſanguinis ſtatus: mor
bi generali vocabulo omnes paſſiones corpo
ris continentur: quod inde veteres morbum
nomīauerūt vt ipſa appellacōe mortis vim
que ex eo naſcitur demonſtrarēt. Inter ſani
tatem autem & morbum media eſt curacō:
que niſi morbo congruat non perducit ad ſa
nitatem. Morbi omnes ex quatuor naſcūtur
humoribus id eſt ex ſanguine & felle melan
colia & flegmate. ex ipſis enim reguntur ſa
ni ex ipſis leduntur infirmi. Dum enim am
plius extra curſū nature creuerūt. egritudi
nes faciūt: ſicut aūt quatuor ſūt elementa.
ſic & iiii. humores. & vnuſquiſq; humor ſu
um elementum imitatur: ſanguis aerem. co
lera ignem: melancolia terrā: flegma aquā
& ſunt quatuor humores ſicut elementa que
conſeruāt corpora noſtra. Sanguis ex greca
ethimologia vocabulum ſūpſit quod vege-
tet. & ſuſtentet & viuat. Colera greci vo-
cauerunt q; vnius diei ſpacio terminetur. vñ
& colera id eſt fellicula nominata eſt, hoc ē
fellis effuſio. greci enim fel colen dicunt. me
lancolia dicta eo quod ſit ex nigri ſanguinis
fece admixta habundācia fellis. greci enim
melan nigrum vocāt fel autem colen appel-
lant. ſanguis latine vocatus quod ſuauis ſit:
vnde & homines quibus dominatur ſanguis
dulces & blandi ſūt: flegma autem dixerūt
quod ſit frigidum. greci enim rigorem fleg
monem appellant: ex his quatuor humorib⁹
vt diximus reguntur ſani ex ipſis ledūtur in
firmi. Dum enim amplius extra curſū natu
re creuerūt. egritudines faciūt. ex ſanguine
autem & felle acute paſſiones naſcuntur q̄s
greci oxea vocāt. flegmate vero & melanco
lia veteres cauſe ꝓcedūt. quas greci cronia
dicūt. Oxea eſt acutus morb⁹ qui aut cito
tranſit aut celerius īterficit. vt pleureſis fre
neſis: axi enim acutū apđ grecos & velocem
ſignificat. Cronia eſt prolixus corporis mor
bus qui multis temporibus remoratur vt po
dagra tiſis: cronon apud grecos tempus di
citur. Quedam paſſiones ex propriis cauſis
nomina acceperūt. febris a feruore dicta. ē
enim abundācia caloris: freneſis appellata ſi
ue ab impedimento mētis. quia greci mētē
frenas vocant. ſeu quod dentibus infrendāt
Medicine curacio ſpernenda nō eſt quia &

# Hrabanus Maurus

## ON THE FITNESS OF WORDS, OR A WORK ON EVERYTHING

Hrabanus Magnentius (776-856) was born of a noble family in Mainz at the end of the Dark Ages. He was a pupil of the famous Alcuin at Tours, where he adopted the name "Maurus" (a favorite disciple of St. Benedict). Later in life he became abbot of the Benedictine monastery of Fulda in Thuringia, Germany. Thanks to Maurus, Fulda achieved fame as a school where long-forgotten classical texts were copied, translated, and studied. Shortly before his death, Maurus became archbishop of Mainz.

Hrabanus Maurus is regarded as one of the first medieval Scholastics. The term "philosophy" was beginning to be applied to the disparate aggregate of learning that was being rediscovered from the writings of classical antiquity. Thus, the period marked a cautious beginning of the great debate between reason and religious dogma.

Maurus's universal knowledge was renowned. In German lands, he became the leader of the first renaissance of art and learning in the western world under the Emperor Charlemagne. He is now remembered chiefly for his encyclopedic dictionary, *De Sermonum Proprietate* (c. 800), which contains one short chapter on medicine, then considered an element of philosophy. Six hundred years later, it was the first encyclopedia to be printed. It consists of twenty-two "books," or essays, combining some classical lore, moralizing, and theological doctrine, on a variety of topics. There are books on man and animals; countries and the world; water and the sea; earth and its composition; magic; stones and metals; measures, weights, and numbers; music; and drugs. Maurus's work is bound with, and follows, *Concordantia Evangelistarum,* by Zacharius Chrysopolitanus.

The section on medicine and diseases occupies only two pages and is a sermon on the subject rather than a factual treatment. It purports to define the physician's art, health, and sickness according to the four humors. It is interspersed with numerous quotations from the Bible and contains many generalizations, such as "health is bodily integrity and temperance," "immoderation brings danger," and "debility of body is debility of mind, as we read in the Book of Leviticus." Leprosy (the main disease discussed) is called a punishment for the spiritual blindness and deafness of heresy and blasphemy.

By 1467, when the encyclopedia was printed, Maurus's ideas had become antiquated. Medicine had made great advances in the later Middle Ages and was progressing even more rapidly in the beginning renaissance of science. Nevertheless, the early printers preferred texts such as this, which were famous and traditional rather than innovative, in view no doubt of their largely clerical clientele.

Hrabanus Maurus. *De sermonum proprietate, sive Opus de universo.* Strassburg, 1467.

A page from Maurus's monumental encyclopedia, which measures seventeen by twelve inches and is over four inches thick. It has an elegant stamped doeskin binding with leather clasps; metal bosses protect the binding when the book lies open. Initial letters throughout are hand-painted red.

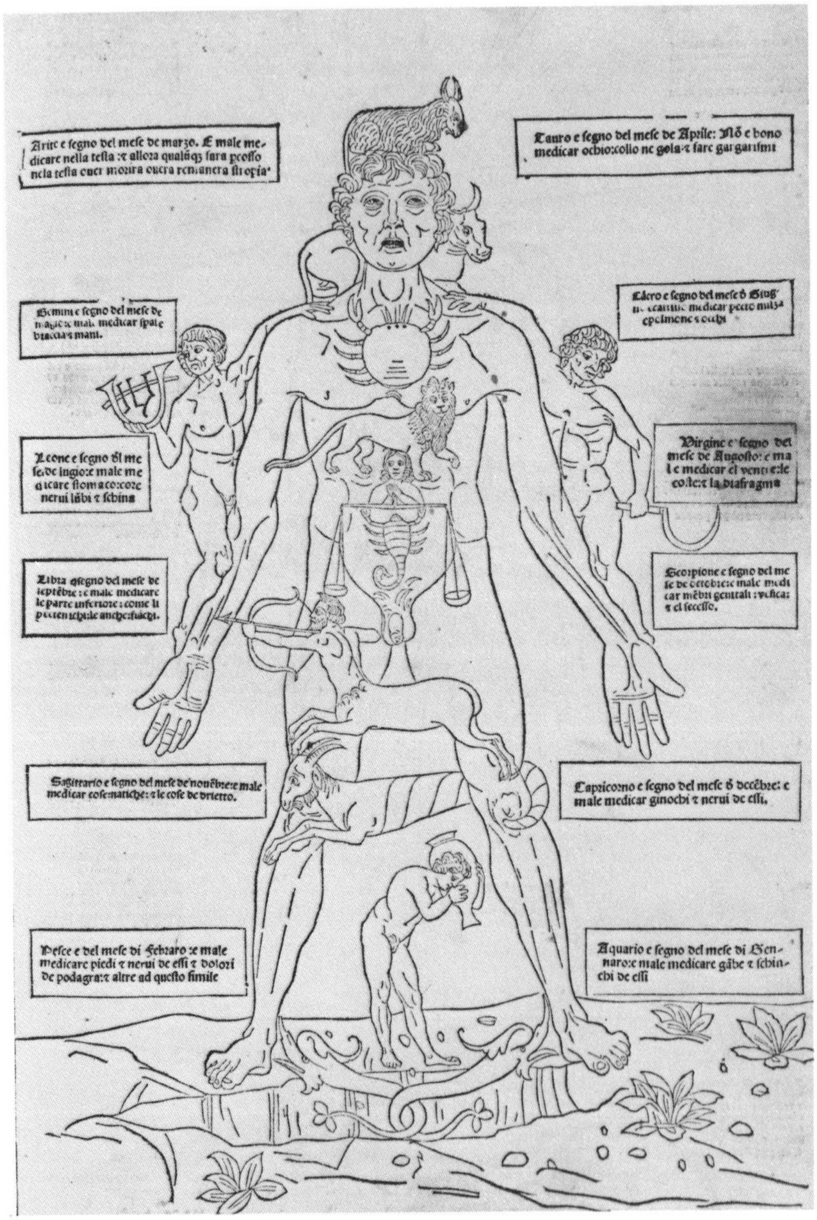
Arite e segno del mese de marzo. E male medicare nella testa: ⁊ allora qualūq3 sara percosso nela testa ouer morira ouera remanera stropia
Tauro e segno del mese de Aprile: Nō e bono medicar ochio: collo ne gola: ⁊ fare gargarismi
Gemini e segno del mese de magio: e male medicar spale braccia ⁊ mani.
Cācro e segno del mese d Giug-
Leone e segno dl mese de lugio: e male medicare stomaco: core nerui lōbi ⁊ schina
Virgine e segno del mese de Augosto: e male medicar el ventre: le coste: ⁊ la diafragma
Libra e segno del mese de septēbre: e male medicare le parte inferiore: come li pecten schiale anche: fianchi.
Scorpione e segno del mese de octobre: e male medicar mēbri genitali: vesica: ⁊ el secesso.
Sagitario e segno del mese de nouēbre: e male medicar cose: natiche: ⁊ le cose de drietto.
Capricorno e segno del mese d decēbre: e male medicar ginochi ⁊ nerui de essi.
Pesce e del mese di Febraro: e male medicare piedi ⁊ nerui de essi ⁊ dolori de podagra: ⁊ altre ad questo simile
Aquario e segno del mese di Gennaro: e male medicare gābe ⁊ schinchi de essi

# Johannes de Ketham

## TRACTS ON MEDICINE

This "little gathering" *(Fasciculus Medicinae)* of short treatises has been called "the first worthy medical text to be printed." Actually, it perpetuates traditional lore but exhibits better than any other book the conditions from which modern medicine arose.

"Johannes de Ketham" is the Latinized form of the name of Johann von Kircheim (?-1490?), who may have written these short guides for his students while he was a professor of medicine and surgery in Venice. Originally published in 1491 in Latin, this later edition is the first translation into the vernacular (Italian).

The treatises contain advice to physicians on conduct in medical practice, prognosis from urine, and techniques of bloodletting, obstetrics, and wound treatment as well as descriptions of common diseases. A paper by Pietro da Tussignano, on precautions against plague, has been included.

Each section of the book carries a traditional diagram: urine glasses arranged in a circle, relating to the influence of the four humors; a male figure marked with the sites for bloodletting; and drawings showing the parts of the body governed by constellations of the zodiac (illustrated) or afflicted by localized diseases ranging from quinsy to gout or by wounds made with various weapons. The treatise on obstetrics originally had a formalized drawing of a half-crouching pregnant woman *(Gravida)*. It was redrawn for later editions and was the first printed representation of the pelvic organs with a fetus *in utero,* as though seen at dissection. This revision may have been influenced by Leonardo da Vinci's anatomic drawings. The book was translated and reprinted several times in the next thirty years.

Four new full-page illustrations were added in the Italian translation of 1493. Of majestic simplicity, these outline wood engravings have been attributed to artists of the school of Gentile Bellini. They are scenes of medical practice in a setting of fifteenth-century Venice. One is of a physician at his desk, with a man, an old woman, and a boy waiting to consult him. Another shows a consultation of five long-robed doctors attended by two youths carrying urine glasses. To illustrate the treatise on the plague, there is a sickroom where a physician holds a sponge over his nose and mouth as he feels a plague patient's pulse. The final picture depicts an anatomy lesson. The professor lectures while the demonstrator prepares to point out to a small audience the organs exposed by the bare-armed dissector.

These formalized pictures and the text they illustrate provide the reader with some understanding of the haughty and rigid attitudes that must have prevailed during the fifteenth century among those who practiced medicine, surgery, and obstetrics. Flasks containing urine, for instance, were not touched by physicians but only by their assistants. The possession and use of books, these pictures seem to show, set medical practitioners apart from common men, who patiently awaited attention while the physician consulted his texts.

Johannes de Ketham. *In comincia el dignissimo Fasiculo* [*sic*] *de Medicina in Volgare. . . .* Venice, 5 Feb., 1493/4.

Woodcut of a "zodiac mannikin."
Medieval medical texts instructed physicians to consult astrologic signs and portents as indicators of prognosis and treatment.

Arm/payn abschneyden hat seyn kunst
Vertreyben sant Anthonien prunst.

Gehört auch nit eym yeden zů/
Er schick sich dann wie ich jhm thů.

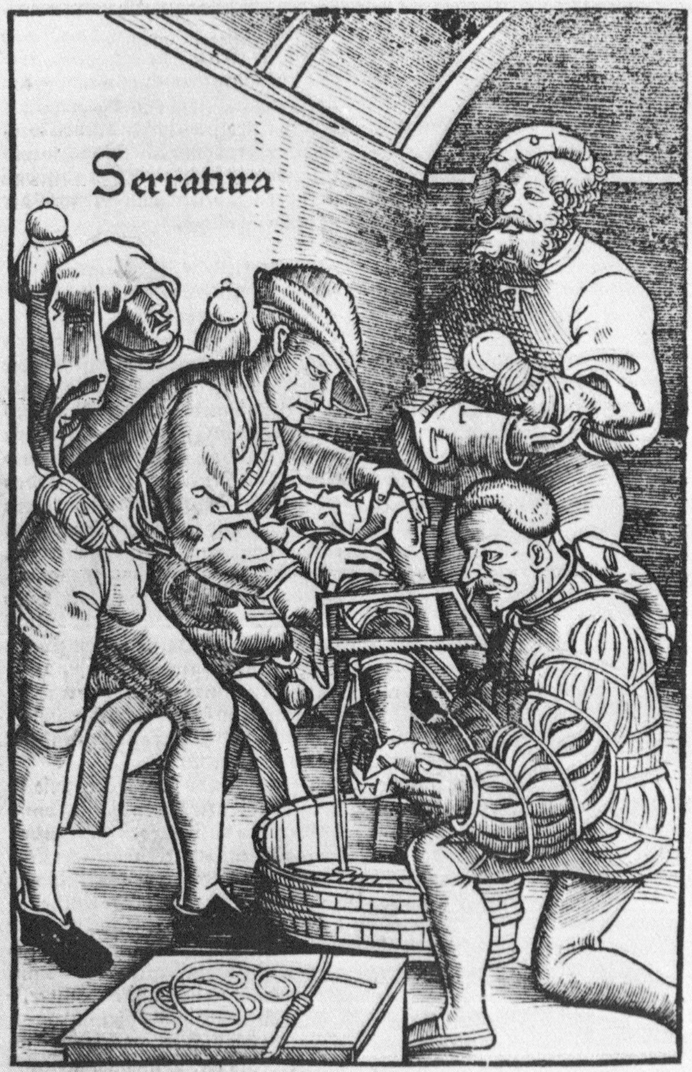

# Hans von Gersdorff

## FIELD BOOK OF WOUND SURGERY

Hans von Gersdorff, a native of Strassburg who lived around the beginning of the sixteenth century, wrote his surgery handbook on the basis of experience gained during forty years as a military surgeon. He was one of the first to discuss gunshot wounds and their treatment; unlike his contemporaries, he did not consider them to be poisonous. It was then common practice to aid removal of bullets by promoting suppuration, but von Gersdorff recommended probing for them with special instruments and then pouring hot oil into the wound. He used a tourniquet when amputating and, instead of cauterizing, checked hemorrhage with a styptic composed of vitriol, lime, alum, aloes, and nutgalls. Finally, he enclosed the stump in "the bladder of a bull, ox, or hog."

His text is divided into four tracts. The first contains a summary of human anatomy based on old Arabic writings and the *Chirurgia Magna* of Guy de Chauliac, physician to several of the fourteenth-century Avignon popes. Such knowledge of anatomy was needed by military surgeons, who had to cope with the extensive tissue and bone damage caused by the low-velocity firearms of the day.

Although most of the second tract deals with surgical treatment of wounds, two of its chapters concern materia medica, including sedatives and analgesics. One preparation is a mixture of aromatic plant juices that, when inhaled preoperatively from a sponge, was said to produce sleep. Another herbal mixture was used following surgery to rouse the patient. The lists of many simples and composita used at the time make this book a forerunner of the dispensatory.

The third tract concerns leprosy. Although most of the text consists of prescriptions employed in its treatment, von Gersdorff did consider the relative merits of cautery in certain cases.

The concluding tract is composed of three Latin-German glossaries—one of anatomic terms, one of diseases, and one of simples (plant, animal, and mineral). Since many medicaments of the time had three or more different Latin names as well as more than one German synonym, this listing of equivalent terms must have filled a need.

The book was so popular that it went through twelve German editions between 1517 and 1606, was translated into Latin and Dutch, and was widely quoted, referred to, and plagiarized in subsequent medical texts. Eminently practical in its instructions on the care and treatment of the wounded, it had admirably graphic wood engravings. The twenty-seven plates show clear diagrams of instruments and prostheses, such as a mechanical iron hand, in addition to scenes of operations, including the first printed picture of an amputation.

Hans von Gersdorff. *Feldtbüch der Wundtartzney.* Strassburg, 1517.

The first published picture of an amputation. The man in the background cradles his stump encased in the bladder of a butchered animal.

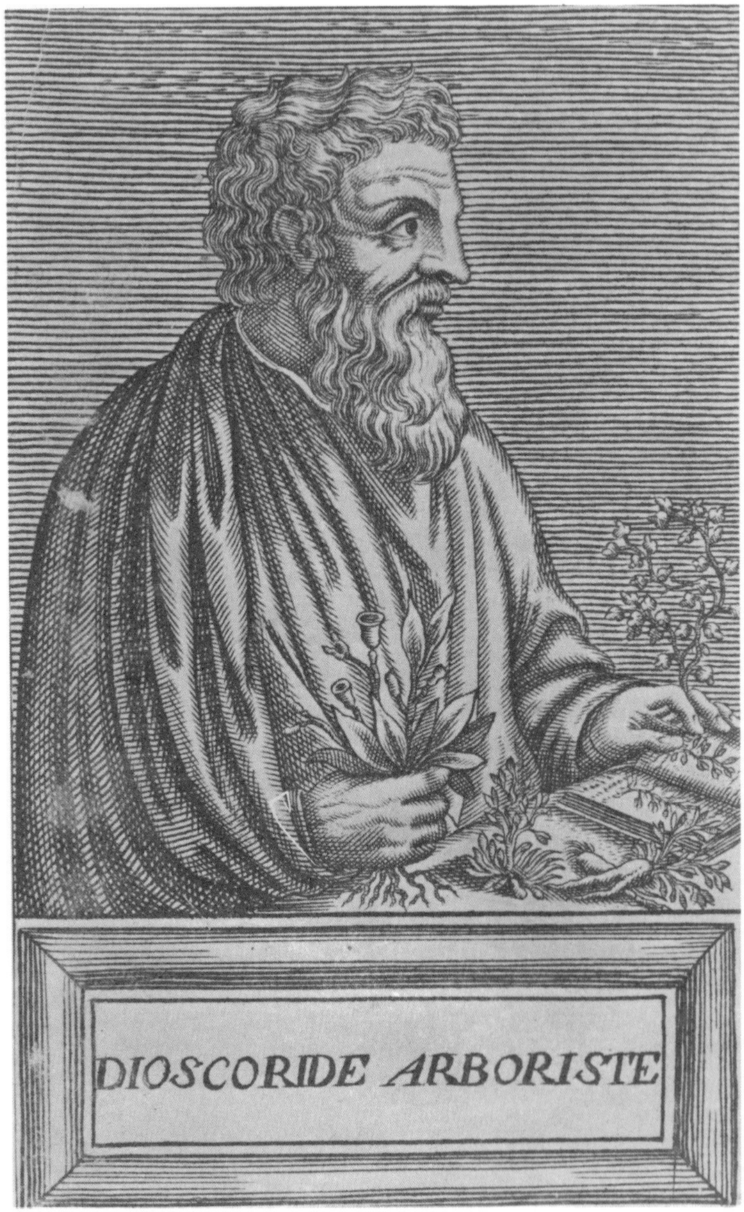
DIOSCORIDE ARBORISTE

# Dioscorides

## MATERIA MEDICA

For fifteen hundred years, the writings of Dioscorides, a Greek physician and surgeon of the first century who served in Nero's army, were regarded as the ultimate authority on materia medica. Dioscorides described more than six hundred plants and plant principles encountered during his army service in the lands around the eastern end of the Mediterranean. The compendium, written in Greek, noted the plants' botanic characteristics and their real or traditional medical properties. Almost one hundred of these plants still serve a pharmaceutical purpose today.

Although opium had been in use for centuries, Dioscorides was the first to write about its virtues, to point out its great benefits in the relief of pain, insomnia, and chronic cough, and to note its dangerous effects, particularly those of overdose. He was also the first to describe the medicinal usefulness of aloes, ammoniac, aconite, and ginger. He invented the name *"hydrargyrum"* (fluid silver) for mercury; he recommended iron for uterine hemorrhage and aspidium for tapeworm infestation; and he was the first to state the need for testing the purity of drugs. Among the methods he advised for detecting adulteration were drug solubility, specific gravity, and reaction to ignition.

Dioscorides also dealt with animal and mineral products useful in medicine and discussed diet and wines. He suggested mandragora wine for insomnia and pain and specifically for analgesia during surgery. An astute observer, Dioscorides recognized family relationships between plants seventeen centuries before Linnaeus.

By the sixth century, the poorly organized compendium had been rearranged alphabetically, illustrations of plants had been added, and a Latin translation had been made. The book was translated during the following centuries into most of the languages of the modern and ancient world, including Arabic in the ninth century. The first printed edition, a Latin version, appeared in Italy in 1478, and the original Greek text was published in Venice in 1499. The revival of the teachings of Dioscorides during the Renaissance laid the foundations for scientific botany and pharmacy. Unfortunately, because all plants were thought to be universally distributed, a great deal of time and ingenuity were wasted in trying to equate western flora with the plants described by Dioscorides.

Pedacius Dioscorides. *De Materia Medica, Libri Sex.* Basel, August, 1529.

Legends prevailed about the "man-shaped" mandrake root (seen lying beside the book in the picture). Said to shriek when pulled from the ground, it was used as an aphrodisiac, soporific, and anesthetic.

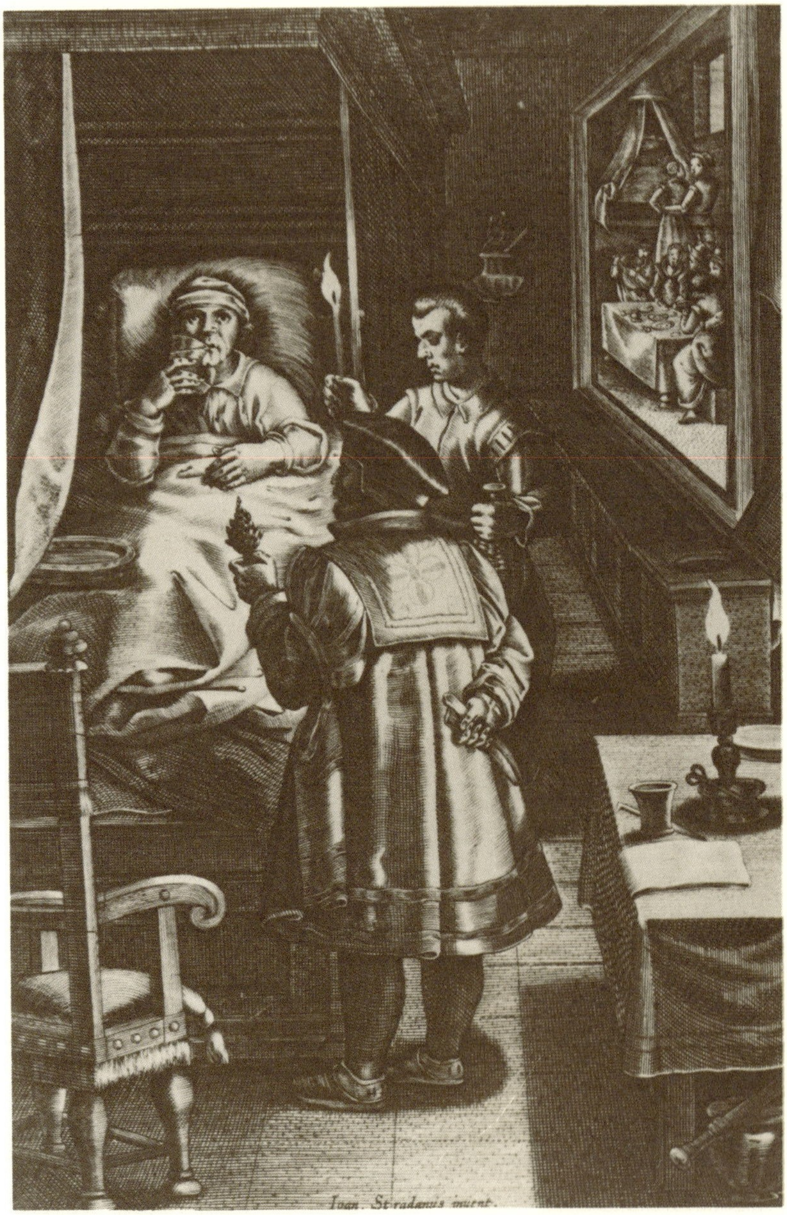
Ioan. Stradanus invent.

# Girolamo Fracastoro

## SYPHILIS and ON CONTAGION

Although Fracastoro (c. 1478-1553) made a truly original contribution to medical knowledge with his book on contagion, he is best known for the word "syphilis," a scholarly frivolity that he coined for the title of his first book.

When the "great pox," or "French disease," swept through Europe, Fracastoro, scholar as well as physician in Verona, composed a mock-heroic Latin poem, *Syphilis*, for his Venetian patron, Cardinal Pietro Bembo. The poem described the course of the disease and its treatment with mercury in the story of an imaginary shepherd, Syphilus. However, by 1525, when the poem was finished, treatment with mercury ointment was in disrepute because of its side-effects. It had been superseded by guaiacum, the "sacred wood" of the American Indian. Guaiacum was imported by Spain about 1508, and three thousand cures had been claimed for it within a decade. Fracastoro therefore added a third section to his poem, telling how Syphilus was cured of the great pox by ritual treatment with the "sacred wood." The title of the poem, *Syphilis*, soon became universally adopted as the name of the affliction.

Fracastoro had wide-ranging interests. Physics and its instruments, geology and maps, and astronomy and telescopes all benefited from his work while he continued to write poetry and practice medicine. In 1546, he published his most important medical treatise, *De Contagione*. This book consists of a short theoretical discourse on sympathy and antipathy in physics and a longer, more practical account of contagion and contagious diseases. Here, for the first time, was a clear description of the spread of disease by "*seminaria contagionum*," the seeds of infection—the suggestion of the germ theory.

*De Contagione* is arranged in three "books." The first explained the mechanism of contagion, how *seminaria* can be carried a distance, and why only some diseases are contagious. In the second book he wrote about a series of contagious diseases. Fracastoro had made careful observations; he differentiated smallpox from measles, gave the earliest precise description of typhus, and showed that tuberculosis was contagious. He discussed rabies and syphilis and dealt with the differential diagnosis of contagious skin diseases. Finally, in the third book, he outlined the treatment of diseases covered in book two and commented on the spread and control of epidemics.

Girolamo Fracastoro. *Syphilis sive Morbus Gallicus*. Verona, 1530.
——. *De Sympathia et Antipathia Rerum, Liber Unus. De Contagione et Contagiosis Morbis et Curatione, Libri III*. Venice, 1546.

A well-attended syphilitic patient, paying the price for a night of indiscretion (recalled by the painting on the wall), sips guaiacum "tea" in this engraving by Philip Gall (1570).

# Der dritt Tractat der grossen wund-artzney Doctors Paracelsi/ lernt aller thier gifft vnd bissz von aussen an beschehen/ hinzůnemen/ auch haylung der baynbrůch/ auch inn einem yegklichen brand/ nach art der handtwercksleüt/ oder nach dem stayn der berckwerck/ als wetter/ saltz sieden/ vitriolpfannen/ püchsenpulver/ vñ dergleichen võ gestandenen blůte/ vnd erfriern.

## Das Erst Capitel/ Vonn den verwündten durch die wůttenden hund/ auch von andern bisszen der hund.

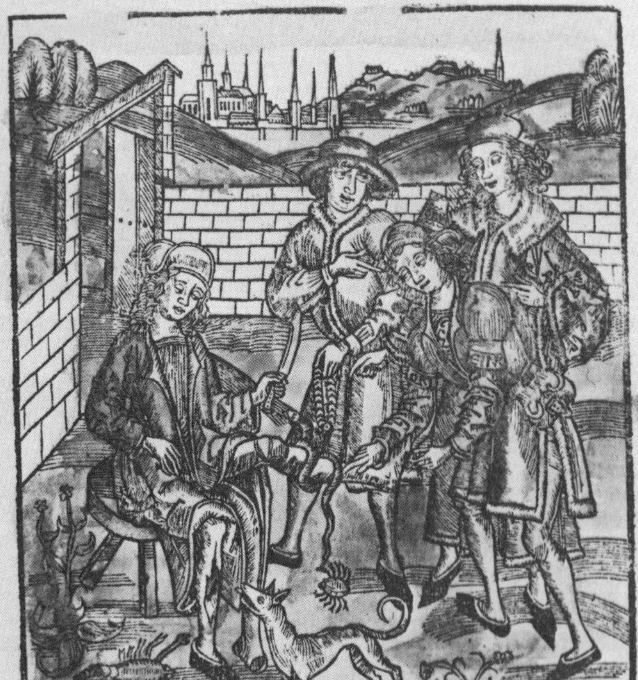

# Paracelsus

## THE GREAT SURGERY

This volatile and versatile Swiss physician, surgeon, and chemist called himself "Paracelsus," meaning "greater than Celsus," the illustrious physician of ancient Rome. Paracelsus (1493-1541) was both an academic and a rebel. After studying at Ferrara, he spent a number of years traveling throughout Europe, collecting information not only from academicians but also from alchemists, gypsies, midwives, astrologers, barbers, and executioners. In this way, he acquired a practical body of knowledge that was in many ways at odds with the traditional medical teaching of his time. Paracelsus was appointed professor of medicine at Basel in 1527 but held the position only one year. During that year, he publicly burned the "Canon" of Avicenna in a campaign to reform medical teaching, lectured in German instead of Latin, and quarreled with the authorities over fees.

The most original medical thinker of the sixteenth century, Paracelsus was perhaps the first to apply chemistry to practical medicine. He rejected the four humors of the Greeks and substituted three alchemical elements—mercury, sulfur, and salt.

Paracelsus taught that medicine could not advance solely by clinging to established ideas but that there must also be "experimentation controlled by authoritative literature." He was the first to note the association between cretinism and endemic goiter, to suggest that syphilis—or, as he called it, "French gonorrhea"—might be congenital in some cases, and to recommend the use of mercury in its treatment. However, he accepted mysticism and occultism, not omitting the astrologic influences.

His first book on surgical techniques was published in two volumes dated 1536. A pirated and unauthorized version of the first volume had been printed earlier in the same year at Ulm by Hans Varnier, who had armed himself with an imperial copyright privilege. Paracelsus justifiably defied this "copyright" and, in his preface, energetically disavowed Varnier's incomplete edition. He dealt with the complete treatment of wounds caused by piercing, shooting, burning, animal bites, bone fracture, and other injuries. Advocating sound surgical techniques, he also recognized the natural power of the body to heal.

Disputatious and loud-voiced, Paracelsus spoke in the coarse words of a peasant rather than the refined language of his academic peers. In his last thirteen years, he resumed the wandering habits of his youth, practicing medicine and surgery throughout Germany. He died at the age of forty-eight in a tavern brawl in Salzburg.

Paracelsus [Theophrastus Bombastus von Hohenheim]. *Der grossen Wundartzney*. Augsburg, 1536.

Lavishly hand-colored, this woodcut appears at the beginning of the first chapter, "About injuries caused by rabid dogs and other dog bites."

# THE CASTEL OF HELTHE,

Gathered, and made by syr Thomas Elyot knight, out of the chief authors of Phisyke, whereby euery man may knowe the state of his owne body, the preseruation of helthe, and how to instruct well his phisition in sicknes, that he be not deceyued.

M. D. XXXIX.

Jho. Twyne me iure possidet

# Sir Thomas Elyot

## THE CASTLE OF HEALTH

Sir Thomas Elyot (c. 1490-1546) was a high official at the court of King Henry VIII of England and served as the king's personal envoy to Emperor Charles V of Spain. Although his career at court began with great promise, he failed to advance beyond the knighthood granted him at the age of forty. Elyot was a humanist and an associate of Sir Thomas More, Lord Chancellor, who fell into disfavor when he opposed Henry's plan to divorce Catherine of Aragon and marry Anne Boleyn. Elyot's friendship with More, who was eventually beheaded, may have raised doubts about Elyot's own loyalty to the king.

An author and lexicographer, Elyot made a point of writing in English rather than in Latin, which was then the customary language for scholarly works, doing this to "augment our Englysshe tongue." He also enriched the language by introducing many new words in his Latin-English *Dictionary,* which was published in 1583, and in his translations of classical and foreign books. In 1531, he had gained recognition as the author of *The Boke Named the Governour,* in which he proposed measures for educating and training young men of noble birth who were expected to assume positions of authority.

Elyot's *Castel of Helthe* is one of the earliest books in the vernacular to propose a scheme for the maintenance of health. Although written by a layman, it is based on a sound knowledge of classical medicine. After an account of the four humors, Elyot discusses diets as they affect different organs, deals with foods in greater detail, and describes repletion and its relief. The last part covers topics of a more strictly medical nature—remedies for "crudity" of digestion, rheums, lassitude, seasonal diseases, the urine, and "preservations in time of pestilence." Elyot recommended marmalade made of quinces "to strengthen a weak stomach or cure a head full of vapors."

Sir Thomas Elyot. *The Castel of Helthe*. . . . London, 1539.

Its antiquity is apparent in the Lilly copy of this four-hundred-year-old rarity, with its damaged title page and a barely legible Latin inscription in the hand of an early owner.

HVMANI CORPORIS OSSIVM CAETERIS QVAS SVSTINENT PARTIBVS LIBERORVM, SVAQVE SEDE POSITORVM EX latere delineatio.

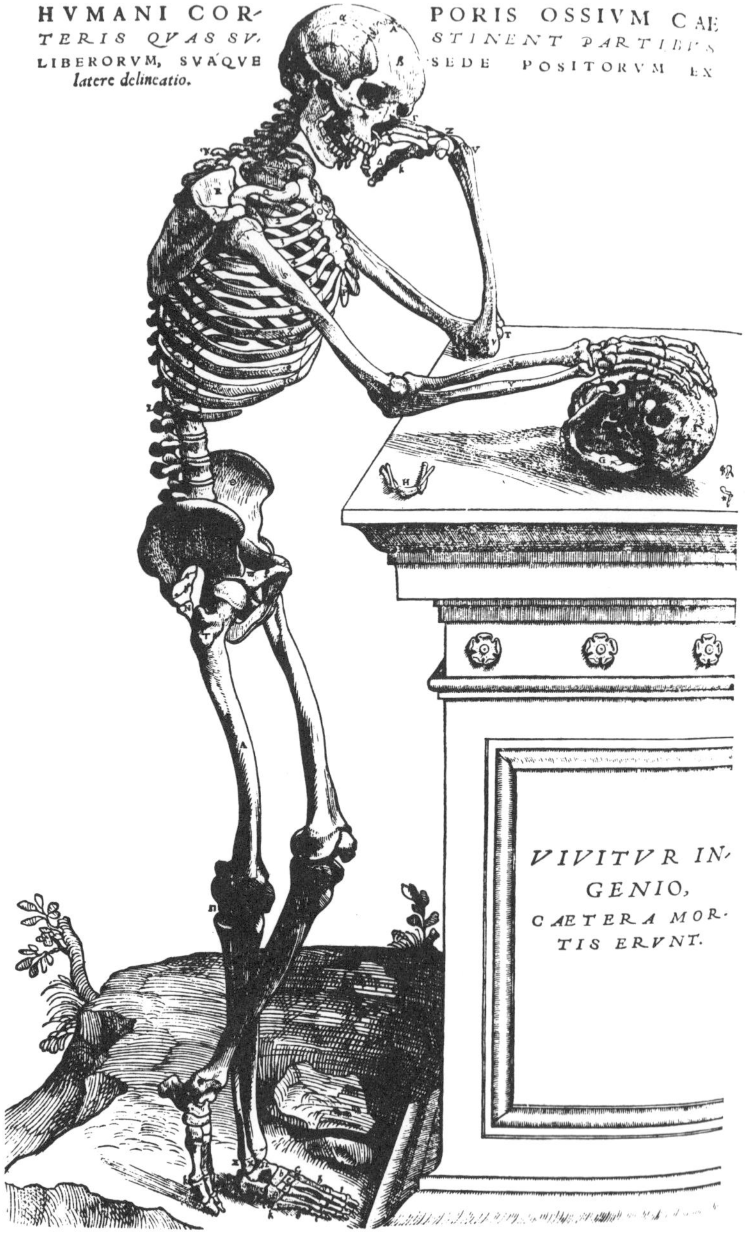

# Andreas Vesalius

## ON THE FABRIC OF THE HUMAN BODY

This magnificent volume entitled *De Humani Corporis Fabrica* successfully explores human anatomy in great detail, an area in which many other explorers had failed. Vesalius (1514-1564) was only twenty-eight when the publication appeared. He took infinite care to insure that everything about his book—paper, type, illustrations, layout, and production—was worthy of its text. The woodcuts by Jan Stephan Kalkar were innovative in that they were designed with a landscape background. Works of greater magnificence and scientific substance exist, but no other single book so successfully combines all these excellencies. Vesalius's confidence that it would be studied and his apprehension that it would be plagiarized led him, as his title page proclaims, to obtain the sponsorship and copyright protection of the three great powers of the time—the emperor, the king of France, and the Grand Council of Venice.

The seven "books" deal in turn with the bones and cartilages, the ligaments and muscles, the blood vessels, the nerves, the abdominal organs, the thoracic organs, and the brain and sense organs. There is a final chapter on vivisection and physiology. This arrangement of material according to the "systems" of the body was in itself revolutionary, for earlier works on anatomy had followed the procedure of the lecturer, who began with the most perishable tissues—the organs in the body cavities—and then continued with other parts, such as the limbs, trunk, and head.

The *Fabrica* is essentially a textbook but one most richly illustrated. Vesalius arranged for it to be published simultaneously with his *Epitome*, which has a briefer text and larger plates. The author had also provided a general atlas in his "Six Anatomic Tables" (Venice, 1538). The plates in all three volumes were the first to combine scientific accuracy with the illusion of three dimensions. The *Fabrica* is famous for its full-page skeletons, but the rest of its illustrations are almost as remarkable, if less striking. Here, for the first time, are presented accurately drawn details of organs, blood vessels, and nerves, designed and placed so as to clarify the descriptions in the text. Vesalius expressed forceful criticisms of the Galenic tradition based on animal anatomy, corroborating them from his own dissections. Some of these criticisms were his own, and some had been voiced by others during the fifty years since the time of Leonardo da Vinci. The illustrations in Vesalius's book were so accurate and clear that anatomists copied them for the next three hundred years. He set a standard for medical textbooks that has never been surpassed.

Andreas Vesalius. *De Humani Corporis Fabrica. Libri Septem.* Basel, 1543.

Anatomic excellence and artistic beauty mark the superb woodcuts of Vesalius's masterpiece.

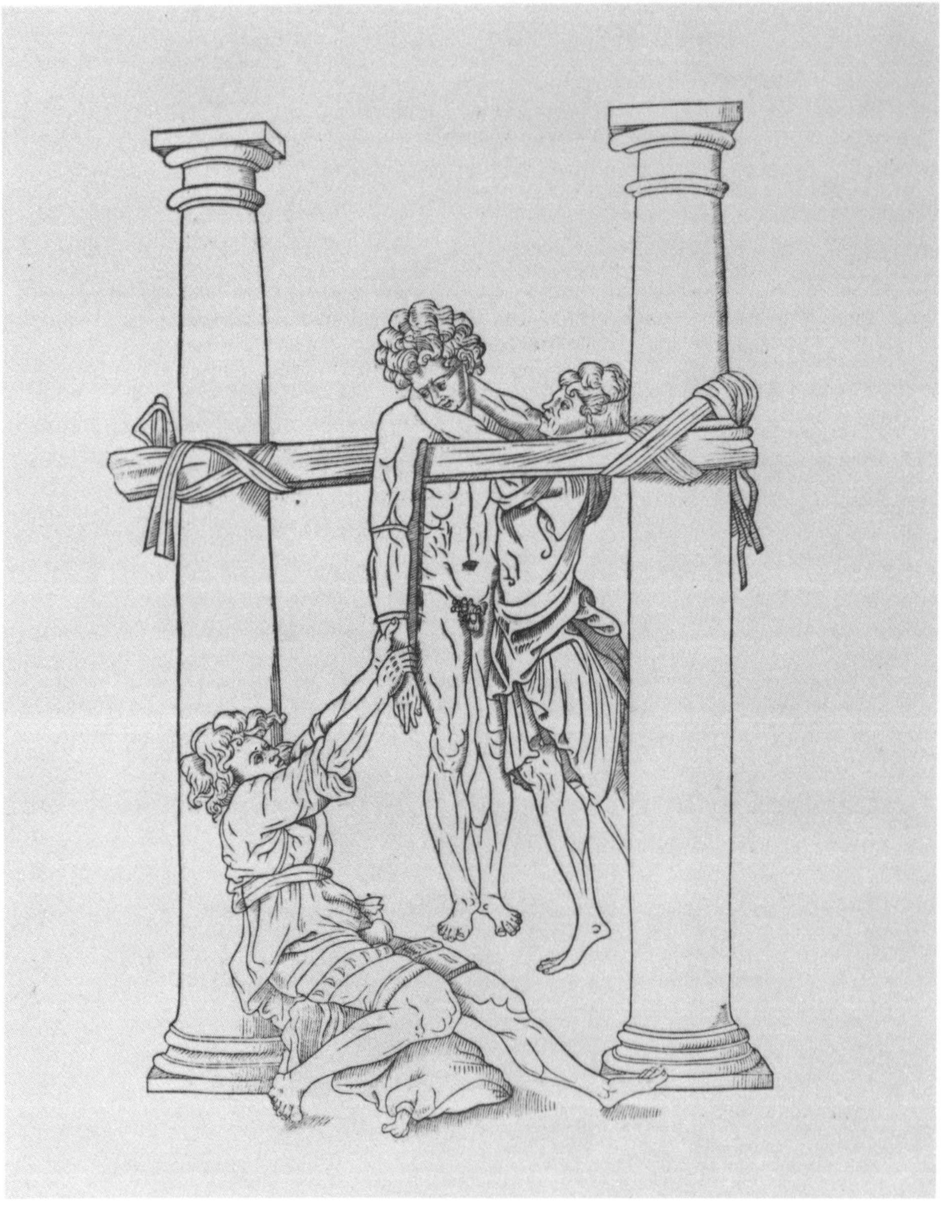

# Guido Guidi

## SURGERY

One year after the publication of Vesalius's book on anatomy, Guido Guidi (1500?-1569), an Italian physician practicing in Paris, made an outstanding contribution to the literature of surgery. When summoned to Paris at the age of thirty-four by Francis I, king of France, who wished to spread the "new learning" of the Italian Renaissance throughout his kingdom, Guidi brought with him a copy of an ancient Greek surgical manuscript as a gift for the king. Guidi's medical and artistic background enabled him to appreciate the importance of this classical book with its illustrations of the manipulative operations devised by the Greek surgeons. Francis I appointed Guidi to organize the medical teaching in his new Collège de France, and under his patronage Guidi published his own Latin translation and commentary on the ancient Greek text, with the figures redrawn by skilled Italian artists.

His book is a splendid oversize volume that has been called "the most beautiful textbook of surgery printed in the sixteenth century" with "woodcut illustrations [that] have never been equaled in this field." The full title, which may be translated as "Surgery Turned from Greek into Latin by Guido Guidi of Florence, Translator, with Some Commentaries by the Same Guidi," conceals the fact that the book provided contemporary Europeans with the best surgical treatises of the whole classical period. The text begins with the writings of Hippocrates on ulcers, fistulas, and wounds of the head and continues with Galen's commentary on Hippocrates on fractures and joints. The large, clear woodcuts reconstruct ancient apparatus, showing a surgeon and his assistants reducing a dislocated shoulder (illustrated), straightening a curved vertebral column on a special bed, and many similar procedures. These drawings were promptly copied by Ambroise Paré, the greatest surgeon of these decades, and often recopied. The book also contained Hippocratic views on the duties of a physician; Galen's on bandaging, as illustrated by more than one hundred small figures; and those of Oribasius on ligatures and mechanical aids to surgery, with more large woodcuts.

In the dedication to Francis I, Guidi wrote: "Our surgeons cannot bandage properly, or fix suitable appliances to align broken bones, or treat wounds of the head adequately, because they lack the Greek authors who excelled in developing this part of medicine." Guidi returned to Italy, where he became professor of anatomy at Pisa, but the results of his research were published only in part and long after his death. The Latin form of his name, Vidus Vidius, is commemorated in the Vidian canal of the sphenoid bone, but the true monument to his influence is his book on surgery with its excellent illustrations.

Guido Guidi [Vidus Vidius]. *Chirurgia è Graeco in Latinum conversa*. . . . Paris, 1544.

Many Renaissance textbooks were embellished by instructional yet elegant illustrations in the classical manner.

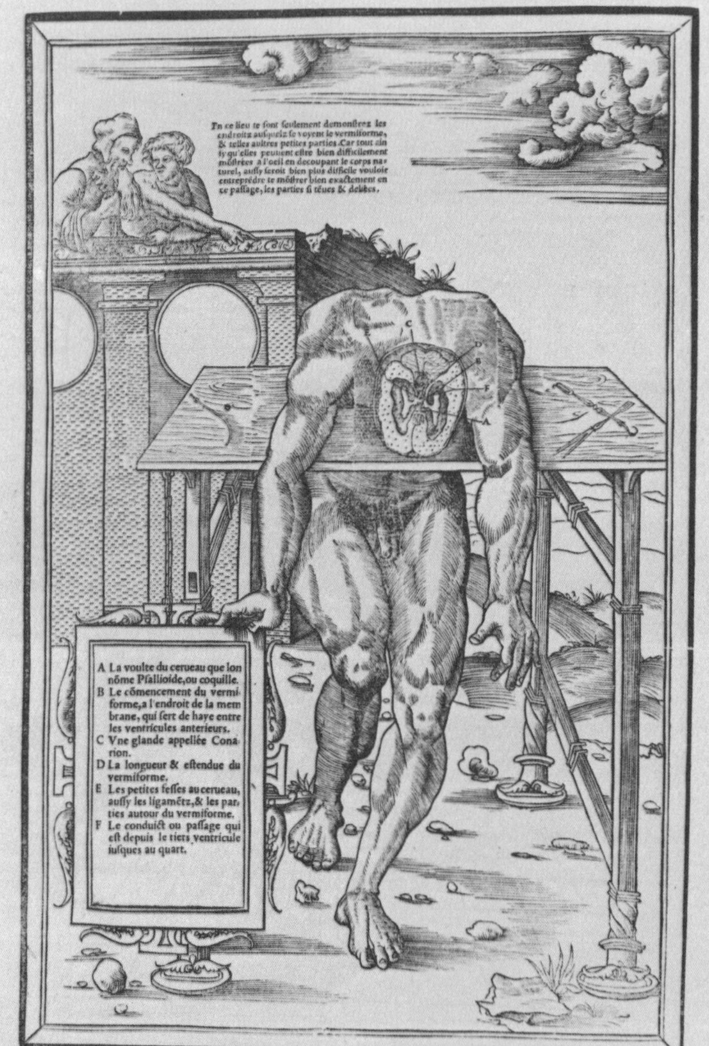
En ce lieu te sont seulement demonstrez les endroitz ausquelz se voyent le vermiforme, & telles aultres petites parties. Car tout ainsy qu'elles peuuent estre bien difficilement mõstrées a l'oeil en decoupant le corps naturel, aussy seroit bien plus difficile vouloir entreprẽdre te mõstrer bien exactement en ce passage, les parties si tẽues & delikes.
A La voulte du cerueau que lon nõme Psallioide, ou coquille.
B Le cõmencement du vermiforme, a l'endroit de la membrane, qui sert de haye entre les ventricules anterieurs.
C Vne glande appellée Conarion.
D La longueur & estendue du vermiforme.
E Les petites fesses au cerueau, aussy les ligamẽtz, & les parties autour du vermiforme.
F Le conduict ou passage qui est depuis le tiers ventricule iusques au quart.

# Charles Estienne and Estienne de la Rivière

## DISSECTION OF PARTS OF THE BODY

It is ironic that a lawsuit should have delayed publication of this book on anatomy and dissection for at least five years. As a result, when the Latin version finally appeared in 1545, it was overshadowed by Vesalius's masterpiece, *De Humani Corporis Fabrica,* which had been issued two years earlier. Vesalius may well have seen Estienne's drawings while he was working in Paris from 1533 to 1536 and may have been inspired to improve upon them. Certainly Estienne's plates, the earliest of which was dated 1530, are lower in quality (especially the skeletons) than those in Vesalius's book.

Charles Estienne (1504-1564), who belonged to a famous family of scholar-printers, began his career as a student of natural history. He turned to anatomy through his association with a surgeon, Estienne de la Rivière, and finally qualified in medicine in 1540. By that time, the text of this book on dissection had been virtually completed. Publication was then delayed, however, because La Rivière sought an injunction from the Paris courts to compel Charles Estienne to display his name on the title page as coauthor. The case dragged on for several years before La Rivière achieved his purpose.

Although the book was surpassed by Vesalius's *Fabrica,* it was not a failure. This French translation appeared a year after the original Latin version, and both editions, it has been said, are "exciting spectacles, even in the shadow of Vesalius." The text and the illustrations, moreover, reflect what was known and taught in Paris, site of the most influential medical school in northern Europe at that time.

The illustrations are of considerable artistic interest, for the authors adapted existing art forms to display their new understanding of anatomy. The first "book" includes fifteen full-page, full-length plates of human figures, depicting skeletons, muscles, and the systems of veins and nerves. Nerves, for instance, hang "in ribbons" around the skeleton. The second section, which describes the male viscera, contains illustrations based on baroque designs with the figures in dramatic poses. In the third book, the plates showing female organs present nudes with the viscera viewed somewhat ludicrously through a window in the abdomen.

Estienne did not reshape anatomic thought as Vesalius did; he presented only what his eyes showed him. His text records many original observations, especially on the bones, nerves, and veins and on the technique of dissection.

Charles Estienne and Estienne de la Rivière. *La Dissection de Parties du Corps humain divisée en trois livres. . . .* Paris, 1546.

This diagram of the brain,
somewhat dwarfed by the artist's dramatic treatment,
is meticulously captioned and labeled.

the deteſtable ſinne of Sodomie in this Monſter.

That of brutes ſuch various ſhapes are borne, it is leſſe wonder therefore, when as *Pliny* reports of living creatures in *Africa* that have ſuch various formes and ſhapes, ſeeing their coupling and conception is of divers creatures.

In the yeere 1512. at *Ravenna* (a City in *Italy*) a Monſter was borne, which had a horne on his head, two wings, no armes, a crooked foot with

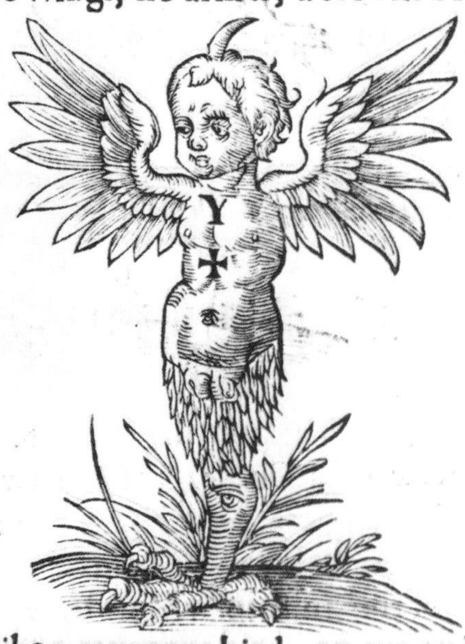


talons, like a ravenous bird, an eye on his knee, of both ſex, in the midſt of his breſt he had the forme

# Jacob Rueff

## THE EXPERT MIDWIFE

Jacob Rueff (1500-1558) practiced as an obstetrician in Zürich, a busy city of forward-looking, independent German Swiss. *The Expert Midwife* is the first English translation of a book written by Rueff in 1554, four years before his death. The work originally appeared in both Latin and German versions *(De Conceptu et Generatione Hominis* and *Trostbüchle* respectively) and contrasted favorably with its predecessors on the same subject, both in the amount and the accuracy of its information and in its illustrations.

Rueff's text comprised six sections, or "books." The first deals with the physiology of impregnation and conception and with the development and nutrition of the fetus. The second describes the uterus and the condition of the fetus within it and includes a chapter of necessary precepts for pregnant women. Book 3 explains parturition, with rules and medicaments for alleviating delay and difficulty of birth and for the care of the mother and infant; it has a chapter on obstetric instruments, such as the speculum and both smooth and toothed forceps for extraction of a dead fetus, which are displayed in clear woodcuts. Book 4 teaches the management of fifteen forms of unnatural birth (including the delivery of awkward presentations and of twins), each illustrated by traditional birth figures in which the fetus looks like a grown child, although the artist has added more anatomic detail than is shown in earlier drawings. Book 5 discusses false conceptions, tumors of the uterus, physically defective infants and monsters, abortion and its treatment, and the signs of conception. Book 6 suggests the causes of sterility and describes the principal diseases of the uterus, once again offering prescriptions for appropriate remedies.

People of the period were morbidly interested in monsters. Remnants of the religious basis of medicine can be seen in the somewhat mythical reports and their interpretation. For example, Rueff's monster illustrated here symbolizes at once sin (sodomy) and virtue (the Greek letter Υ and the cross of Christ, or salvation, on the infant's torso).

Rueff's book kept its usefulness for nearly a century and was often reprinted. The title page of the English translation of 1637 announced that the book had been "translated into English for the generall good and benefit of this Nation."

James Rueff. *The Expert Midwife, or An Excellent and most necessary Treatise of the generation and birth of Man... Six Bookes....* London, 1637.

"It may be demanded here whether beasts may conceive by men...." Rueff stated, "We affirm this may come to pass."

*Cautere, Scie, Couteau courbé.*

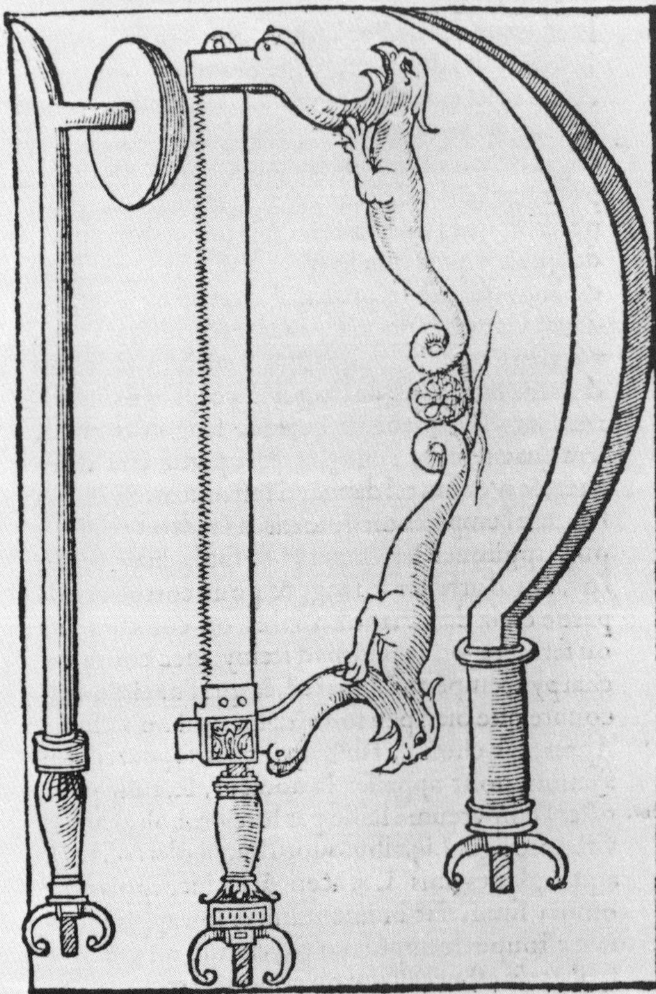

# Pierre Franco

## TREATISE ON HERNIAS, STONES, AND CATARACTS

Pierre Franco (1500-1561), a native of Turriers in Provence, practiced as a surgeon in the south of France. In the sixteenth century, men like him who operated for stones or repaired hernias were usually itinerant surgeons, often regarded with some doubt by the apothecaries and physicians, who considered them mercenaries. Franco, however, apart from an interval spent in Switzerland as a Huguenot refugee at the time of the Waldensian massacres, spent most of his life in Orange, where he established himself as a respected professional. His books also helped greatly to elevate the status of the humble practitioners who performed lithotomy and were forerunners of the modern surgeon.

In 1556, Franco published a "Little Treatise on Surgery Such as the Hernia Surgeons Perform." It was followed five years later by this more complete and useful small, thick book. Although the treatise on hernias is dedicated to Jacques Roy, "Lieutenant of the Master-Surgeons of Lyons," it also contains a nine-year copyright privilege from the king of France and a license to print from the provost of the Sworn Surgeons of Paris. These legal authorizations suggest that Franco wished to make his book known not only in the south, where he lived, but all over France.

Written in the vernacular, the book provides the first practical and precise account of the surgery of hernias, stones in the bladder, and cataracts. It is well illustrated with full-page woodcuts, including clear diagrams of instruments and three drawings of skeletons copied from Vesalius but reduced in size. Franco was the first surgeon to record operative cure of a strangulated hernia and the first to perform suprapubic cystotomy. There is a kind of genius in his pioneering achievements.

Pierre Franco. *Traité des hernies . . . et autres excellentes parties de la Chirurgie, assavoir de la Pierre, des Cataractes des yeux, & autres maladies . . . .* Lyons, 1561.

Cautery, saw, and curved knife
as illustrated in the treatise. Surgical instruments were
handwrought with skill and artistry.

# GABRIELIS FALLOPPII MEDICI MVTINENSIS OBSERVATIONES *Anatomicæ.*

AD PETRVM MANNAM medicum Cremonensem.

Cum Priuilegio Summi Pontificis, Regis Philippi, Senatusque Veneti.

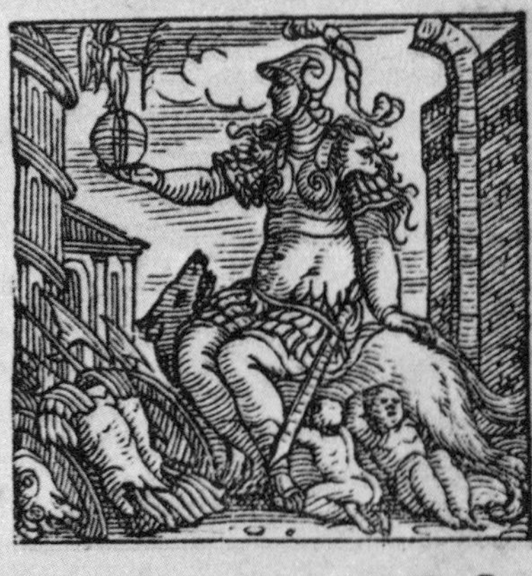

VENETIIS,
Apud Marcum Antonium Vlmum
M D LXI.

# Gabriele Falloppio

## OBSERVATIONS IN ANATOMY

Falloppio, or Fallopius (1523-1562), of Modena, was an influential teacher of anatomy at Padua, where for eleven years he occupied the famous chair not long vacated by his teacher, Vesalius. The year before his death, he published this one book, *Observationes Anatomicae.* The small, thick volume is mainly a commentary on some points made by Vesalius in the *Fabrica* rather than a formal treatise. However, it did present many new discoveries and thus displayed Falloppio's independent achievement. In form, it is a long, continuous narrative without summary, index, or illustrations. (The text includes a tabular classification of the different kinds of joints.)

Although a great admirer of Vesalius, whom he called "divine"—or, as we might say, "inspired" —Falloppio did not hesitate to point out where his own dissections had shown the master to be wrong. He sent a copy of his book to the famous anatomist, then at the Spanish court, where he had gone as physician to Emperor Charles V, and Vesalius wrote a courteous reply dated December 17, 1561. Vesalius, who was then still under fifty, hoped to return to research again at Padua. Falloppio died of tuberculosis before receiving Vesalius's answer, and Vesalius died on the Greek island of Zante in the Ionian Sea in 1564 on his way home from a pilgrimage to Jerusalem. The text of his answer to Falloppio was published by friends later that year.

Falloppio's most original contribution was made in his dissections and discussions of the female reproductive organs. He first clearly differentiated and named several special structures and, in particular, described the oviducts named for him. He himself employed the Latin term *tuba*, a trumpet, to indicate their trumpet-shaped lateral extremities.

Falloppio added to knowledge of the centers of ossification and described the primary teeth and their replacement. He improved on earlier accounts of the muscles of the head and face and also made numerous discoveries concerning nerve pathways. He was the first anatomist to delineate precisely all three ossicles of the ear, and he provided a full description of the kidney.

Gabriele Falloppio. *Observationes Anatomicae.* Venice, 1561.

Title page of *Observationes Anatomicae.*
The classical embellishment depicting mythologic figures
is characteristic of sixteenth-century book design.

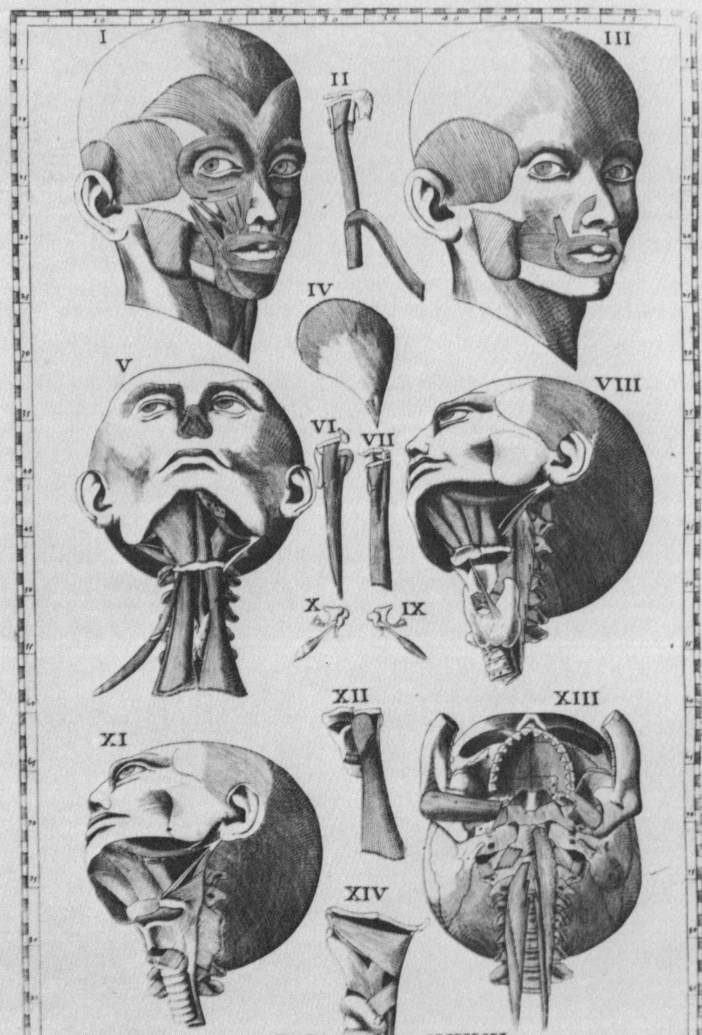


TAB. XXXXI.

# Bartolommeo Eustachio

## ANATOMIC TABLES

Eustachio, or Eustachius (1520-1574), is considered to have been the most scientific anatomist of the High Renaissance. Although the plates that illustrated his distinctly original observations were engraved by 1552, they remained unprinted for 160 years. Early in the eighteenth century, they were found in the Vatican Library and presented by Pope Clement XI to his physician, Giovanni Maria Lancisi, who in 1714 published the forty-seven plates with his own notes.

Whereas Vesalius designed his illustrations to exhibit nature as he had observed it (however artistically the figures were posed), Eustachius drew anatomic types based on study of many different cadavers. Although he, too, arranged his figures in lifelike poses, he was more interested in accurate proportions. This is emphasized by the frame and scale of measurement around each plate. Thus, the whole picture is both representational and mathematically exact. Vesalius's artist had employed wood engraving with its strong contrasts, but Eustachius preferred the newer copper engraving, which permitted a more delicate delineation of detail. By juxtaposition of drawings, he also contrived to show front-and-back and left-and-right views of the same figure. Among the best plates are those displaying the base of the brain and the sympathetic nervous system, the relationships of blood vessels and muscles, and the structure of the larynx. Many of the illustrations present the component parts of a particular system; each part is identified by a Roman numeral that corresponds to a discussion in the text.

Eustachius himself had published an important small volume, *Opuscula Anatomica* ("Little Works on Anatomy"), which contained chapters on the kidneys, the organs of hearing, the bones, the motions of the head, the azygos vein, and the common deep vein of the arm. A companion treatise on the teeth gave the first accurate account of their structure. Eustachius's essay on the veins shows advanced knowledge of the heart's structure. The eustachian tube, named for him, was first described in the section on the organs of hearing. The treatise on the kidney is his best work and is illustrated by eight excellent small plates which, like his large anatomy plates, were designed with a graduated border. Among his other original observations is the first account of the adrenals.

Bartolommeo Eustachio. *Tabulae anatomicae*. Rome, 1714.

Scale drawings of the anatomy of the head.
Eustachius's drawings were the first anatomic plates
to be engraved on copper.

# DOS LIBROS, EL V-
## NO QVE TRATA DE TODAS LAS COSAS

*que traen de nueſtras Indias Occidentales, que ſiruen al vſo de la Medicina, y el otro que trata de la Piedra Bezaar, y de la Yerua Eſcuerçonera.*

*Cōpueſtos por el doctor Nicoloſo de Monardes Medico de Seuilla.*

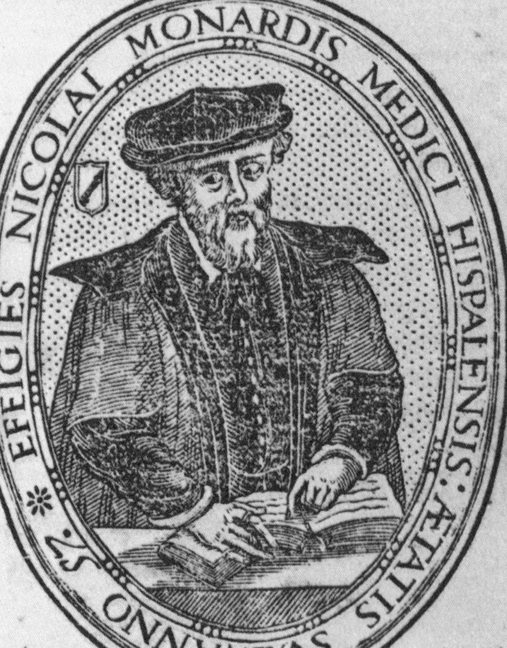


IMPRESSOS EN SEVILLA EN CASA DE
*Hernando Diaz, en la calle de la Sierpe.*
*Con Licencia y Priuilegio de ſu Mageſtad.*
*Año de 1569.*

# Nicolás Monardes

## THINGS BROUGHT FROM OUR WEST INDIES WHICH CAN BE USED IN MEDICINE

Nicolás Monardes (1493-1588) belonged to an Italian family established in business in Seville, the city in southern Spain most involved in trade with "New Spain" in the Americas. An imaginative entrepreneur as well as a physician, he was the first to introduce the herbal products of Central America to the pharmacopoeias of Europe. Although he never left Seville, Monardes obtained specimens of all plants imported from Central America and established a museum for them. Part of it was a botanical garden in which he managed to cultivate every plant that had been brought to him from the New World.

Monardes was the first physician to write about the arrow poison curare and about tobacco, which the West Indians used medicinally. He imported tobacco in 1558 and was growing it in his garden in Spain while Sir Walter Raleigh was still a child in England. Monardes first described these drugs in 1565 in *Historia medicinal que trata de las cosas que se traen de nuestras Indias occidentales.* The book was then expanded and published in three sections, of which the Lilly collection contains the first. Its subtitle anticipates the second volume and reads (in translation): "Two Books. One deals with all things brought from our West Indies which can be used in medicine, and the other deals with the bezoar stone and scorzonera grass." A third section was published in 1574, and three years later all three parts appeared in an English translation entitled *Ioyfull Newes Out of the New-founde Worlde.*

Monardes recorded many native Indian plant names. He described the sacred wood guaiacum, thought to be a cure for syphilis; chinaroot and its cognate, sarsaparilla; and, more particularly, the purgative "white rhubarb." His second volume made a special impact on Europe because of its account of tobacco. He tells of its various medicinal uses—as a treatment for toothache and carbuncles and as an antidote for some types of poison. "Some time ago," he wrote, "some Caribbean Indians set out in canoes for San Juan de Puerto Rico...and they came to a plantation and killed a few Indians and Spaniards and wounded many. Since the foreigners did not have corrosive sublimate to cure them, it was decided to treat them with tobacco juice...and God willed that...the pains, ravings and fainting spells, from which they used to die, were relieved. Thus the power of the poison was removed...and the islanders, being acquainted with this cure, are now using it for wounds received when fighting the Caribs. And they are no longer afraid, for they have found such a great remedy for such a desperate menace."

Nicolás Monardes. *Dos libros, el uno que trata de todas las cosas que traen de nuestras Indias Occidentales, que sirven al uso de la medicina....* Seville, 1569.

Title page with portrait of the author at the age of fifty-seven.

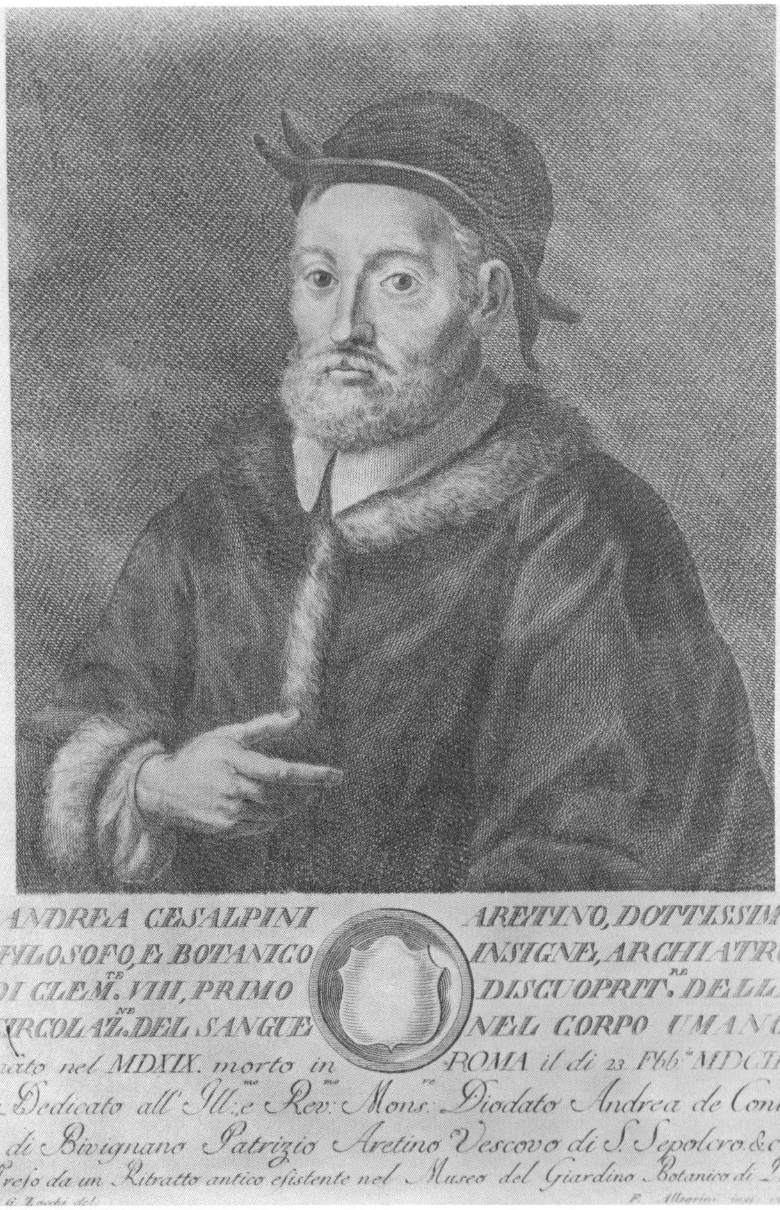

ANDREA CESALPINI ARETINO, DOTTISSIMO FILOSOFO, E BOTANICO INSIGNE, ARCHIATRO DI CLEM.TE VIII, PRIMO DISCUOPRIT.RE DELLA CIRCOLAZ.NE DEL SANGUE NEL CORPO UMANO, nato nel MDXIX. morto in ROMA il dì 23. Febb.ro MDCIII.

Dedicato all' Ill.mo e Rev.mo Mons.re Diodato Andrea de Conti di Bivignano Patrizio Aretino Vescovo di S. Sepolcro. &c.

Preso da un Ritratto antico esistente nel Museo del Giardino Botanico di Pisa.

G. Zocchi del. F. Allegrini inci.

# Andrea Cesalpino

## BOOKS OF ARISTOTELIAN QUESTIONS

Cesalpino (1519-1603), a physician and naturalist, was not so much an innovator in Renaissance medicine as a man of philosophic outlook. In this volume, "Five Books of Peripatetic [i.e., Aristotelian] Questions" (1571), he attempted a general survey of the medical and anatomic research of his contemporaries. Cesalpino had been a student at Padua under Matteo Realdo Colombo and may even have heard Vesalius lecture. He was only a few years younger than his teachers but long outlived them and practiced for many years in Rome.

Aristotle's doctrines had been discussed in Italy since at least the thirteenth century, and Cesalpino tried to recapture Aristotle's spirit of scientific inquiry, although he himself was a classifier rather than a discoverer. His best achievement as a naturalist was the introduction of a logical arrangement of plants based on their organs of fructification. This scheme of classification appeared in his *De Plantis, Libri XVI*, published in Florence in 1583. He then revised the "Peripatetic Questions," producing an expanded edition in 1593, and followed it with a more thorough medical textbook in two parts: "The Art of Medicine—Universal Diseases" in 1602 and "The Hippocratic Mirror [Speculum] of the Art of Medicine" in 1605. In that work, Cesalpino recorded observations he had made on the blood vessels; these to some extent anticipated William Harvey's exposition in 1628 of the circulation of the blood.

For instance, in the *Quaestionum* he made the first published statement concerning the centripetal flow of blood in the veins. Elsewhere, he describes "continuous motion from the veins to the heart and from the heart to the arteries." In another place, he says that the very hot blood from the heart passes through the lungs to be cooled by the air. From these scattered observations it is possible to build up a theory of the circulation, but Cesalpino did not make the necessary synthesis, nor did he provide any experimental evidence to support his theory of blood circulation. It has been noticed that Harvey, who acknowledged indebtedness to hints from Colombo, Fabricius, and others, never once mentioned Cesalpino as a forerunner.

Andrea Cesalpino. *Peripateticarum Quaestionum, Libri Quinque*. Venice, 1571.

In this engraved portrait, Cesalpino is cited as "learned philosopher and famous botanist, court physician of Pope Clement VIII, first to discover circulation of blood in the human body."

*Autre cornue auec le recipient aßiſe en vn mortier de fer ou de marbre pour pareillement diſtiller au ſoleil.*

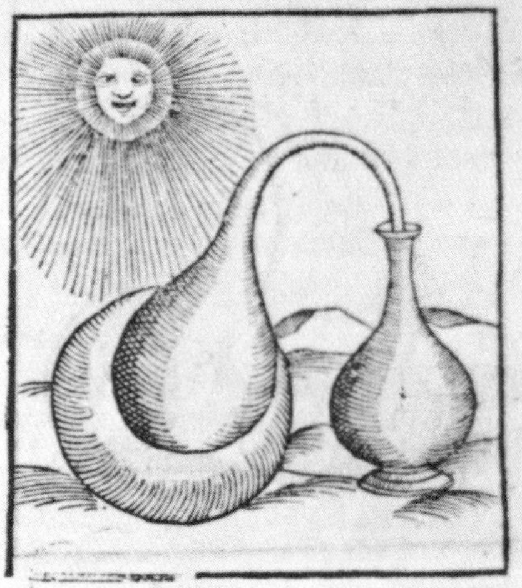

*Vaiſſeau ſublimatoire lequel peut außi ſeruir à donner vne euaporation aux oreilles & à la matrice.*



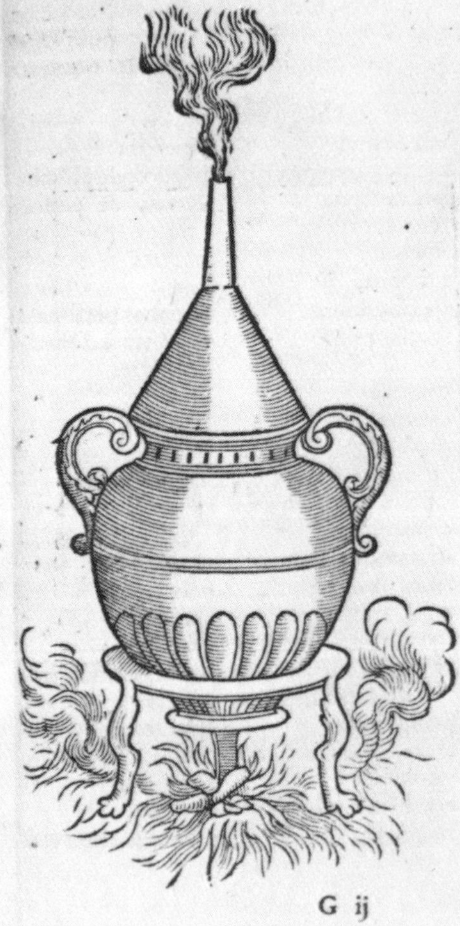

# Ambroise Paré

## FIVE BOOKS ON SURGERY

Ambroise Paré (1510-1590) rose to fame as an army surgeon during the foreign and civil wars that ravaged France in the sixteenth century. His books are notable for his vivid case histories, but he himself relied less on book learning than on his own experience and on learning by example. In his first work, a short treatise on the method of treating gunshot wounds (1545), he recommended that surgeons give up their traditional cauterizing of wounds with boiling oil, a treatment as dangerous as it was cruel. Paré's second book, on anatomy, appeared in 1549, and by 1561 or 1562 he had completed another on the care of wounds and "fractures of the head." His major surgical message, however, was detailed in two practical volumes, elegant in design but small enough for the field surgeon's knapsack—the *Dix livres* ("Ten Books") of 1564 and the *Cinq livres* ("Five Books") of 1572.

In *Dix livres,* Paré discussed war surgery, involving the treatment of gunshot and arrow wounds, fractures and dislocations, contusions, and burns; bone caries and gangrene; and urinary tract infections and strictures, kidney and bladder stones, and renal failure. There are many illustrations of instruments and appliances for reducing dislocations, a few illustrations of operations, and a picture of an artificial hand with articulated fingers.

The *Cinq livres* of 1572 deal again with bandaging, fractures, and dislocations but also with animal bites, gout, and fluxions. They are illustrated with drawings of instruments, appliances, and ligatures.

A year later, Paré published a similar volume, *Deux livres de chirurgie* ("Two Books on Surgery"). The *Deux livres* discuss procreation and monsters and, in fact, concern obstetrics. Paré revived podalic version and had induced artificial labor in a case of uterine hemorrhage. Among his surgical innovations were an exarticulation of the elbow joint, union of a fracture of the neck of the femur, and ligature instead of cauterization for amputations.

All these works were published in 1575 in a single large volume containing the twenty-six "books" of his *Oeuvres*. This compendium was later translated into Latin and several modern languages, including English.

Paré's medical writings, published without the permission of the faculty of medicine of the University of Paris and in the common tongue instead of learned Latin, provoked the anger of the physicians, who feared rivalry from surgeons. The physicians sought legal injunction against him in 1575, but he was again protected by the king, who had granted Paré a ten-year privilege in 1572 "to employ such printers as seems good to him."

Ambroise Paré. *Cinq Livres de Chirurgie*. Paris, 1572.

Woodcuts of vessels used for distillation. "Things of nature" from which medicaments were made included herbs, plants, trees, horns, feathers, and blood.

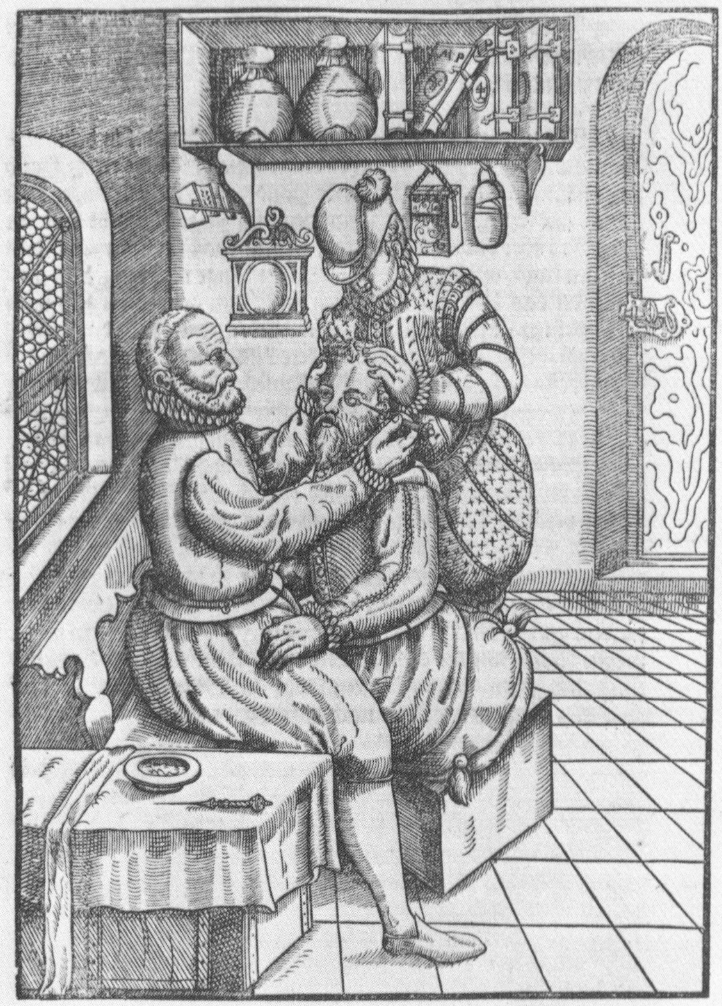

# Georg Bartisch

## CARE OF THE EYES

Georg Bartisch (1535-1606), of Königsbrück, who describes himself on his book's extraordinarily verbose title page as "Citizen, Oculist, Cutter, and Surgeon in the Ancient Ducal Town of Dresden," published the most comprehensive treatise that had yet been compiled on the care of the eyes. It was profusely illustrated with large woodcuts made from the writer's own colored drawings. In his role of "cutter," Bartisch wrote a similar treatise on lithotomy, which did not appear in print until modern times.

His work resembles that of other German surgeons, such as Hieronymus Brunschwig or Caspar Stromayr, whose "Copious Practice in the Treatment of Hernia" had been issued in 1559. Each was a complete picture book of practical methods of treatment. The pictures were drawn from life and crowded with detail; they represent individual cases, in contrast to the generalized prototypes that appear in contemporary French and Italian books. Where a modern artist would depict only the particular part of the body subject to the operation, Bartisch displays a whole face, the full-length figure of the patient, or a group scene with the surgeon and his assistant in attendance. Some of these portraits are repeated with slight variations to depict different conditions of the eyes. A few anatomic plates with hinged overlays show successive depths of dissection. Vesalius had introduced this method in 1543, although it was not much exploited until the seventeenth century. Bartisch also pictures instruments and masks for treating strabismus.

This oversize book is divided into sixteen sections that cover anatomy, defects and diseases of the eyes and sight (especially strabismus, cataract, running or pustulent conditions, and corneal damage), the eyelids and eyelashes, external injuries, pain in the eyes, and injuries caused by witches or the devil. In each case, the surgical or medical treatment is clearly explained. Bartisch concluded with sections on the care necessary to maintain health of the eyes, the effects of venesection and diet, methods of preparing the necessary medicines and ointments, a survey of instruments, and forms of religious thanksgiving for cure. In addition to its remarkable range, the book is notable for recording in detail the bold and dangerous operations undertaken by sixteenth-century surgeons.

Georg Bartisch. *Ophthalmodouleia. Das ist, Augendienst. . . .* Dresden, 1583.

Bartisch's graphic illustrations included this one of proper cataract operative procedure. He recommended that, to insure a steady hand, the physician stay continent for two days before the operation.

Sum liber Willi: Copland

# A TREATISE OF MELANCHOLIE.

CONTAINING THE CAVSES thereof, & reasons of the strange effects it worketh in our minds and bodies: with the phisicke cure, and spirituall consolation for such as haue thereto adioyned an afflicted conscience.

*The difference betwixt it, and melancholie with diuerse philosophicall discourses touching actions, and affections of soule, spirit, and body: the particulars whereof are to be seene before the booke.*

By T. Bright Doctor of Phisicke.

Imprinted at London by Thomas Vautrollier, dwelling in the Black-Friers. 1586.

# Timothy Bright

## A TREATISE OF MELANCHOLIE

Timothy Bright (1551-1615), physician to St. Bartholomew's Hospital, London, for four years, was dismissed in 1591 for neglecting his duties and became a clergyman in Yorkshire. When his memorable *Treatise* appeared, he had already published four medical books between 1580 and 1584. The *Treatise* was printed in 1586 by Thomas Vautrollier, a reputable but somewhat careless printer. Consequently, the book contained many misprints and was not registered as the law required. Bright transferred the book to John Windet, who produced a more correct edition in October of the same year and later printed other books for him.

*A Treatise of Melancholie* was the first thorough study of a psychosomatic condition, for Bright recognized that this peculiar affliction was primarily an illness of the mind that, in turn, profoundly affected the health of the body. His approach, indicative of his dual professions, was both medical and religious. Shakespeare later drew on this book for his characterization of Hamlet, not only using the medical matter but also echoing Bright's phrases in Hamlet's speeches. Furthermore, the *Treatise* inspired Robert Burton to write his large and more famous book on the same subject, *The Anatomy of Melancholy* (1621).

Bright's *Treatise* is closely printed on small pages and divided into forty-one chapters. The word "melancholie" retained its first significance —a disease produced by an excess of "black bile"—but Bright's treatment introduced the psychologic connotation it has since held. After debating whether it is congenital and therefore unpreventable "by fault of body," Bright describes how melancholy "worketh fearful passions in the mind," "how the body affecteth the soul," and how melancholy "procureth fear, sadness, despair," and he notices "how sickness and years alter the mind." He discusses the physical symptoms of melancholy—tears and sighing, weeping and laughing together, bashfulness, and the alteration of "natural actions." He differentiates melancholy from "the affliction of conscience for sin" and shows that they can occur together.

Treatment and cure occupy the last quarter of the book. Bright maintains that patients must "order themselves" in mind, in sense and motion, in affections, and in choice of air, meat, and drink; their houses are to be kept cheerful and "lightsome," trim and neat; and their apparel should be light, clean, and well fitting. He prescribes suitable medicines and advises "the manner of strengthening melancholic persons after purging."

Timothy Bright. *A Treatise of Melancholie*. London, 1586.

Title page, bearing a Latin inscription identifying this as a book belonging to one William Copland.

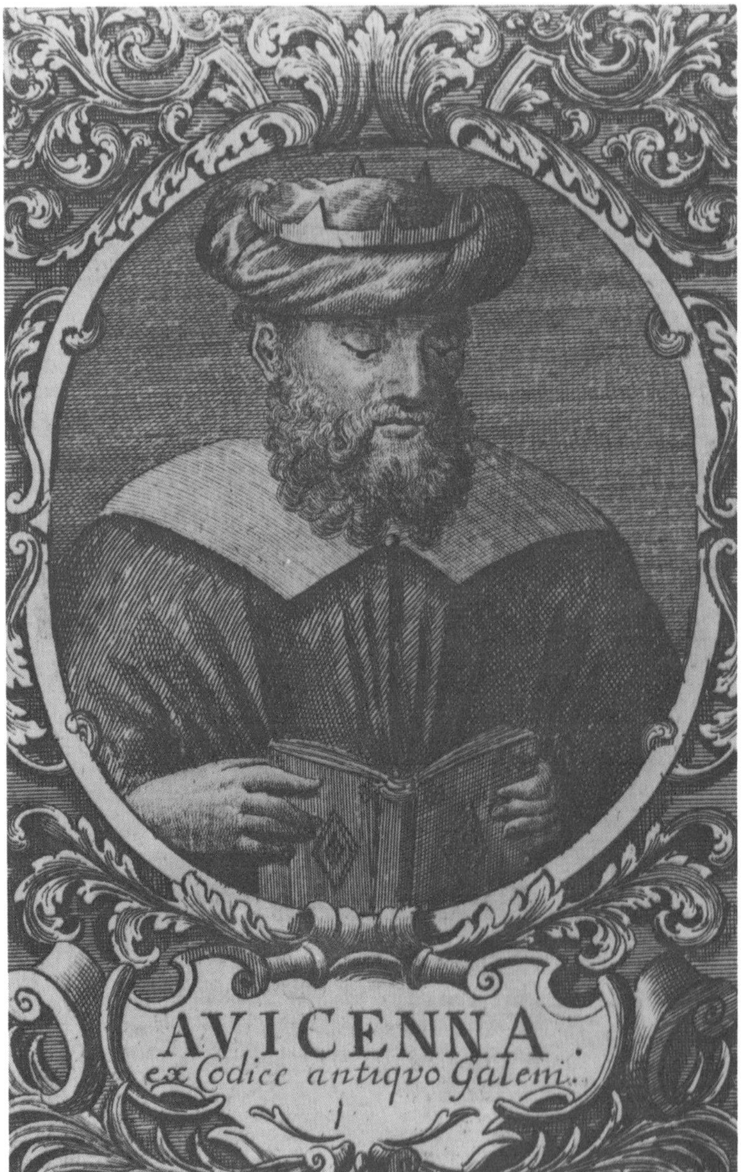
AVICENNA.
ex Codice antiqvo Galeni..
1

# Avicenna

## CANON OF MEDICINE

Avicenna (980-1037), Persian by birth and Mohammedan by religion, was a child prodigy who had memorized the Koran by the age of ten. Avid for knowledge, he became well versed in mathematics, jurisprudence, philosophy, and poetry. In fact, several quatrains ascribed to Omar Khayyam are believed to have been written more than a century earlier by Avicenna. At sixteen, he took up the study of medicine and, by eighteen, had already gained renown as a physician. He became court physician and vizier to several caliphs in the Persian city of Isfahan and was chief physician to the great hospital at Baghdad.

Avicenna's most influential work was the "Canon of Medicine," written in Arabic, in which he summarized the experience of the Greco-Roman physicians Hippocrates and Galen and added many personal observations. Avicenna realized that certain illnesses, such as tuberculosis and dysentery, are communicable. Of the latter he wrote, "Disease is transmitted from person to person....The traveler is more exposed to illness from the diversity of the drinking water than he is from the diversity of foods. Hence it is necessary to be particular about correcting the bad qualities of the drinking water, and expend every effort in purifying it. Boil the water, for as we have already pointed out, boiling sometimes clarifies the water and separates off the impurities which are admixed with the intrinsic substance of the water." Avicenna also recognized the genetic nature of certain conditions, stating, "Hereditary transmission includes premature baldness and gout."

This massive and encyclopedic book of almost a million words was used throughout the Arabic-speaking world until relatively modern times. No author, after Galen, enjoyed so wide and durable a reputation.

The "Canon" was translated into Latin for European physicians and reprinted many times in that language from the fifteenth to the seventeenth century. Only during the Renaissance, when Western physicians gained direct access to the medical writings of the ancient Greeks, did the "Canon" begin to decline in influence.

The magnificent two-volume "Canon" in the Lilly collection is in the original Arabic (although a Latin title page has been added) and includes some of Avicenna's other scientific writings.

Avicenna [Abu Ali al Husain ibn Abdullah ibn Sina]. *Libri quinque Canonis Medicinae... Arabice nunc primum impressi.* Rome, 1593.

In an autobiography
of his first twenty-one years, the self-assured
Avicenna wrote: "Medicine is not a difficult subject, and
in a short space of time, of course,
I excelled in it."

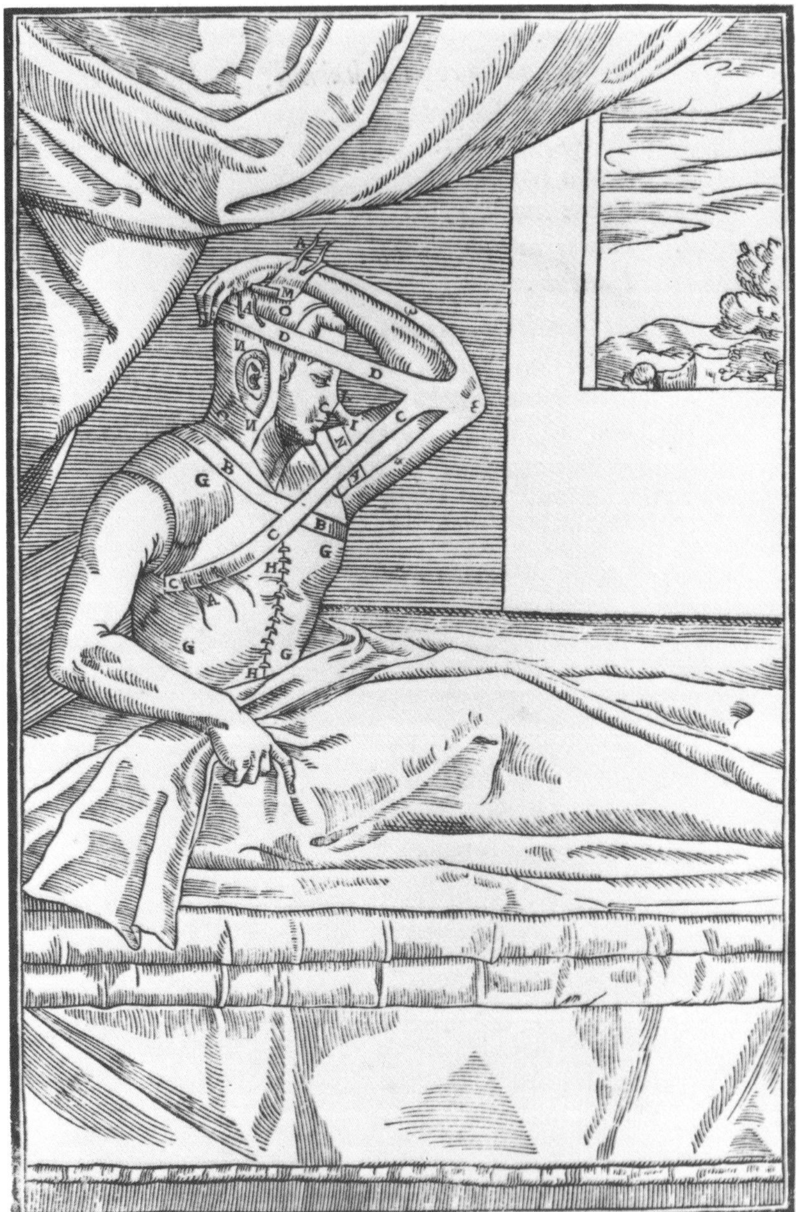

# Gasparo Tagliacozzi

## SURGERY OF THE MUTILATED

"Two books on the Surgery of the Mutilated by grafting, in which all things which seem to appertain to the Theory and the Practice of this surgery of restoration by grafting of Noses, Ears and Lips are most completely explained in the clearest method. Portraits and plates are added of all the instruments and bandages for the skin graft, with a most convenient quadruple index of the separate chapters, authors, controversies, and finally memorable matters and words." Such is the full title of this handsome and thorough book, the first on the subject of plastic surgery. The author's method of transplanting the patient's own tissue met a very real need, because the dueling and violence that were widespread in Italy at that time frequently resulted in mutilation of the face.

Tagliacozzi (1546-1599) was a professor and successful surgeon at Bologna. Nevertheless, his methods were not adopted by his contemporaries, who probably feared complications. With the revival of plastic surgery in the early nineteenth century, his book was rediscovered and was reprinted in Berlin in 1831.

The first twelve chapters of Book 1 deal with the philosophic background and pertinent observations from ancient and contemporary writers. The author explains the reason for preferring a skin graft to reattachment of the amputated part: that the latter shrinks and hardens before union is achieved. Finally, he discusses the revival of life in the graft while union is taking place.

Book 2 presents the actual stages of surgery and the care of all the parts concerned, both before and after the operations, e.g., for raising a skin flap on the arm and grafting it in situ to a deformed nose. There are also descriptions of an operation for forming new nostrils and of another for reconstructing damaged lips. Tagliacozzi expounds his ideas for preventing hemorrhage, gangrene, and scar formation.

The twenty-two carefully styled illustrations are well designed and are arranged in a logical sequence. They depict the principal instruments and methods of bandaging, with a demonstration of how bandages may be used to anchor the arm to the head during the grafting stage. The final plates show the separation of the flap and removal of the bandages. The linear woodcuts give instructive detail. Although the patient appears as a full-length figure, the emphasis is clearly placed on the site of operation.

Gasparo Tagliacozzi [Gasparus Taliacotius]. *De Curtorum Chirurgia per insitionem, Libri Duo.* Venice, 1597.

This well-composed woodcut depicts an early skin-grafting procedure. Before Tagliacozzi, plastic surgery was a haphazard and uncertain art.

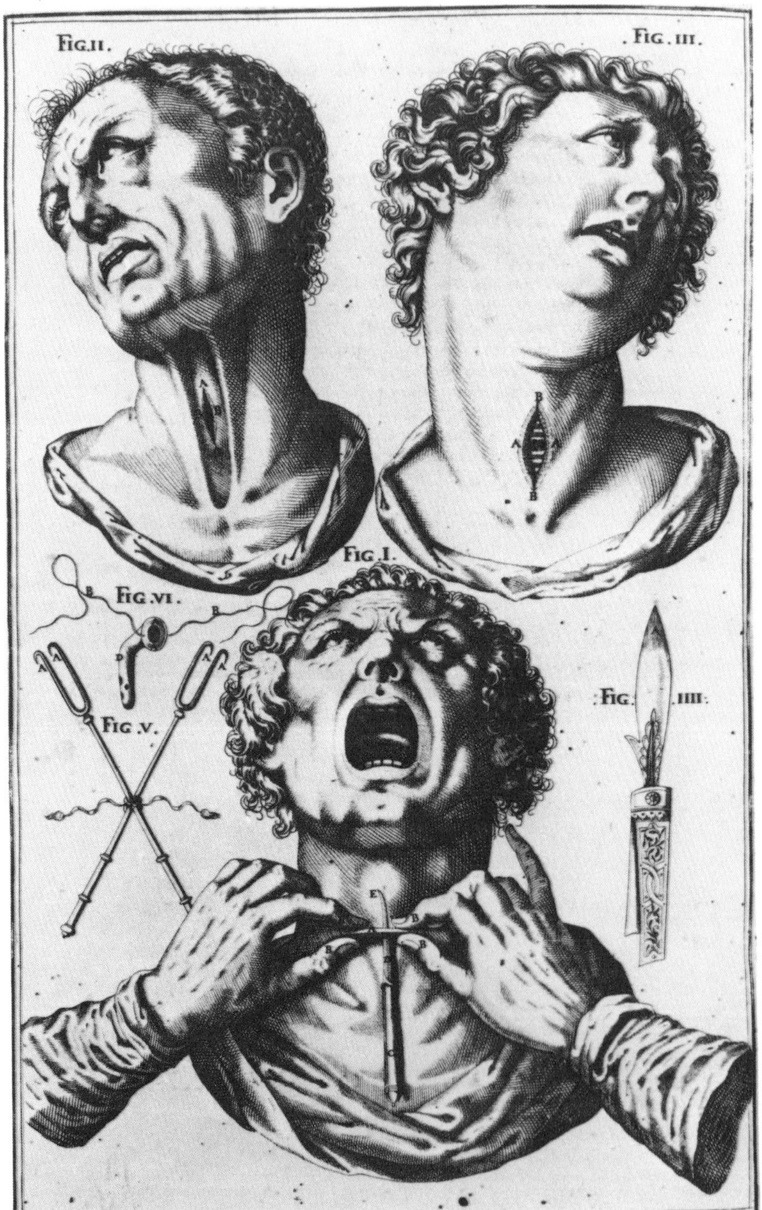
FIG.II.
FIG. III.
FIG.I.
FIG.VI.
FIG.V.
FIG. IIII.

# Giulio Casserio

## ON THE ORGANS OF SPEECH AND HEARING

Casserio (1552-1616) was pupil, assistant, and finally deputy of the famous Fabricius (q.v.) at Padua for nearly forty years. He might well have succeeded Fabricius to the chair of anatomy if his sudden death at the age of sixty-four had not preceded that of Fabricius by three years. Casserio was a keen comparative, as well as human, anatomist and also a successful surgeon. His fame rests on his anatomic study of the organs of speech and hearing, *De Vocis Auditusque Organis Historia,* in which the orientation is clinical and, to a lesser degree, physiologic. The drawings for this work were based on his extensive human and animal dissections and were exceptionally well executed by Joseph Maurer, whose plates have been called "the model for the copperplate illustrator."

This volume is composed of two separate books that were issued together, although the second, on the subject of hearing, is dated a year earlier than the first. Each book is divided into three sections—fabric (anatomy), function (phonation or acoustics), and uses (physiology). They record many original observations and correct deductions, especially on the innervation of the parts described. Most valuable is the detailed account of the larynx, in which Casserio's dissections of a wide range of animals—mammals, birds, amphibians, and even insects—are compared with his human material. He gives the first accurate description of the laryngeal muscles and nerves.

Later he published a longer book on the organs of the five senses, *Pentaestheseion* (1609), illustrated with thirty-three plates. This work was considered authoritative until more detailed studies were made by anatomists of the later seventeenth century, some of whose "discoveries" he anticipated. For instance, he described both the antrum named for Highmore (1651) (q.v.) and the conjunctival glands named for Meibom (1666). Seventy-eight plates that he had prepared for an atlas of general anatomy were published after his death. These splendid and accurate drawings were made by Fialetti, a pupil of Tintoretto. They include clear delineations of the abdominal muscles and viscera, the blood vessels of the liver, and the peritoneum. Many of these structures had never been illustrated before.

Casserio was one of the representatives of the golden age of the school of anatomy at Padua.

Giulio Casserio [Julius Casserius]. *De Vocis Auditusque Organis Historia Anatomica . . . Tractatibus Duobus Explicata.* Ferrara, 1601. Part II: *De Auris Auditusque Organi, Historia Anatomica.* Ferrara, 1600.

This example of Joseph Maurer's drawings is a striking illustration of a laryngotomy, exemplifying anatomic and artistic excellence.

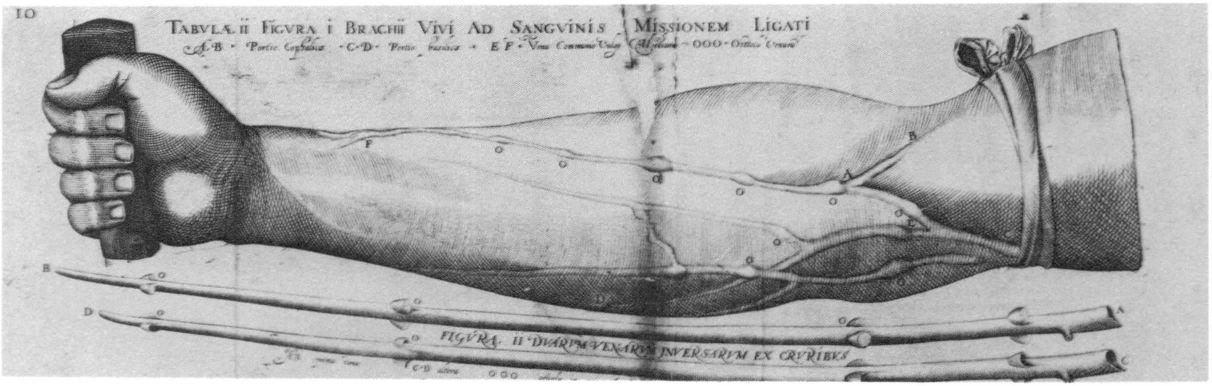
10
TABVLÆ II FIGVRA I BRACHII VIVI AD SANGVINIS MISSIONEM LIGATI
FIGVRA II DVARVM VENARVM INVERSARVM EX CRVRIBVS

# Hieronymus Fabricius

## THE VALVES OF THE VEINS

Geronimo Fabrizio d'Acquapendente (1537-1619), better known by his Latinized name, Hieronymus Fabricius, taught anatomy in the famous medical school of Padua for nearly fifty years. He was also a successful practicing surgeon. His work on veins undoubtedly inspired his pupil William Harvey to study the functioning of the cardiovascular system, although Fabricius himself did not draw far-reaching physiologic conclusions from his own anatomic observations of the circulation.

The presence of valves in the veins had been known from at least the middle of the sixteenth century, but Fabricius gave the first complete description of them in his brief essay. Printed in very large format, the book's twenty-three pages include eight full-page illustrations. The second occupies a two-page spread and shows the veins at the inner surface of the arm, which is stretched out as if for bloodletting. Harvey adapted this plate in reduced size for the illustrations in his epoch-making treatise published in 1628, in which he announced and expounded his discovery of the circulation of the blood.

Although he was an indefatigable worker whose accurately recorded observations give him high rank as a medical biologist, Fabricius was a traditionalist. He dissected a great variety of animals and birds without comparing their homologies. He postulated a local, almost entirely structural, purpose for the organs he dissected and did not extend his opinions to wider physiologic horizons as did Harvey and the later seventeenth-century anatomists. The term he used for the valves, *"ostiola,"* implies small sluice gates in a stream, and he thought of them as serving to slow down the blood flow and maintain an even distribution of blood to the parts of the body.

Fabricius intended to prepare a survey of the whole animal "fabric," to repeat Vesalius's term. Toward this he gathered colored illustrations of comparative anatomic subjects, which still remain on view in Venice. He published instead a series of special studies between 1600 and 1618 on anatomic and physiologic subjects and on embryology. This book is the fourth of ten such monographs.

It is significant that there is a direct teacher-student line from Vesalius to Fallopius to Fabricius to Harvey.

Hieronymus Fabricius ab Aquapendente. *De Venarum Ostiolis*. Padua, 1603.

Fabricius's illustration of the valves of the veins was adapted by his pupil William Harvey (see page 63), who acknowledged his indebtedness to his mentor.

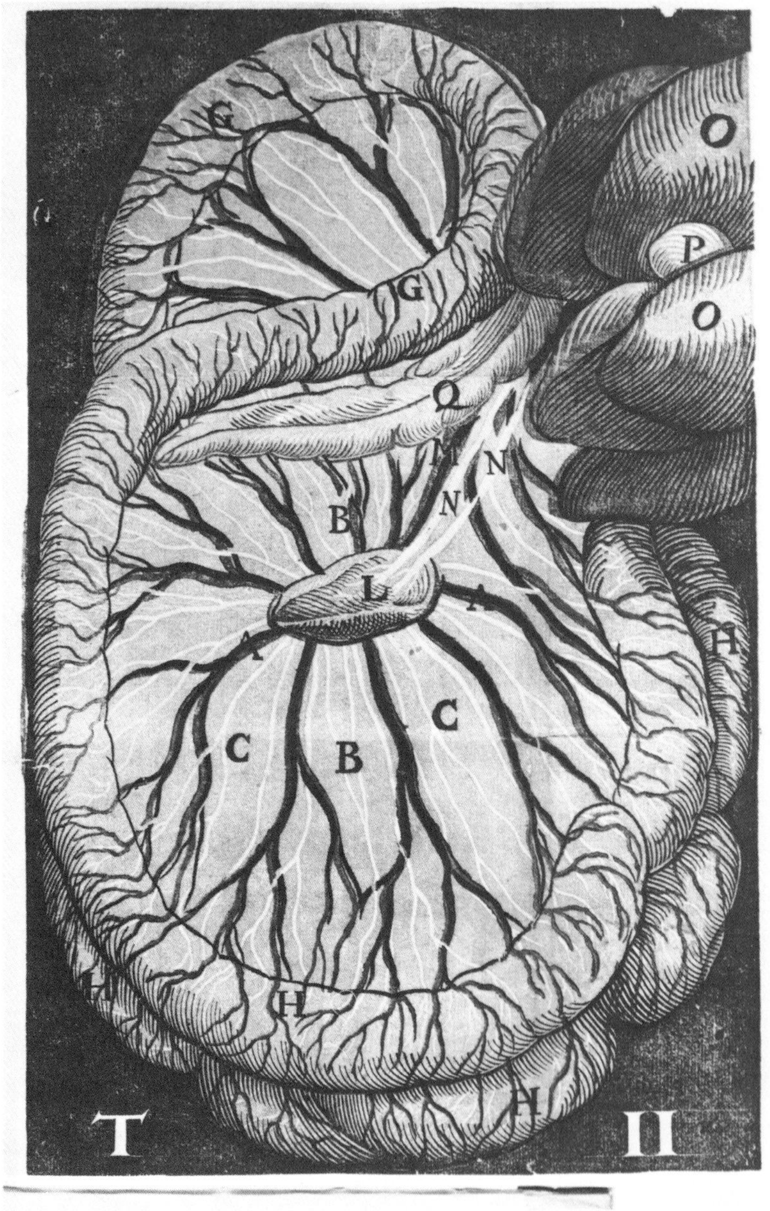
G
O
P
G
O
Q
M
N
N
B
L
A
A
H
C
C
B
H
H
H
T
II

# Gasparo Aselli

## THE LACTEAL VESSELS

Aselli (1581-1626), who had been a pupil of Fallopius, practiced as a surgeon in Milan. There he continued his anatomic research and wrote in a more dynamic manner and with greater physiologic insight than had his predecessors, whose approach had been essentially teleologic and descriptive. Although Aselli's notebooks and jottings for lectures have never been published, he is renowned for this small volume, which was published two years after his death at the age of forty-five.

The book records his chance discovery of the lacteal vessels in 1622 while he was displaying the mesenteric nerves of a dog at an anatomic demonstration. In this fed animal, he noted a network of mesenteric vessels that contained a whitish fluid. Because such engorgement was absent in a fasting animal, he concluded that it was related to recent feeding.

Writing before the publication of Harvey's work on the circulation, Aselli maintained that the liver was the center of the venous system and believed, as did Galen, that the intestinal veins carried chyle to the liver. Harvey knew that the Galenic account was wrong and remained skeptical about the existence of lacteals; the contradiction was cleared away when Jean Pecquet announced his discovery of the thoracic duct in 1651.

In his text, which comprises thirty-five chapters, Aselli took up the intestines in general, their veins, arteries, nerves, and a "fourth, new kind" of vessels. He explained why he had named the vessels he discovered "lacteal," or milky, vessels and asked why they had remained undiscovered for so long. He presented their anatomy in great detail and wondered whether they were supplied with chyle or blood. He also described the transit of chyle to the liver and discussed the contribution of the new vessels to the formation of blood.

The book was illustrated with a copperplate portrait of the author at the age of forty-two, when he made his discovery, and with four large foldout plates showing the lacteals in animal dissections. These are most remarkable woodcuts, both for their display of the dissections and for the method in which they were produced.

Gasparo Aselli. *De Lactibus Sive Lacteis Venis*. Milan, 1627.

The original woodcut is printed in black, red, and two shades of brown. The Aselli plates were the first colored illustrations in an anatomic text.

uide harũ figurarũ explicationem supra. fol. 58. 57

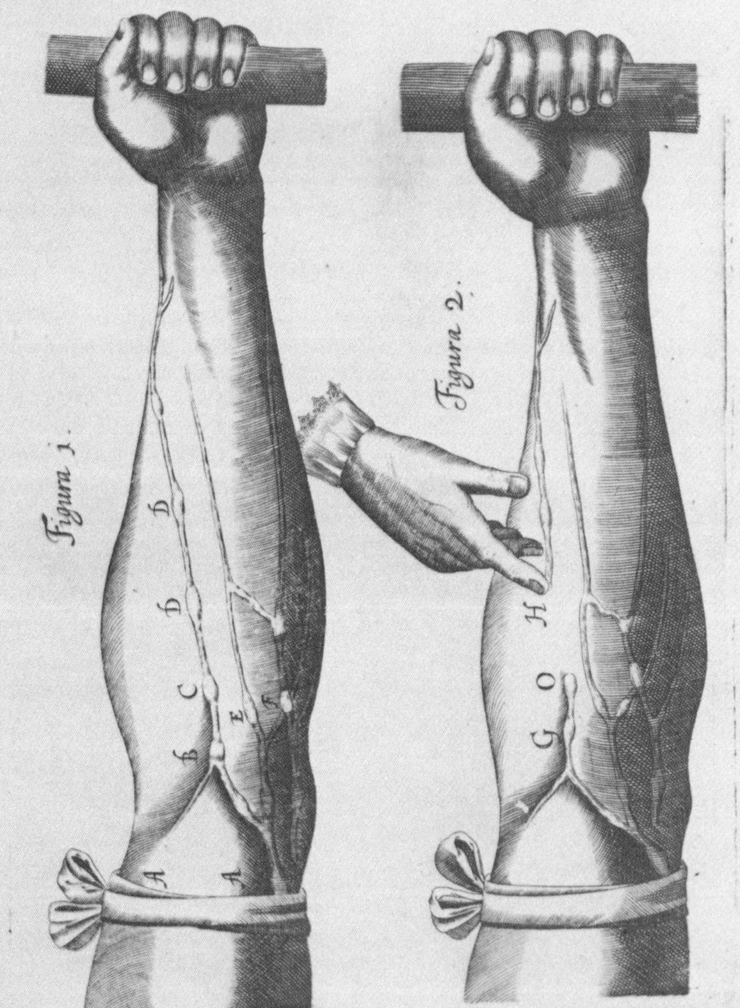

# William Harvey

## THE MOVEMENT OF THE BLOOD

Harvey's small book is usually considered the most important single medical work ever published. It was written in Latin and issued in Frankfurt by William Fitzer, an English printer residing in Germany. In this book, Harvey (1578-1657) announced his discovery of the circulation, gave a clear description of the heart's action, and reported the experiments that provided proof for his assertions. He had performed these studies by himself over a period of several years on many classes of vertebrate and invertebrate animals. He had become convinced of the truth of his conclusions several years before this book appeared; in the first chapter, he wrote that he had previously announced his opinion in lectures which the president and Fellows of the College of Physicians in London had attended and approved.

Harvey's book comprises, in seventy-two pages, an introduction and seventeen chapters. The introduction records some "manifest errors" of current teaching on the arteries, pulmonary circulation, and heart structure, and in the first chapter Harvey gave his reasons for writing, acknowledging the work of Fracastoro and Fabricius. The book goes on to describe vividly the heart's expulsion of the blood during systole, its passive refilling during diastole, and the filling of the arteries during systole. The heart's movement and function are presented in detail, together with experimental evidence that was derived from the dissection of mollusks, insects, and cold-blooded animals, in which the slow motions of the heart can be readily observed. Harvey also reported on the heart muscle's ability to recover from fatigue. The account of the movement of the blood into the right heart from the vena cava, its passage through the lungs, and its arrival in the left ventricle establishes the reality of the pulmonary circulation and postulates the presence of invisible capillaries in the lungs. Harvey recounted his timed measurements of the volume of blood that returned to the heart and the amounts entering the aorta during systole. This was a major part of his evidence for the uninterrupted stream of the circulating blood. He admitted that the peripheral anastomoses of the arteries and veins were still to be clarified. The valves in the veins are correctly described and their function explained with records of his classic centripetal-flow experiments. Two illustrations are provided, reproducing four figures of the veins in the forearm, from Fabricius. The last chapter summarizes the whole argument.

Harvey's clear reasoning from the observations and precise measurements made during his purposeful experiments supplied the key for advancing knowledge of physiology and was also a model for future scientific procedure.

William Harvey. *Exercitatio Anatomica de Motu Cordis et Sanguinis in Animalibus*. Frankfurt, 1628.

This dramatic illustration of the function of the valves should be compared with that of Fabricius (page 58), which shows their anatomy.

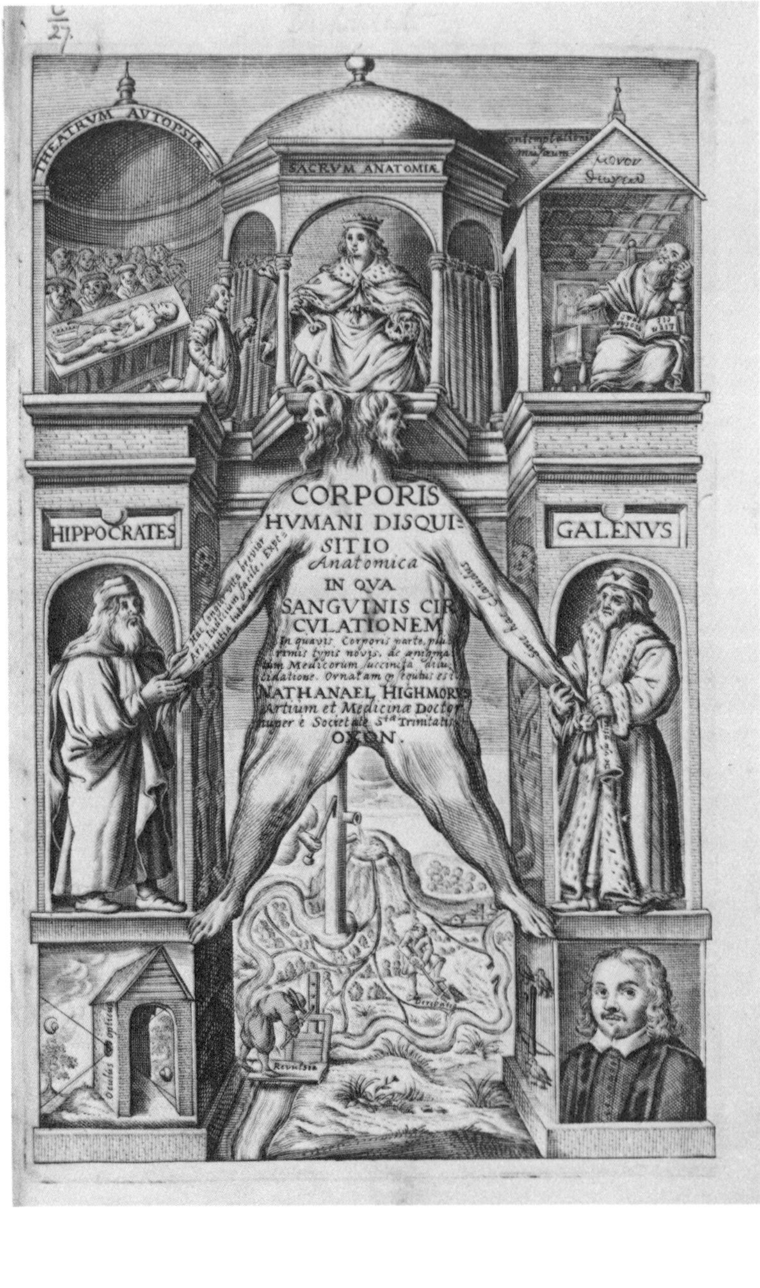
THEATRUM AUTOPSIÆ
SACRUM ANATOMIÆ
HIPPOCRATES
GALENUS
CORPORIS
HUMANI DISQUI-
SITIO
Anatomica
IN QUA
SANGUINIS CIR
CULATIONEM
In quavis Corporis parte, plu
rimis typis novis, ac ænigma
tum Medicorum succincta dilu
cidatione. Ornatam
NATHANAEL HIGHMORUS
Artium et Medicinæ Doctor
nuper è Societate Sta Trinitatis
OXON.
Revulsio

# Nathanael Highmore

## ANATOMIC INVESTIGATIONS OF THE HUMAN BODY

Highmore (1613-1685), a country surgeon at Sherborne in Dorset, was a devoted follower of Harvey, whom he had known at Oxford and to whom he dedicated this book. It has the distinction of being the first anatomy textbook by an Englishman to give an account of the circulation of the blood and to credit Harvey for his discovery. Highmore describes his book on the title page, which may be translated as follows: "Anatomic Investigations of the Human Body, in which he follows the circulation of the blood into every part of the body, ornamenting it with many new examples and a brief explanation of medical problems." The book was published in Holland by S. Broun, an English bookseller at The Hague in 1651. Highmore's little *History of Generation* appeared in London in the same year, which also saw the publication of Harvey's second great book, *De Generatione*.

The text of "Anatomic Investigations" is arranged in three "books," following the traditional dissection order of discussing the organs of the three body cavities—the abdomen, thorax, and head. Apart from the full treatment of the circulation, the book, though not very original, contains a number of new descriptions, most notably one with a good illustration of the antrum of the upper jaw, which has been named for Highmore. His attention was drawn to the cavity in the superior maxillary bone by a woman who had an abscess there that was drained by extraction of a tooth. The seminal ducts and the epididymis are also described. There are copper-engraved plates and text illustrations.

Publication abroad brought recognition from Continental anatomists, and the book must have been welcome to students in England, since it was one of the best of its day.

Nathanael Highmore. *Corporis Humani Disquisitio Anatomica in Qua Sanguinis Circulationem In quavis Corporis parte, plurimis typis novis, ac anigmatum Medicorum succincta dilucidatione Ornatam prosequutus est.* The Hague, 1651.

This allegorical and architectural title page, even then old-fashioned for a scientific book, brought together many elements of seventeenth-century medical knowledge.

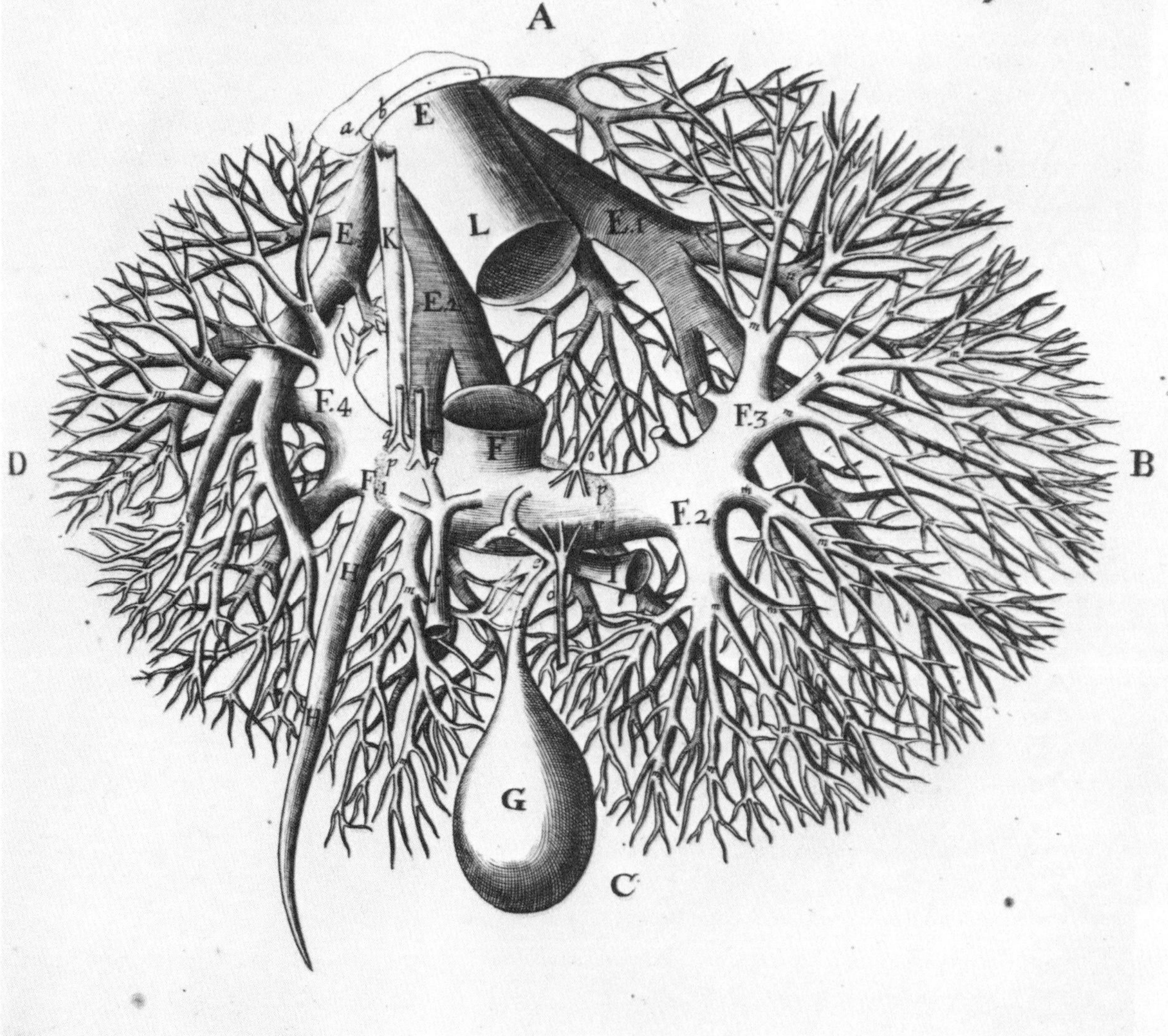
A
B
C
D
E
E.1
E.2
E.3
F
F.1
F.2
F.3
F.4
G
H
K
L

# Francis Glisson

## ANATOMY OF THE LIVER

Glisson's treatise on the liver was the first book printed in England to give a detailed account, based on original research, of a single organ. Glisson (1597-1677) was associated with the "natural philosophers" who founded the Royal Society in 1660, and he was also active among the physicians who wished to keep medical research within the College of Physicians, of which he was president from 1667 to 1669. He was regius professor of physic at Cambridge for forty years but practiced continuously in London, even during 1666—the year of the plague.

His book on the liver is in Latin. There are ten chapters on general anatomy and forty-five on the liver, which give an admirable description of the gross anatomy of that organ. However, because microscopic study had scarcely begun and biochemistry was still to be born, his account of the liver's function is necessarily primitive. The research was done twelve or more years before the book was published. Glisson recorded that he discovered the "common capsule," now named for him, while preparing a lecture in 1642. This "capsule of Glisson" is the envelope of fibrous tissue that encloses the portal vein and hepatic artery (the two vessels carrying blood to the liver) and becomes continuous with the fibrous scaffolding of the whole organ.

Glisson made use of injection and casts and included a good engraving of a cast of the liver vessels. He also reported in detail his experiment to show the passage of the blood from the portal vein to the vena cava and demonstrated that the color of the liver derives from the contained blood. In the final chapters, he proved that the lymph flows, not to the liver, as had been taught, but from it and passes to the then recently discovered "common receptacle."

Four years earlier, Glisson had published the first clear description of infantile rickets, which was called "Glisson's disease." Many years later, in his book on the stomach and intestines (1677), he demonstrated the mechanism of muscle contraction, substituting the theory of inherent "irritability" for the prevalent idea of "vital spirits."

Francis Glisson. *Anatomia Hepatis....* London, 1654.

Glisson's book contains a number of striking illustrations, such as this one, based on his dissections and on injected models of the liver.

P. 132

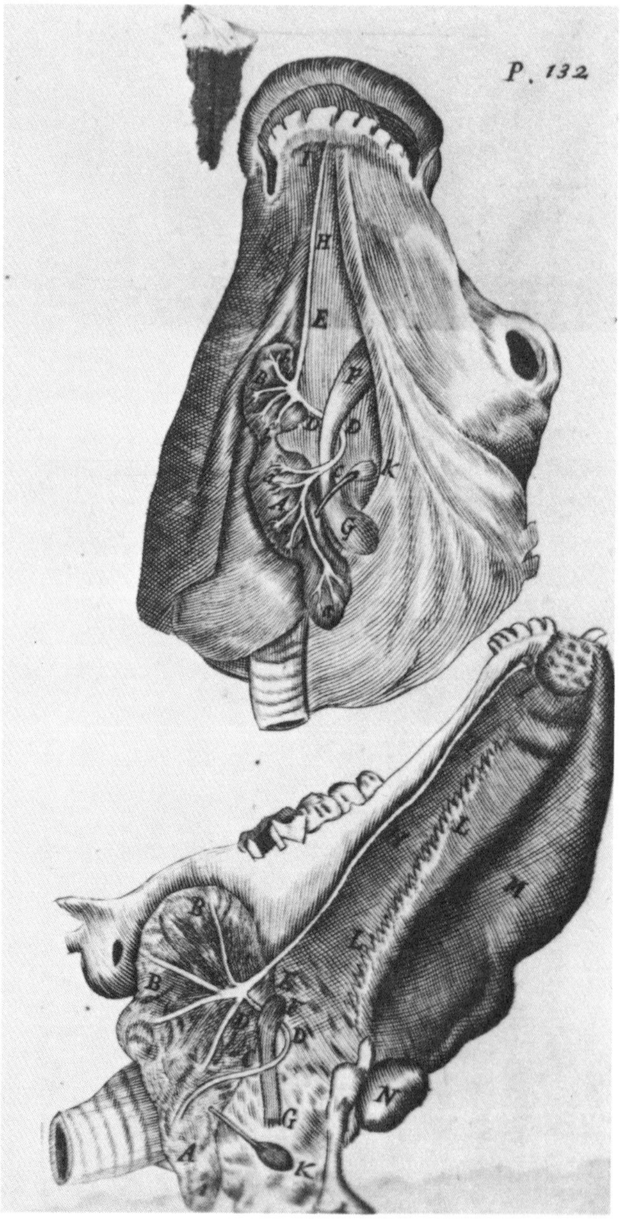

# Thomas Wharton

## DESCRIPTION OF THE GLANDS

Thomas Wharton (1614-1673) presented the first comprehensive report and classification of all the glands in the human body. In differentiating the glands from the viscera, he also explained their relationship. His name has been particularly associated with the duct of the submaxillary salivary gland, called "Wharton's duct," and he accurately expounded the role of saliva in mastication and digestion. Even more valuable were his descriptions of the "renal glands" (adrenals) and the thyroid, to which he gave the first adequate treatment, providing its name, "thyroid" (shield-shaped), in place of the former vague "laryngeal gland."

His explanations were sometimes teleologic, as when he stated that the purpose of the thyroid was, among other functions, to fill the neck and make it shapely. Elsewhere he attempted a physiologic judgment, suggesting, for instance, that the adrenals act "to restore to the veins some humors imbibed from the spleen which were not profitable to the nerves." He gave a good account of the spleen and pancreas and furnished the original description of the mucoid matrix (Wharton's jelly), which keeps the umbilical cord supple and cushions the fetal vessels.

The book is arranged in the traditional order (abdominal, thoracic, and cephalic), to which Wharton added a section on the reproductive glands. He worked closely with his colleagues at St. Thomas's Hospital and with Francis Glisson (q.v.); like Glisson, he stayed in London through the plague but lost his house in the Great Fire of London in 1666. He was one of the conservative physicians who resented the new Royal Society for trespassing on the preserves of the long-established College of Physicians in biologic research. Nevertheless, he was one of many investigators whose individual contributions greatly advanced anatomic research in seventeenth-century England.

Wharton's work on the endocrine glands was continued by the next generation of anatomists, but the subject was then neglected until the mid-nineteenth century.

Thomas Wharton. *Adenographia: sive, Glandularum Totius Corporis Descriptio.* London, 1656.

Wharton's duct as portrayed by its discoverer. The illustration is a narrow foldout inserted between two pages of text.

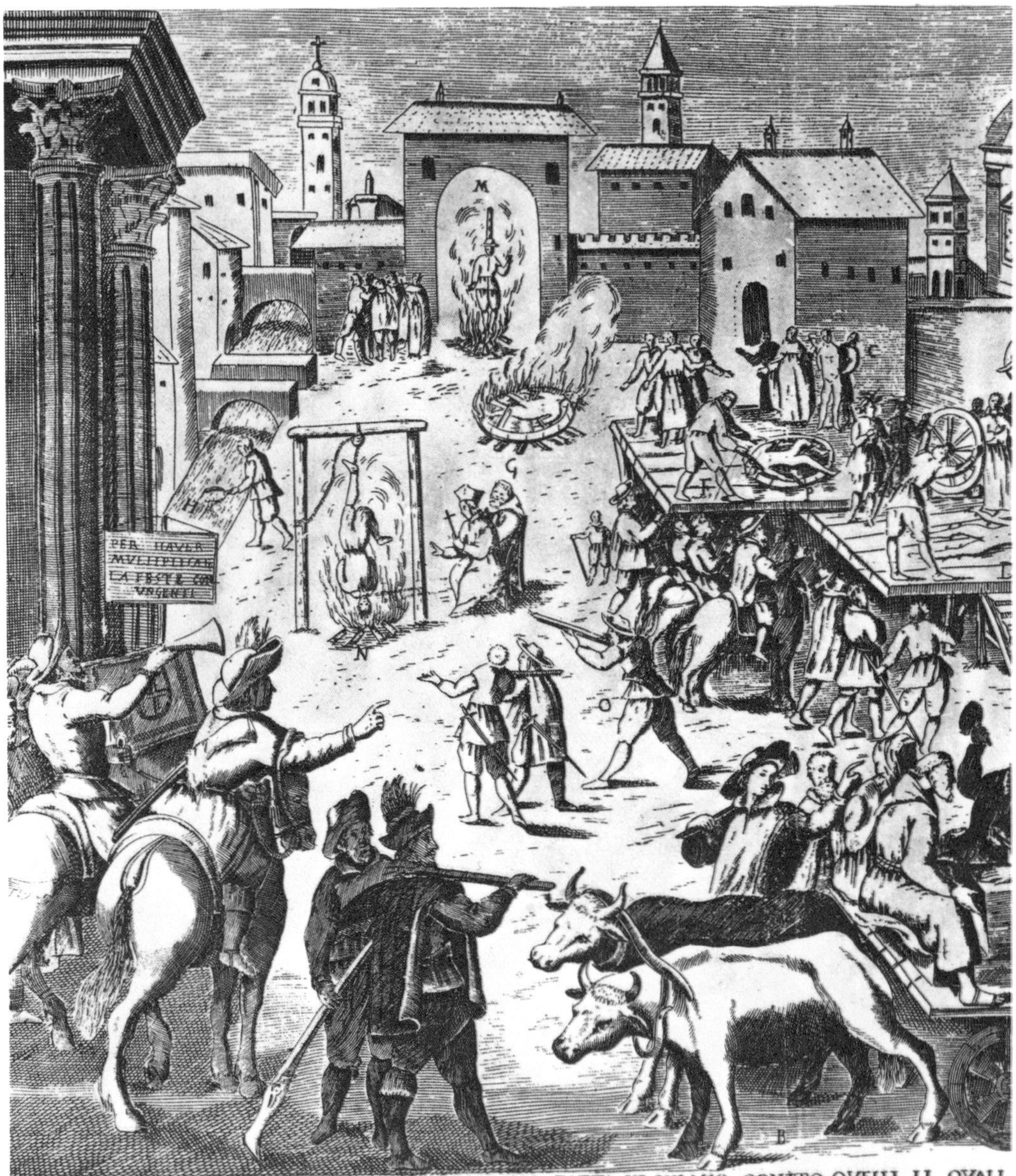


DESCRITTIONE DELLA ESECVTIONE DI GIVSTITIA FATTA IN MILANO CONTRO QVELLI LI QVALI

# Athanasius Kircher

## SCRUTINY OF CONTAGIOUS PLAGUE

Just as Galileo's telescope revolutionized astronomy, so did the microscope open a window to the study of body tissues. Probably the first to employ the microscope in the investigation of disease was the Jesuit priest of Fulda, Athanasius Kircher (1602-1680), contemporary with but slightly older than van Leeuwenhoek. This learned man was a virtuoso musician, orientalist, mathematician, and physicist and had some knowledge of medicine. His study of plague is valuable for its well-understood and carefully explained theory of *contagium vivum,* or the infection by living matter. In his *Scrutinium,* published in Rome in 1658, he describes his studies on putrefaction, during which he saw maggots and other creatures develop in necrotic tissue. He found the blood of plague patients full of "little worms which propagate plague, so very small and unperceivable except with a very fine microscope."

This description occurs in the central section of his book, where he dealt with the "contagion or kindling of plague" at some length. The earlier chapters discussed the causes and effects of plague, its prognosis, and the signs of its course, with some experiments on infected air. After the chapter on contagion, there is a thorough account of "therapeutics and prophylaxis, or the cure and preservation from contagion of the plague."

It seems unlikely that Kircher could have seen bacilli in the blood of plague patients with the simple low-power microscope available at that time. What he actually saw is less important than his realization of the association between disease and bacteria. Though he was probably wrong in identifying the objects under his crude microscope, his concepts led to a correct appreciation of the cause of infectious disease.

The last twenty pages of his book provide a chronologic table of historic plague epidemics, including the Great Plague of Athens (430 B.C.) and the Black Death (A.D. 1350).

Athanasius Kircher. *Scrutinium physico-medicum Contagiosae Luis, quae Pestis dicitur.* Rome, 1658.

Engraving of the Square of Justice in Milan in 1630, showing the torture and execution of persons accused of violating precautions against the spread of plague.

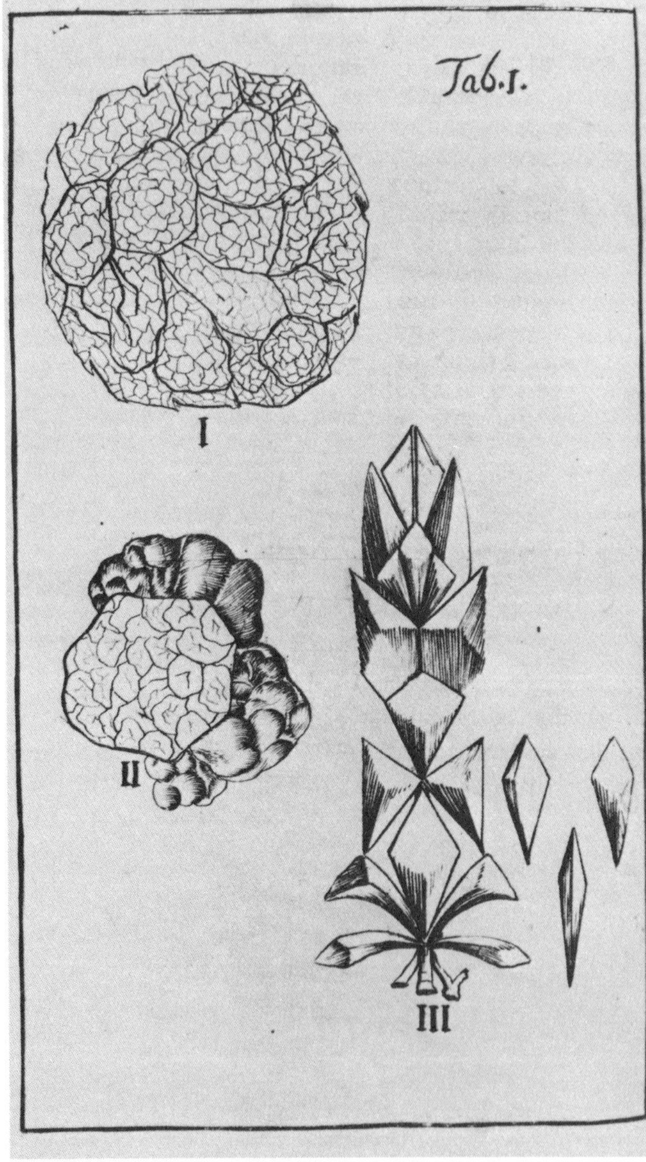
Tab. I.
I
II
III

# Marcello Malpighi

## ON THE LUNGS

Malpighi (1628-1694), the founder of histology, was physician to Pope Innocent XII and professor of anatomy at Bologna, Pisa, and Messina. He was remarkable for the range of his research in comparative anatomy, embryology, and physiology and for his innovative studies of plant tissues. His most original contribution to medicine is contained in his *De Pulmonibus*, or "On the Lungs."

That work, originally published in 1661 as a pamphlet of twenty-three pages, is exceedingly rare. Written in the form of two letters to G. A. Borelli, his colleague at Pisa, it was reissued in 1663 in book form with Bartholin's *De Pulmonum*. In the first letter, Malpighi showed that the pulmonary tissues are vesicular and that the trachea ends in bronchial filaments; this supplied the anatomic basis for respiratory exchange in the lungs. The second letter recorded his discovery of the capillary link between the arteries and the veins, which complemented Harvey's experiments and theory on the circulation of the blood. Malpighi later described the red blood cells as "fat globules looking like a rosary of red coral."

Another book, on the viscera, was first issued in 1666 as three essays—on the liver, the cerebral cortex, and the kidneys. Later in the same year, two more essays were added, on cardiac polyp and on the spleen. All of them are notable for their original descriptions of histologic structure, in which Malpighi was a pioneer. Here, Malpighi elaborated Lorenzo Bellini's account of the uriniferous tubules and noted that the glomeruli are attached to the tips of the arterial branches, which have been called the "Malpighian bodies." His name has also been applied eponymically to the Malpighian bodies of the spleen and the Malpighian layer of the skin.

His later studies on embryology and plant physiology, though carried out in Italy, were encouraged by the Royal Society of London, which also published most of this work. The illustrations in *De Formatione Pulli in Ovo* (1673) and *De Ovo Incubato* make him the founder of modern descriptive embryology. Better than those of all other contemporary embryologists, his detailed observations were also the first accurate reports of the development of the aortic arches, the head fold, the neural groove, and the cerebral and optic vesicles.

This gentle, fair-minded man's life was marred by the personal attacks of his former colleague Borelli and by a long-standing feud between his family and a neighboring clan. Some of his major work was destroyed in manuscript form and never rewritten.

Marcello Malpighi. *De Pulmonibus Observationes Anatomicae*. In Thomas Bartholin's *De Pulmonum Substantia & Motu Diatribe*. Copenhagen, 1663.

Malpighi's remarkable ability to interpret and communicate his observations is represented by these drawings of the alveolar structure of lung tissue and his stylized schematic diagram of the respiratory tree.

Fig: 1

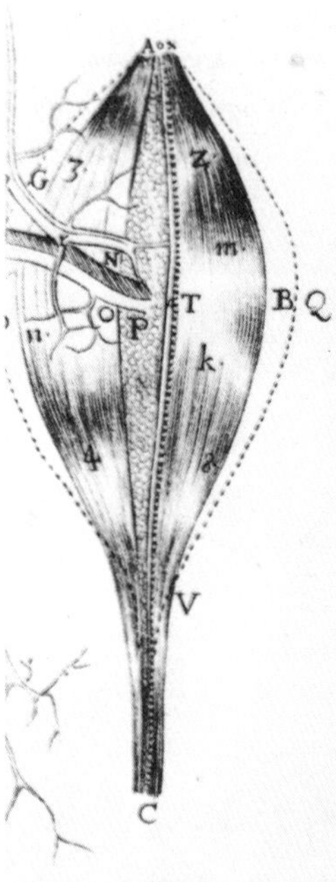


Fig: 2

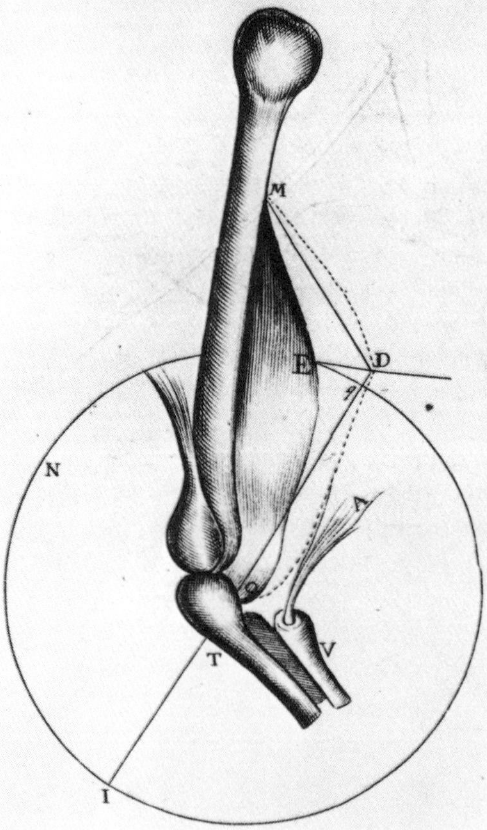

# William Croone

## THE MOVEMENT OF MUSCLES

William Croone (1633-1684), a London physician, was an associate of the great Robert Boyle (q.v.) and an original Fellow of the Royal Society. He was lecturer on the anatomy of the muscles to the Company of Surgeons in London, a position he held for the last fourteen years of his life. His most notable contributions to medicine were his monographs on muscle physiology and on the embryology of the chick, both of which were published after the essay on muscular movement.

The treatise on muscular motion was an attempt to give a rational account of muscle contraction. Accepting the then-current belief that the action of the nerves was affected by "nervous spirit," he suggested that this fluid was a "spirituous liquor," a rectified and "enriched juice," which interacted with the blood and other substances in the muscle to produce contraction. Yet he hinted that the nerve impulse consisted of vibrations along the nerve that was in a state of tension.

The year after the publication of his essay, Croone met Nicolaus Steno (q.v.) and learned of a new—and still unpublished—discovery: that muscles do not enlarge when in contraction. In spite of this new knowledge, Croone proceeded to develop his theory of contraction, suggesting that each individual muscle fiber contained small bladders to receive the increased fluids supplied from the nerves. The series of lectures in which this refined theory was presented was delivered in 1674-1675 but was not published until 1681. Before the lectures appeared in book form, Francis Glisson stated, in 1677, that muscle does not increase in volume when it contracts. Glisson's conclusion, made with the authority of long experience, overshadowed Croone's theory even in his lifetime. Croone is perhaps best remembered from the famous Croonian Lectures; these were endowed by his widow from the fortune that she inherited at his death in 1684.

William Croone. *De Ratione Motus Musculorum.* London, 1664.

Diagram illustrating the interaction of "spirituous liquor" and blood in the muscles (Figure 1), producing muscular contraction in the flexion of joints (Figure 2).

Figura Iª

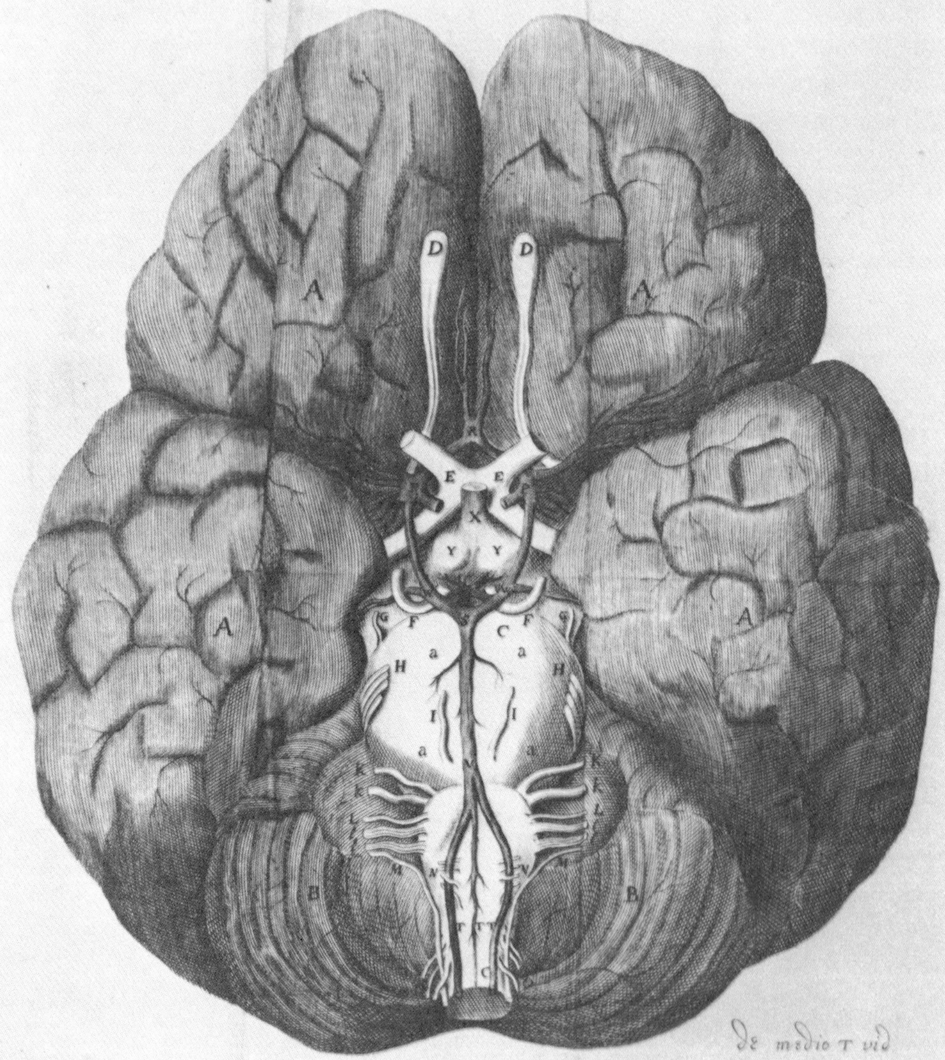

# Thomas Willis

## CEREBRAL ANATOMY

Willis (1621-1675), who was Sedleian professor of natural philosophy at Oxford, wrote the most thorough account of the anatomy of the brain (with a clear classification of the cranial nerves) in that era. With this contribution, he was entitled to be a member of the notable group of seventeenth-century anatomists that included Valsalva, Malpighi, Leeuwenhoek, and others.

In his preface, Willis acknowledged the help of Richard Lower (q.v.), Thomas Millington, and particularly Christopher Wren, who, "with the singular kindness for which he is esteemed, made light of drawing many figures of the brain and skull with precise skill and his own highly trained hands." Wren's plates are not signed, but he is credited with the drawing of the base of the human brain that exhibits the "circle of Willis" (see illustration). Since they show a wealth of detail, the plates are clearer than Willis's text.

The book is divided into twenty-nine chapters that are partly anatomic and partly physiologic; it includes comparative studies. One chapter, for instance, describes the brains of birds and fish; another, the cerebral arteries "in the various animals." A plate shows human and equine carotid arteries as well as the rete mirabile and pituitary of the calf. The sequence of chapters covers the posterior parts of the brain, the cerebellum, the cranium, and the dura and meninges; the blood supply; and animal spirits and animal faculties. In the final chapter, the blood supply to the spinal medulla is traced.

Willis moved from Oxford to London in 1666 and was successful in medical practice there for the nine years before he died at the age of fifty-four. His important contributions to clinical medicine included differential descriptions of epidemic typhoid and puerperal fever and two books on nervous diseases. The *Pharmaceutice Rationalis* contained the materia medica of his time. Willis made an exhaustive study of urine and was the first to report that the urine of patients with diabetes mellitus has a sweet taste (distinguishing it from the urine in diabetes insipidus). Typical of his powers of observation is his report of a deaf woman who could hear only when a drum was beating. Her condition was named for him, *paracusia Willisii.*

Thomas Willis. *Cerebri Anatome: cui accessit Nervorum Descriptio et Usus.* London, 1664.

Willis studied the cerebral arteries by injecting the brain with saffron-stained water. This engraving is thought to be the work of Sir Christopher Wren.

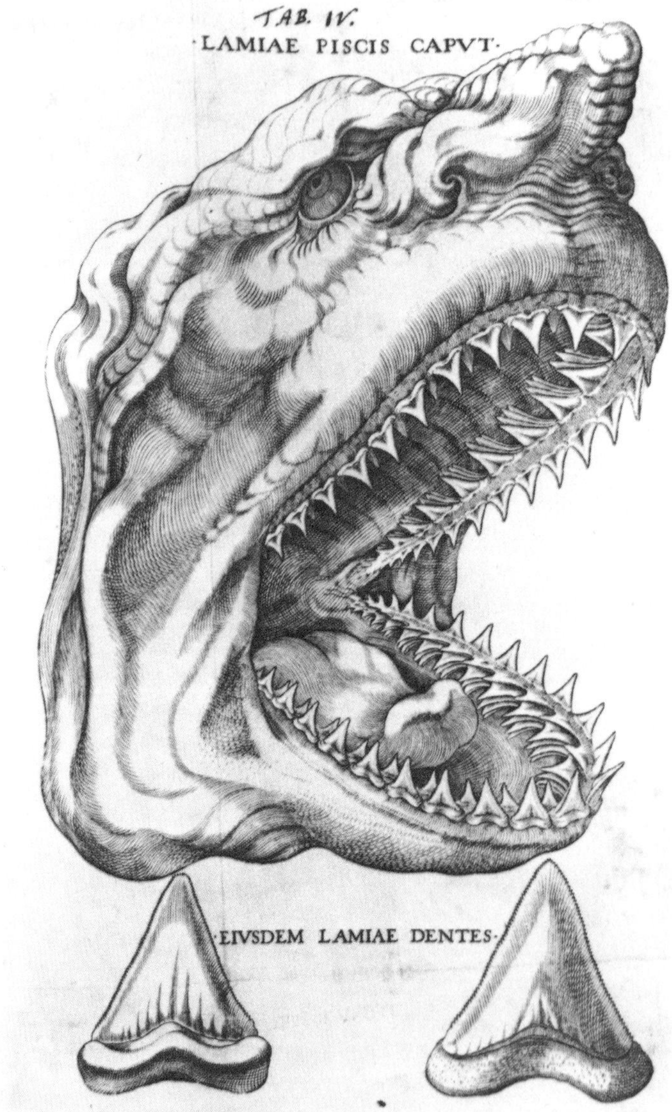
TAB. IV.
·LAMIAE PISCIS CAPVT·
·EIVSDEM LAMIAE DENTES·

# Nicolaus Steno

## ELEMENTS OF MYOLOGY

Nicolaus Steno, or Niels Stensen (1638-1686), was taught in Copenhagen by the renowned Dane, Thomas Bartholin, and then spent four years in Holland; there, at the age of twenty-four, he published his "Anatomical Observations on the Vessels of the Mouth, Eyes and Nose," which included his discovery of the parotid duct (named for him). Upon returning to Copenhagen in 1664, he published his pioneer work on muscles and glands. This was supplemented three years later by his "Elements of Myology, a Geometric Description of Muscles," printed in Florence, where he had settled in 1666.

In the book on muscles and glands, Steno advanced his theories on the muscles of the digestive organs, followed by a description of muscle fibers. In this, he explained how the tensile strength of each fiber contributes to the action of the whole muscle and demonstrated that the heart is a muscle. He discussed the glands of the oral cavity, the lymphatics, the tear glands, and the milk glands.

"Elements of Myology," expanding his concepts, provides a mechanistic explanation of muscular physiology. From the histologic appearance of muscles and of the nerves supplying them, Steno deduced that the apparent increase in muscle size during contraction represents a change in shape rather than an increase in bulk. Earlier writings on this topic, which postulated the flow of fluid from the nerves into the muscles during contraction, Steno termed "mere words, meaning nothing!" In a two-part appendix to this book, he described dentition of the shark and made an important correlation between the ovaries of the viviparous shark and the human.

Willis had correctly deduced that the cerebrum is the center for thought, but he arbitrarily assigned perception to the corpora striata, imagination to the corpus callosum, and instinct to the midbrain. Steno denounced Willis for having thus speculated without experimental evidence or knowledge of the anatomic connections involved. Steno's criticisms of Willis and other anatomists appear in an important discourse on the anatomy of the brain (Paris, 1669). He contributed anatomic papers to *Acta Medica et Philosophica Hafniensia,* the earliest medical periodical, and examined the fossil content of sedimentary rock strata, which he described in *De Solido intra Solidum* in 1669. For that monograph he is regarded as one of the founders of geology.

Late in his life, he gave up science for religion. Having been converted from his Lutheran faith to Catholicism, he was consecrated a bishop and went to a diocese in northern Germany, where he died at the age of forty-eight.

Nicolaus Steno. *Elementorum Myologiae Specimen, seu Musculi descriptio Geometrica*.... Florence, 1667.

The artist strikingly combines realism and fancy in this awesome drawing of the shark's jaw.

FIG. 12

PAG. 45.

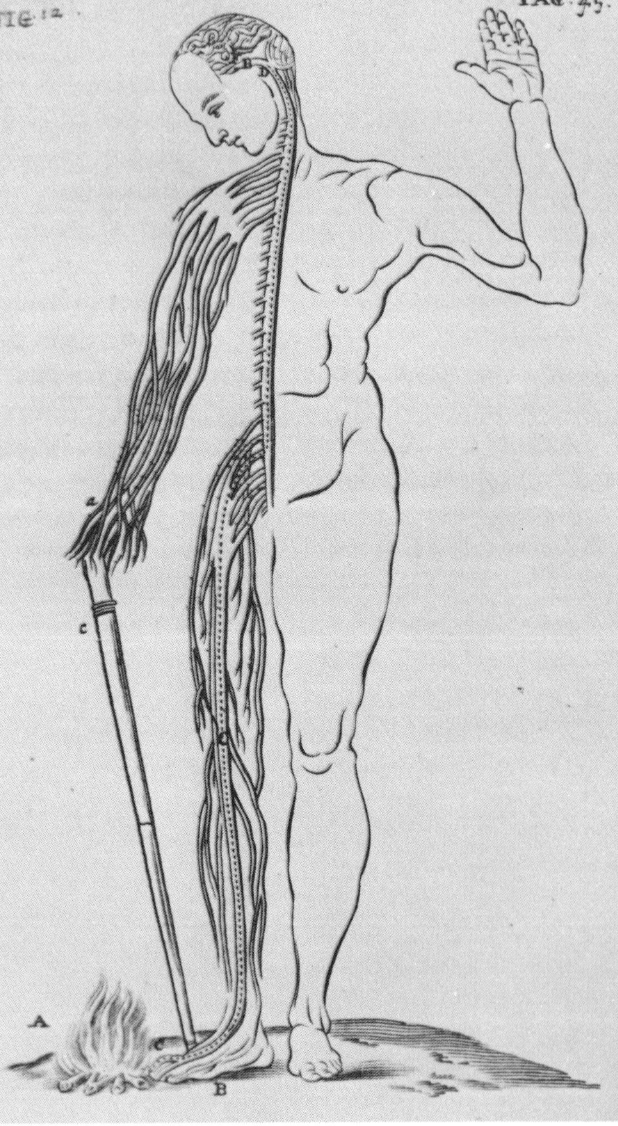

# René Descartes

## ON MAN and MAN AND THE FORMATION OF THE FETUS

"On Man," considered by many to be the first important textbook on physiology, reflects the firm conviction of Descartes (1596-1650) that all physiologic processes were consequences of the laws of mathematics and physics. Organs were compared to machines, biologic functions to mechanical processes. Descartes's interpretations of his observations were speculative; he set out from what he knew to find the cause of what he saw. Although he performed a wide range of animal dissections and chemical manipulations, he never fully grasped the scientific method of hypothesis tested by experiment. Nevertheless, most of the experimentalists who made such great advances in knowledge late in the seventeenth century were deeply influenced by his mechanistic approach, which allowed them to discard traditional conceptual explanations.

These two treatises were published posthumously. "On Man" (*De Homine*) was translated from the French manuscript into Latin by Schuyl, who took some liberties with the text and the illustrations. The French edition two years later was an accurate representation of Descartes's original manuscript and artwork and included his essay on the fetus.

The volume on man considers the organism as an automaton and discusses "the machine of the body" and "how the machine moves." The workings of the interior and the external senses, particularly vision, are explained. The book ends with a discourse on "animal spirits" and the function of brain and nerves.

The treatise on the formation of the fetus is more speculative and dogmatic. It is based on a conceptual picture of the corpuscles of the male and female seeds fermenting together to create the heart and lungs, the blood, sense organs, and nerves; later these coalesce to make the tissues that grow together to form the solid parts.

From his mother, Descartes is said to have inherited both weak lungs and enough property to free him for philosophic pursuits. He learned mathematics and physics from Jesuit teachers, whose school he entered at the age of ten. After finishing his formal education (he graduated in law at the age of twenty), he lived in Holland and Germany, traveled in Italy, and sought intellectual stimulation among the natural scientists and philosophers of Paris. Some of his interests in physics and mathematics come to us in such expressions as Cartesian geometry, Cartesian coordinates, and Cartesian diver.

He lived in Holland from 1628 to 1649 and then moved to Sweden at Queen Christina's invitation. The harsh weather of Stockholm was too severe for his weak lungs, and he died at the age of fifty-three, a great philosopher, mathematician, and scientist.

René Descartes. *De Homine Figuris et Latinitate Donatus a Florentio Schuyl.* Leyden, 1662.
——. *L'Homme . . . et un traitté de la formation du foetus. . . .* Paris, 1664.

Impulse triggered by burning toes travels through hollow nerves to the brain, where Descartes thought the "soul" resided in the pineal gland (1662 edition).

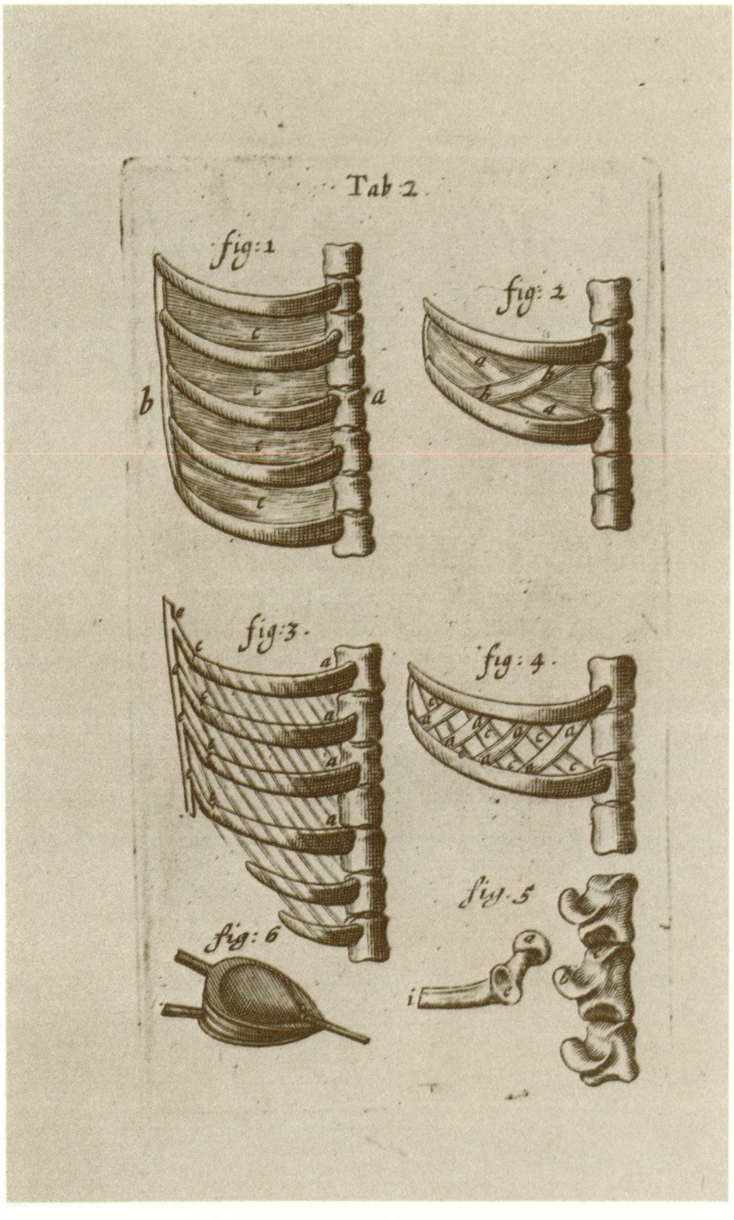

Tab 2
fig: 1
fig: 2
fig: 3
fig: 4
fig: 5
fig: 6

# John Mayow

## FIVE TREATISES ON MEDICINE AND PHYSIOLOGY

John Mayow (1641?-1679) as a young Oxford lawyer became interested in physics and medicine through the influence of Robert Boyle (q.v.) and his circle. Although there is no record of his having gained a medical degree, he studied physics and practiced medicine in London and in Bath and was familiar with Malpighi's work. At twenty-seven, he published a small book, "Two Treatises on Respiration and on Rickets," in Latin. The second edition was "Five Treatises," containing the original two along with additional papers on "Aërial Spirits of Nitre," "Respiration in the Foetus," and "Muscular Motion and Animal Spirits."

The early essay on respiration is the most important of Mayow's writings, for he demonstrated the part played by movement of the ribs in respiration; he first noted the double articulation of the ribs with the spine and the arrangement of the intercostal muscles that control the movement of the thoracic cage. He also observed that blood changes in color from blue to red during its passage through the lungs. He ascribed this change quite correctly to the taking up by the blood of a certain portion of the air, which he called the "igneo-aerial particles" of the "aërial spirits of nitre." Mayow, it seems, had an intuitive understanding of the gaseous interchange that occurs during respiration between blood and the inspired air. Thus, he was very close to the discovery of oxygen. He may have owed the concept to Boyle but was certainly the first to demonstrate it by ingenious experiments. The identification and isolation of oxygen had to wait for Priestley and Lavoisier.

Mayow showed also that animal heat is generated in the muscles themselves and realized that the maternal blood, besides nourishing the fetus, gives it "aërial spirits of nitre" through the placenta.

Mayow was elected a Fellow of the Royal Society in 1678. He died the next year, still a young man. It is unfortunate that his writings, which were in Latin, were so unskillfully translated for the Royal Society that the English version could not be properly understood and hence was disregarded.

John Mayow. *Tractatus Quinque Medico-Physici....* Oxford, 1674.

Schematic drawings of the ribs, the intercostal muscles, and (Figure 5) the double articulation of the ribs with the spine.

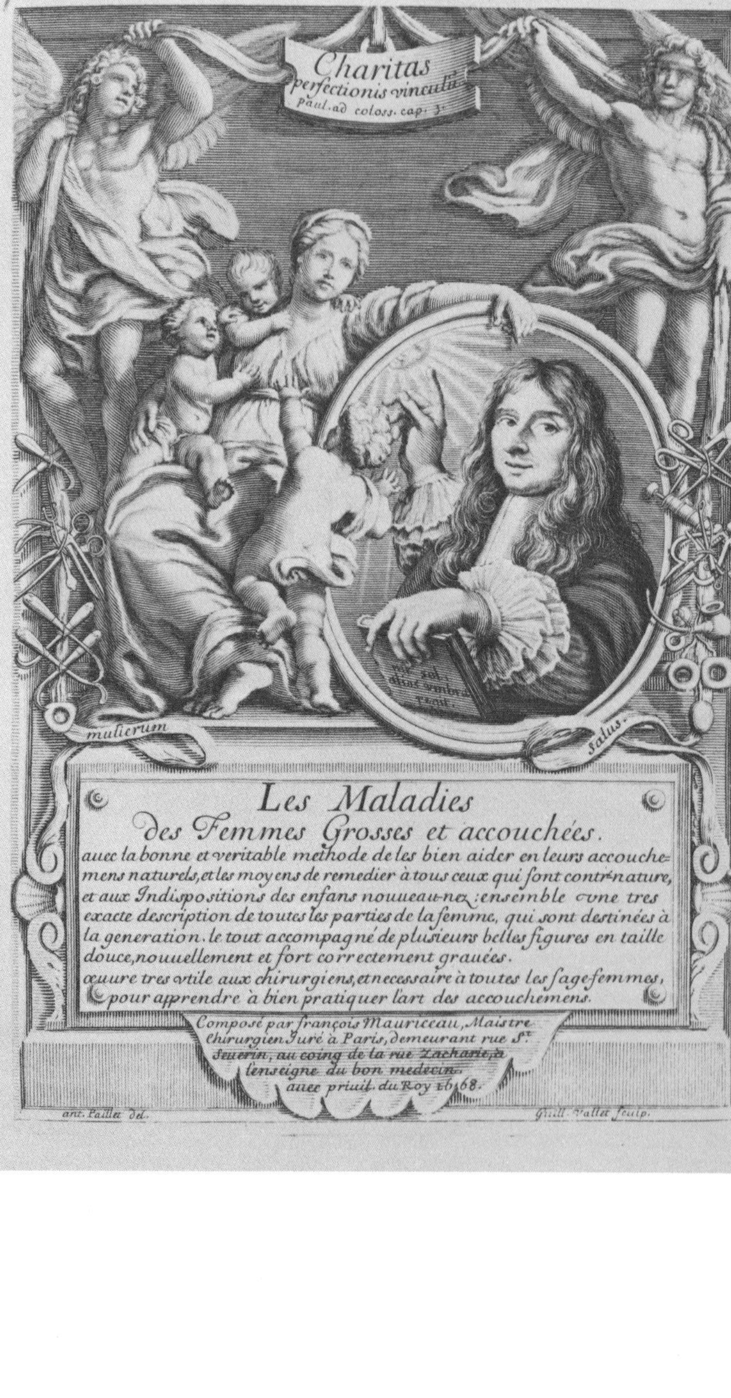
Charitas
perfectionis vinculū
Paul. ad coloss. cap. 3.
mulierum
salus.
Les Maladies
des Femmes Grosses et accouchées.
auec la bonne et veritable methode de les bien aider en leurs accouchemens naturels, et les moyens de remedier à tous ceux qui sont contre nature, et aux Indispositions des enfans nouueau-nez: ensemble vne tres exacte description de toutes les parties de la femme, qui sont destinées à la generation. le tout accompagné de plusieurs belles figures en taille douce, nouuellement et fort correctement grauées.
œuure tres vtile aux chirurgiens, et necessaire à toutes les sage-femmes, pour apprendre à bien pratiquer l'art des accouchemens.
Composé par françois Mauriceau, Maistre Chirurgien Iuré à Paris, demeurant rue St. Seuerin, au coing de la rue Zacharie, à l'enseigne du bon medecin.
auec priuil. du Roy 1668.
ant. Paillet del.
Guill. Vallet sculp.

# François Mauriceau

## DISEASES OF WOMEN WITH CHILD

It was in the seventeenth century, when physicians were beginning to take over the practice of obstetrics from untrained midwives, that Mauriceau's book was published. The work, which received approbation from Daquin, first physician to the king of France, contains the best summary of the knowledge and practice of obstetrics of the era. It is beautifully illustrated with copperplate engravings of birth figures and obstetric instruments and became a standard of excellence for book publishers in its time. Mauriceau (1637-1709) mentioned the several generations of the Chamberlen family, who had kept their obstetric forceps secret for over two hundred years. After the Huguenot Chamberlens had migrated to England, one of them, Hugh Chamberlen, translated Mauriceau's book into English.

The book has a long subtitle that recommends it as useful for surgeons and necessary for midwives. After an anatomic introduction, it is divided into three sections that deal with diseases and abnormalities from the moment of conception to the end of childbirth, normal childbirth, and care of the mother and the newborn infant, including the choice of a suitable wet nurse.

Mauriceau recommended delivering patients in bed rather than on the traditional "birthstool" and described normal labor, version, and the management of placenta previa. He was the first to dispute the old beliefs that the pelvic bones were separated during normal labor and the amniotic fluid was an accumulation of milk and menstrual blood. He was also the first to write on tubal pregnancy, epidemic puerperal fever, and the complications that arise in labor from misplacement of the umbilical cord.

Mauriceau became accoucheur-in-chief of the Hôtel-Dieu in Paris, where he published the first edition of this work in 1668. The third edition was translated into nearly all the languages of Europe and greatly contributed to the spread of good obstetric practice throughout the Continent. Mauriceau himself made a Latin translation, and the book continued to be revised and reissued for some seventy years.

François Mauriceau. *Les Maladies des Femmes Grosses et accouchées*. . . . Paris, 1668.

The title page artistically combines a portrait of the author, the tools of his profession, and an idealized maternal scene.

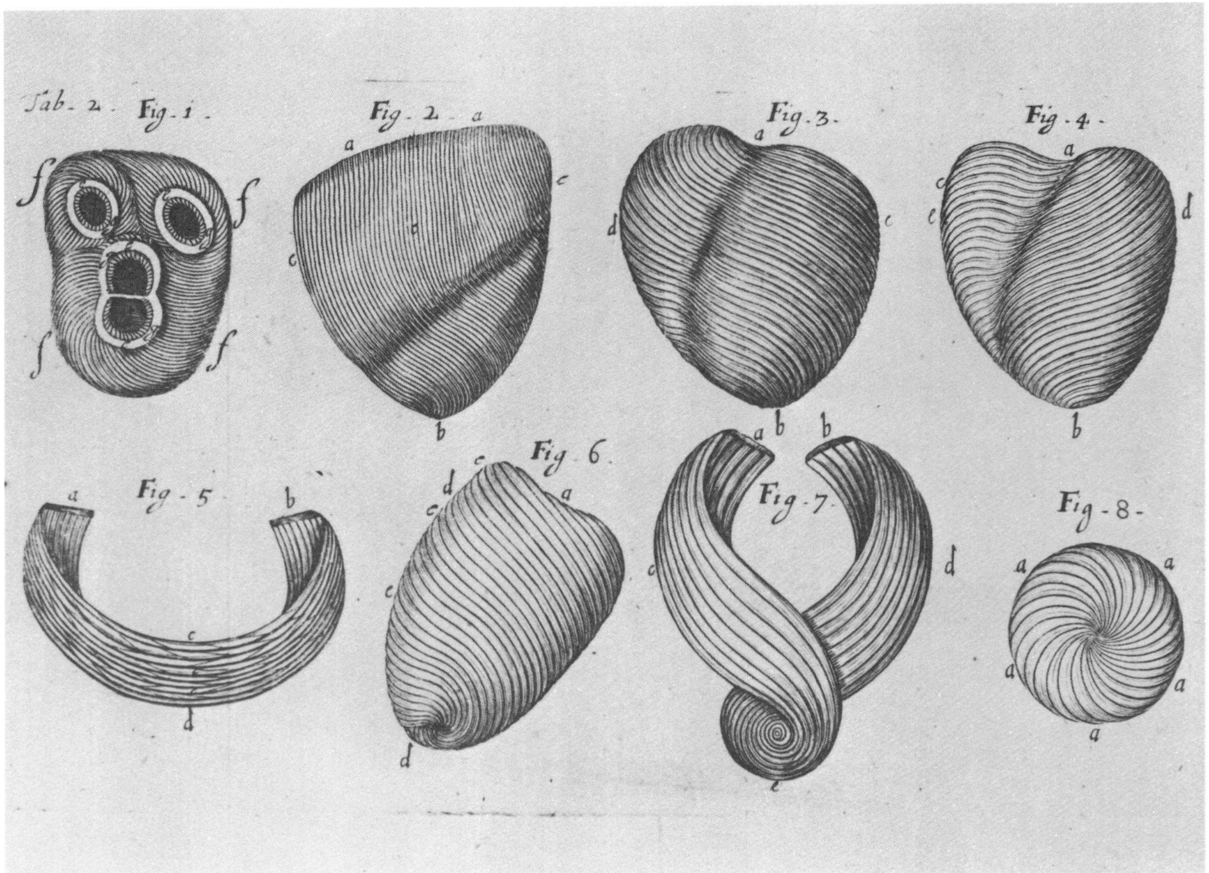
Tab. 2.
Fig. 1.
Fig. 2.
Fig. 3.
Fig. 4.
Fig. 5
Fig. 6.
Fig. 7.
Fig. 8.

# Richard Lower

## TREATISE ON THE HEART

Richard Lower (1631-1691), a native of Cornwall, belonged to the group of young Oxford scientists led by Robert Boyle and Thomas Willis. From the time he took his arts degrees in 1655, he collaborated in the dissections on which Willis based his book on the brain, published in 1664. Lower was the first man to effect the intravenous transfusion of blood (through a quill cannula) from one animal to another. The first human transfusion was performed by J. B. Denys in Paris in 1667, two years later; shortly after that, Lower made the first one in England.

He received his medical degree in 1665 and moved to London, where he carried out physiologic research, was active as a member of the Royal Society, and practiced with great success as a physician. He tried to explain the function of anatomic structures through his experiments and, in dissecting the cardiovascular system, made significant observations that virtually completed Harvey's work on the heart.

His book, *Tractatus de Corde*, is in five sections: the site and structure of the heart, its movements, the movements and colors of the blood, blood transfusion, and the chyle and its transition and transmutation into blood. Lower's most original contributions, recorded in the book, were his concept of the heart muscle (illustrated) and his explanation of the heartbeat as a muscular mechanism, his description of the change in color of the blood from dark to bright as it passes through the lungs, and his conclusion that this was caused by the absorption of air. Soon after the observation, John Mayow, another Cornishman, made the correct observation that only part of the inspired air is absorbed by venous blood in the lungs.

In a second edition, in 1670, Lower incorporated a chapter, "De Catarrhis," in which he showed that catarrh does not come from the pituitary, as had been believed, but is secreted in the respiratory passages of the nose and sinuses. It was courageous of him to oppose the traditional Galenic belief that even Vesalius had upheld. This discovery ended the practice of "purging the brain."

Richard Lower. *Tractatus de Corde. Item de Motu & Colore Sanguinis et Chyli in eum Transitu.* London, 1669.

Lower's concept showed the heart muscle as a scroll-like figure-eight structure, viewed here from various angles.

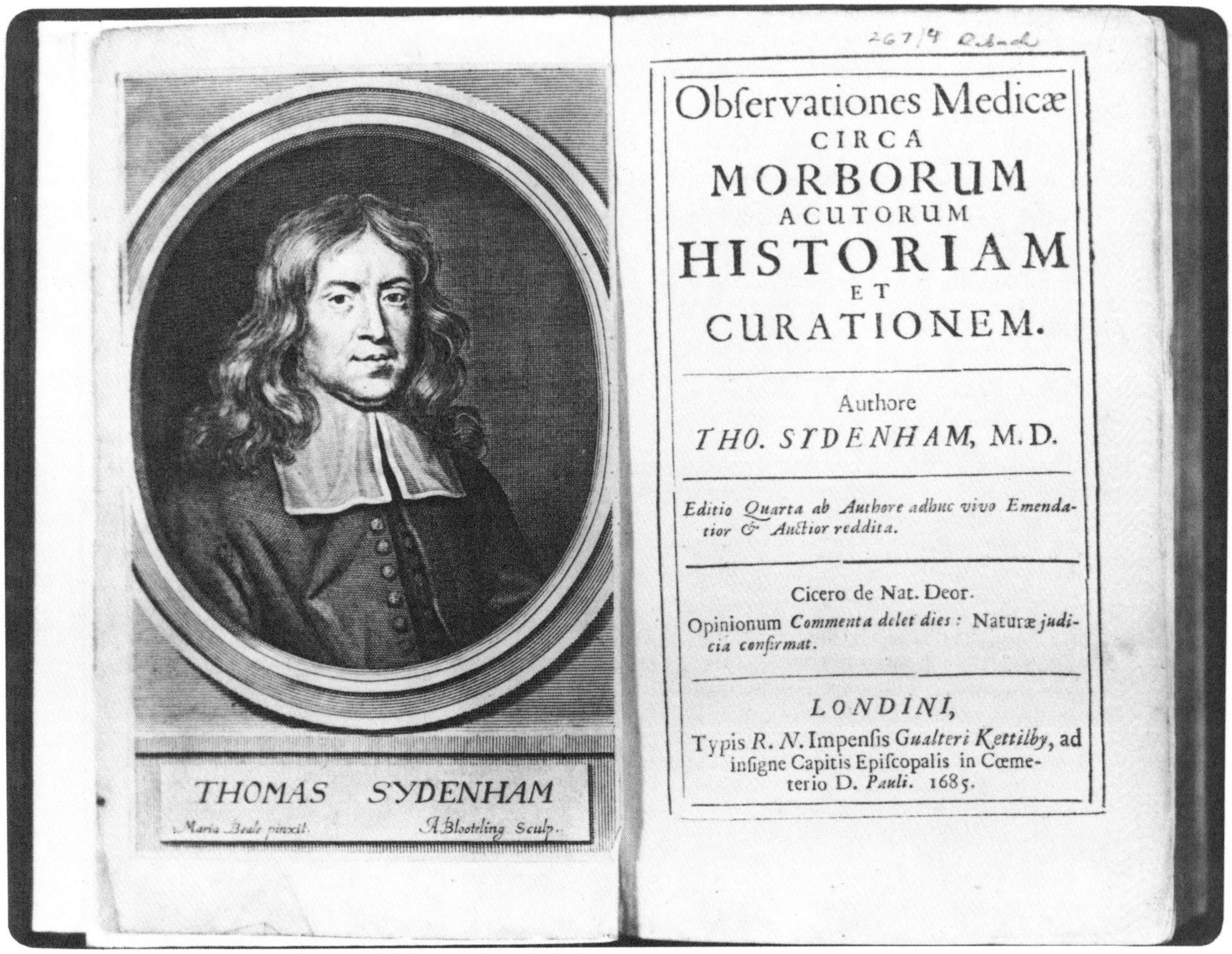


Obſervationes Medicæ
CIRCA
MORBORUM
ACUTORUM
HISTORIAM
ET
CURATIONEM.

Authore
*THO. SYDENHAM*, M.D.

*Editio Quarta ab Authore adhuc vivo Emendatior & Auctior reddita.*

Cicero de Nat. Deor.
Opinionum *Commenta delet dies:* Naturæ *judicia confirmat.*

*LONDINI*,
Typis *R. N.* Impenſis *Gualteri Kettilby*, ad inſigne Capitis Epiſcopalis in Cœmeterio D. *Pauli.* 1685.

# Thomas Sydenham

## MEDICAL OBSERVATIONS

Among the notable medical books in the Lilly collection, this work by Thomas Sydenham (1624-1689) stands out because it does not announce a major original discovery or the foundation of a new development in medicine. Instead, Sydenham's contribution was the reintroduction of the Hippocratic method of careful clinical observation based on wide personal experience. As a recorder of the natural history of disease, he had few equals. For example, even today one can read his description of an acute attack of gout with profit and pleasure.

His medical education was interrupted twice by military service under Cromwell. Although his formal education in medicine was somewhat limited, he was a most successful clinician. Conservative and even distrustful of scientific innovations, Sydenham approached the treatment of disease with empiricism. His personal influence was so strong that most of the leading clinicians of the next generation may be considered directly or indirectly his pupils. His contributions, however, were not truly appreciated until after his death, when he came to be known as the "English Hippocrates."

It is interesting that the original *Observations* were written in English and published in 1676. The translation into Latin (the proper language of science at the time) was printed nine years later by John Mapletoft, to whom Sydenham dedicated the book. It includes sections on diseases, especially those seen in London epidemics between 1661 and 1675, and the characteristics and treatment of continuous and intermittent fevers, for which he introduced cinchona bark into general use in England. He discussed "pest" (bubonic plague) and smallpox, recommending a regimen of cooling drinks for the latter, and described cholera, dysentery, bilious colic, epidemic cough, pleurisy, pneumonia and "false pneumonia," rheumatism, and quinsy.

Although Sydenham's notions of the causes of fevers and epidemics were traditional (he believed in "epidemic constitutions" and the influence of atmospheric "miasma"), he did note the rhythmic periodicity of the recurrence of epidemics. He also recognized precise "species" of disease, made a distinction between small-pox and measles, and gave the first diagnostic account of scarlatina. He continued to advocate bloodletting in moderation, but his other treatments were simple and sensible: fresh air in the sickroom, exercise for consumptives, iron tonics for anemia, and liquid opiates (laudanum) for pain.

Sydenham gained fame through his "Treatise on Gout and Dropsy" (1683), in which he differentiated gout from rheumatism, but his most enduring work was the *Observationes Medicae.* His classic account of hysteria appears in *Dissertatio Epistolaris* (1682).

Thomas Sydenham. *Observationes Medicae circa Morborum Acutorum Historiam et Curationem.* London, 1685.

"The light of day effaces
the contrivances of fancy but confirms
the decisions of nature" are the words of Cicero
quoted on Sydenham's title page.

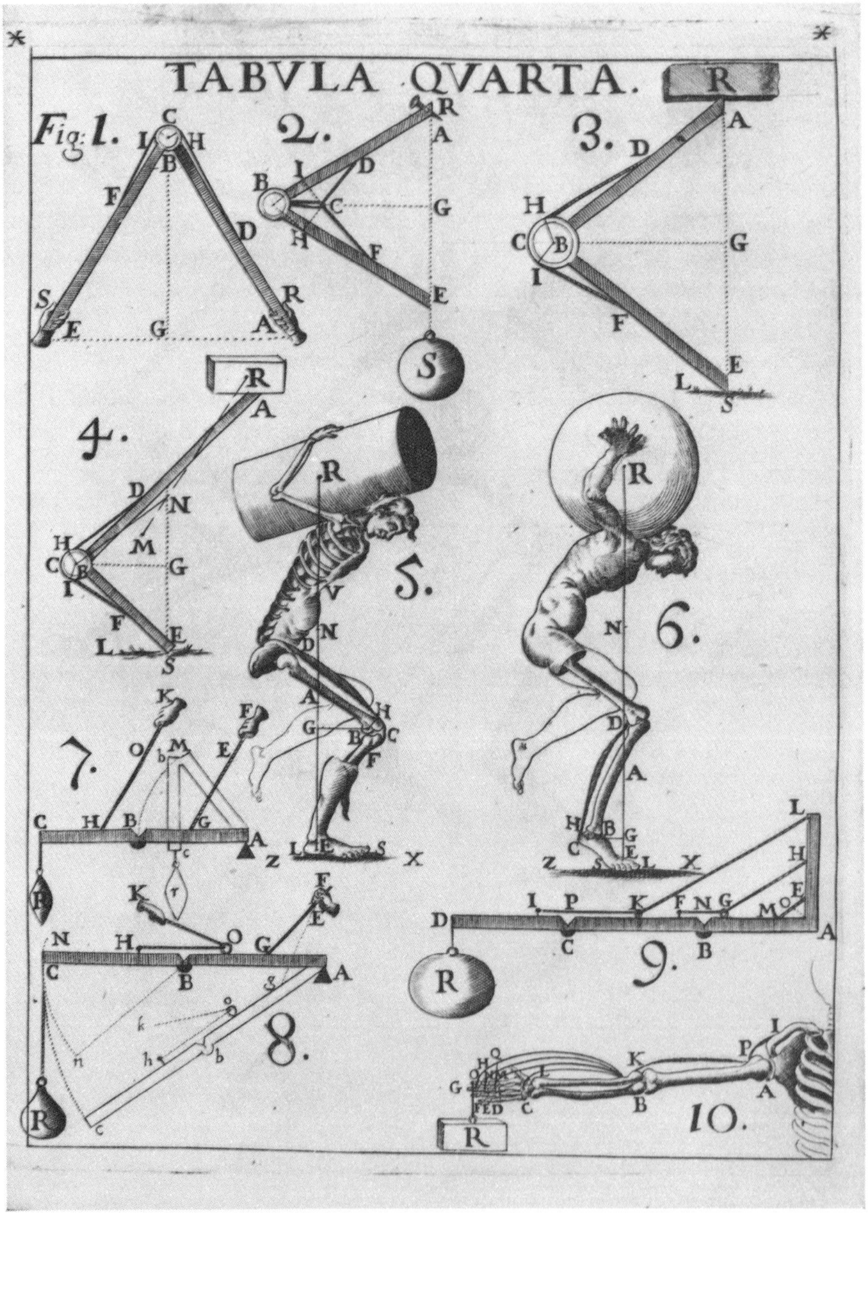
TABVLA QVARTA.

# Giovanni Alfonso Borelli

## ON MUSCULAR MOTION

Born in Naples, Borelli (1608-1679) was primarily a mathematician, a pupil of Galileo. He spent some years in Rome and, in 1635, became lecturer in mathematics at the University of Messina. He stayed there for twenty years, extending his interests into many fields. There was an epidemic of malarial fevers in Sicily in 1647 and 1648, the cause of which he was commissioned to investigate. He concluded that they were caused by the entrance of some chemical substance into the body with the food and not, as was generally believed, by influence of the weather or the stars. He then became interested in the chemical aspects of digestion.

Later he served as professor of mathematics at Pisa for ten years. This brought him into contact with many investigators, notably Malpighi. Although Borelli was still mainly interested in mathematics, physics, and astronomy, he also studied the mechanics of physiology, investigating the kidney with his pupil Lorenzo Bellini and preparing this large volume on muscular activity. He returned to Messina in 1667 and there produced books on percussion and gravity, novel at the time but soon superseded by Newton's work. He fled from Messina after involvement in a patriotic uprising against Spanish rule and spent his last years teaching at a boys' school in Rome. Until his death in 1679, Borelli was also physician to the former Queen Christina of Sweden, in voluntary exile after her abdication. His great book on muscular motion was published posthumously.

Borelli based this work on Harvey's mathematical demonstration of the circulation of the blood, treating movements of the limbs and the internal organs and vessels in mechanical terms. However, he retained a hypothetical theory of "nervous juice," *succus nerveus;* this fluid, he thought, caused muscle contraction by coursing through the nerves and producing fermentation with the liquids in the muscles. He erroneously believed that the process increased the bulk of contracting muscle, a view already disproved by Steno and Glisson. In spite of this error in hypothesis, Borelli's observations contributed to the understanding of body movements.

His theory led him to explain the heart-beat as a simple muscular contraction activated by the nerves and to describe the circulation in simple hydraulic terms. He also contributed to the understanding of flight by calculating the mechanical relationship of the bird's wingbeat to the resistance of the air.

Giovanni Alfonso Borelli. *De Motu Animalium. Opus posthumum.* 2 vols. Rome, 1680-1681.

Primarily a mathematician,
Borelli used principles of physics to illustrate
the movement of both skeletal and visceral muscles and to
show the complementary roles of flexor
and extensor muscle groups.

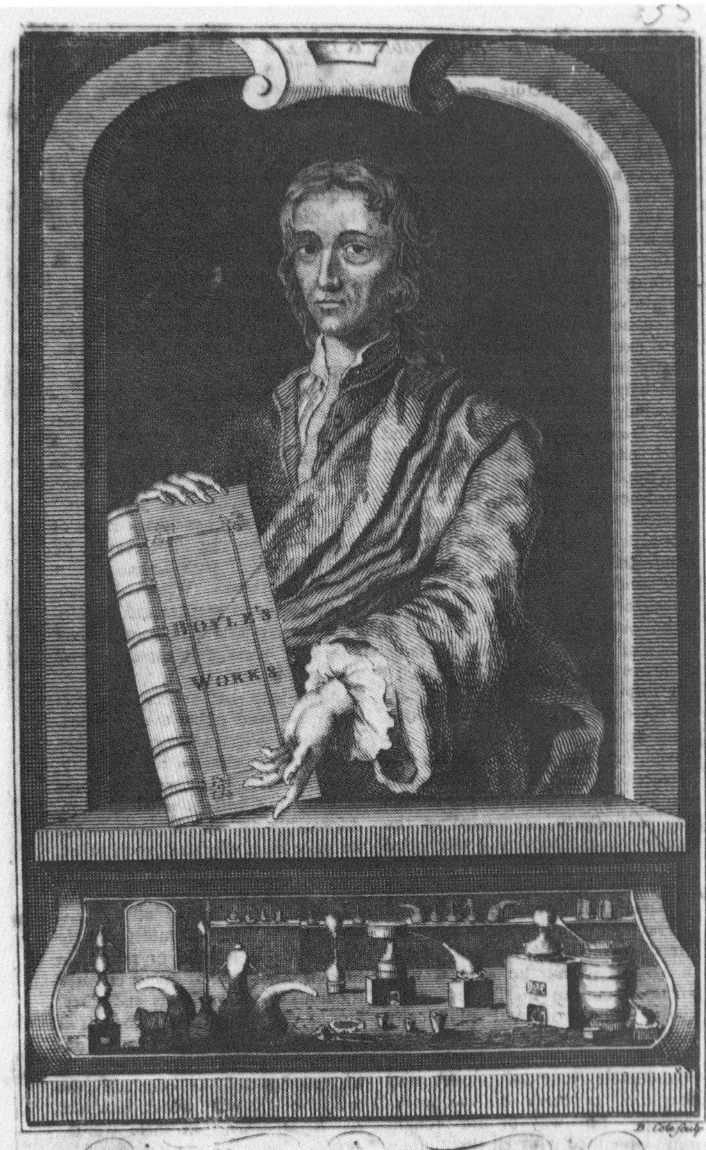


B. Cole sculp.

The Hon$^{ble}$ ROBERT BOYLE, Esq$^{r}$.

# Robert Boyle

## THE NATURAL HISTORY OF HUMAN BLOOD

Robert Boyle (1627-1691) was the moving spirit in the group of English scientists who formed the Royal Society in 1660. He was a self-taught scientist, philosopher, theologian, and writer. His medical degree was not actually earned but was awarded by the Royal Society in recognition of his achievements. His interests were chiefly in chemistry, and his name remains familiar in Boyle's law on the relationship of temperature, pressure, and volume of gases. In 1656, he assisted Sir Christopher Wren in the first intravenous injection, an experiment in which they injected opium and crocus metallorum into the veins of dogs. The procedure was not generally adopted, however, because it often led to thrombosis and embolism. Boyle published more than forty books or pamphlets and contributed nearly as many papers to the *Philosophical Transactions.* In the field of biology, his experiments with flames and with animals *in vacuo* demonstrated that an unidentified element in the air was necessary for combustion as well as for life. A century later, Lavoisier discovered the element to be oxygen.

In this book on the blood, Boyle set forth a list of problems pertaining to whole blood, the serum, and the corpuscles. He then described his experiments and conclusions. He made a chemical analysis of human blood and discussed its affinity with the blood of "quadrupeds, birds, fishes, and sanguineous insects." Boyle easily obtained human blood for his experiments from the barbers' shops, where bloodletting was a daily practice.

He announced a similar list of problems concerning urine, but the subject is not pursued further. Medically, this volume is the most important of Boyle's writings. It summarizes contemporary knowledge of the chemical content of the blood and is the first scientific study in physiologic chemistry.

There is an interesting point about the printing of the book. It was first issued over the date 1684, but Boyle later reissued it with a new title page dated 1683/4 to establish its time of publication precisely. In accordance with the usage of the period, the commercial New Year began on the March "quarter day," whereas the people's New Year was observed on January 1; thus, the first quarter of the layman's 1684 was the last quarter of the businessman's 1683.

In his will, Boyle left part of his estate for the advancement of the Christian religion. His executors implemented this by a bequest to "the corporation for propagating the Gospel amongst the heathen natives in New-England and other parts of America." By a circuitous route, the College of William and Mary in Williamsburg, Virginia, became the major beneficiary.

Robert Boyle. *Memoirs for the Natural History of Humane Blood, Especially the Spirit of that Liquor.* London, 1684.

The chemical apparatus below the portrait may remind chemistry students of Boyle's law: When temperature is held constant, the volume of a given quantity of a gas varies inversely with the pressure.

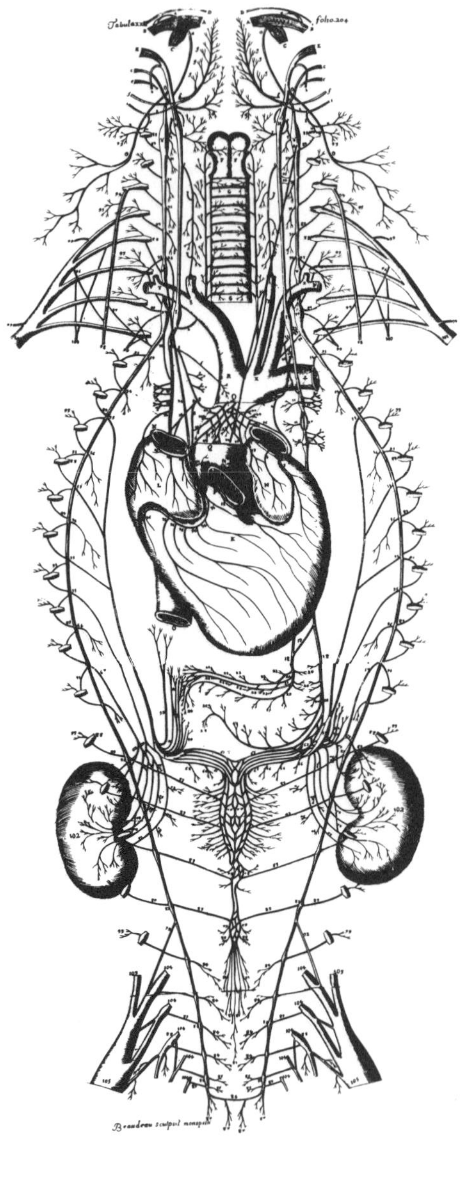

Tabula xx
folio 204
Beaudrau sculpsit monspelii

# Raymond Vieussens

## UNIVERSAL NEUROGRAPHY

Vieussens (1641-1715), professor of medicine at Montpellier, published a detailed study of the nervous system that was regarded as the best account written in the seventeenth century. It was illustrated with thirty particularly fine engravings by Jean Beaudeau, most of them on foldout pages larger than the pages of the book. It also contained a splendid portrait of the author by Boulanger. Vieussens was an untiring dissector, and his work revealed the structure and arrangement of the nervous system better than that of any predecessor in addition to recording new and correct observations. For example, he showed that the spinal cord was an independent structure, not merely an appendage of the brain, and he first defined the centrum ovale.

The book, which is divided into three parts, discusses the brain, the spinal cord, and the nerves. It was based on 500 dissections of postmortem material. The words "Editio Nova" on the title page indicate a new and original publication rather than a "new edition" in the modern sense.

Vieussens was physician to the royal court in Paris from about 1688 to 1698. During this period, he became interested in chemical physiology and was among the first to study the chemistry of the blood and saliva. His exploration of the heart and blood vessels was recorded in three volumes issued late in his life. He also published an important, though less original, monograph on the structure of the ear. His investigations on the cardiovascular system resulted in many new anatomic and pathologic observations—for instance, the correct structure of the left ventricle of the heart, the course of the coronary vessels, and the coronary sinus. He was the first to record the symptoms of aortic insufficiency and mitral stenosis, describing the character of the pulse and the pathologic features with clarity and thoroughness.

He was part of that golden age of anatomy which produced such eponymic contemporaries as Wirsung, Glisson, Wharton, Cowper, Malpighi, Brunner, and de Graaf.

Raymond Vieussens. *Neurographia Universalis....* Lyons, 1685.

The autonomic nervous system. The illustration appeared as part of a four-page foldout.

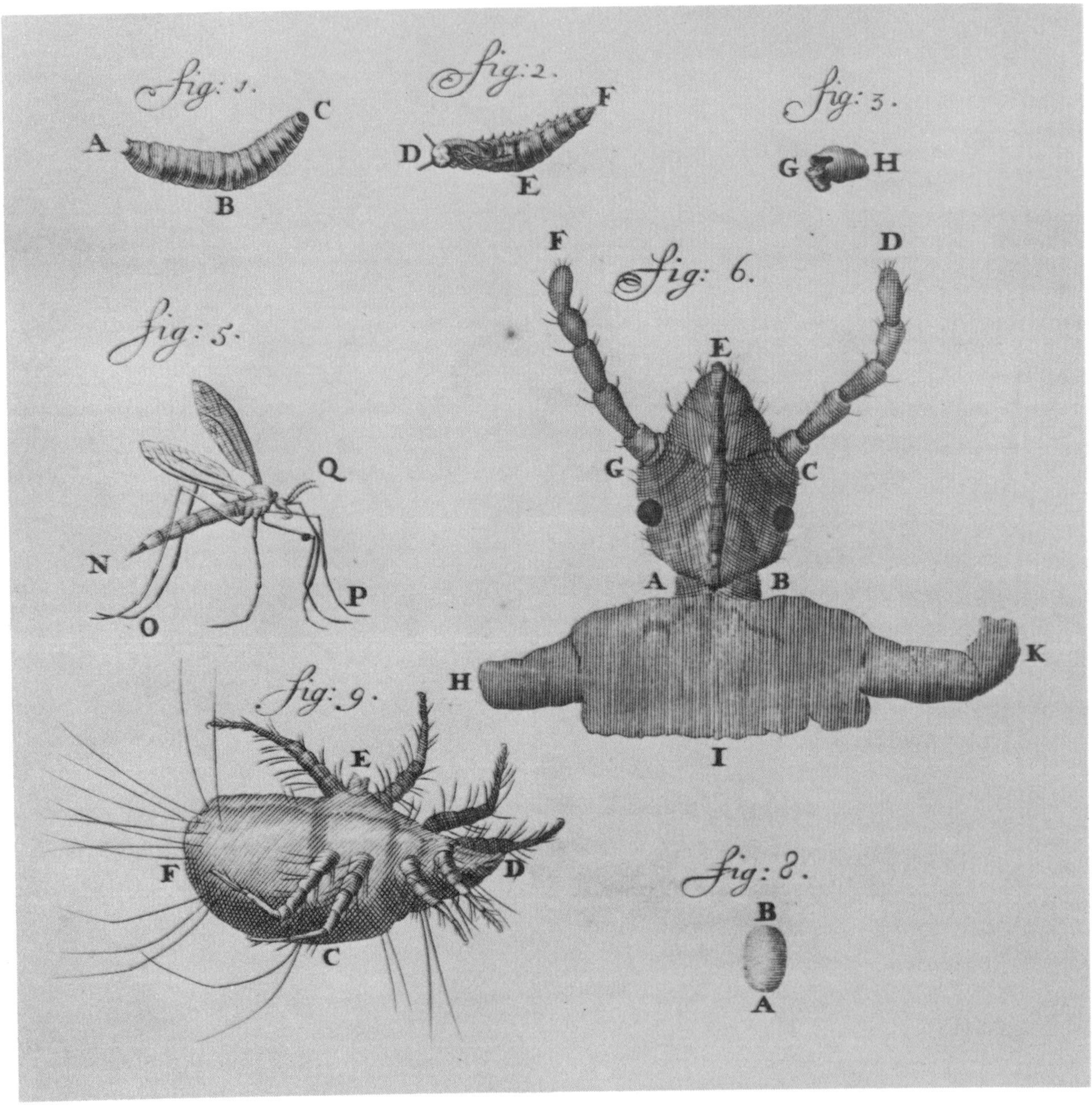
fig: 1.
A
B
C
fig: 2.
D
E
F
fig: 3.
G
H
fig: 6.
F
D
E
G
C
A
B
H
K
I
fig: 5.
Q
N
P
O
fig: 9.
E
F
D
C
fig: 8.
B
A

# Anton van Leeuwenhoek

## NATURE'S SECRETS UNCOVERED

A draper by trade and a municipal official in the city hall of Delft in Holland (a sinecure position he held all his life), van Leeuwenhoek (1632-1723) turned to microscopy as a hobby. He devised a microscope with one small, strong objective lens that avoided the distortions and color refraction of previous types of instruments. He made over two hundred microscopes, for which he himself ground most of the lenses, and once sent twenty-six of them as a gift to the Royal Society in London, of which he became a Fellow in 1680. His industry and important observations attracted such wide attention that even Peter the Great, Czar of All the Russias, paid him a visit in 1689 to see his microscopes, and the directors of the East India Company sent him specimens for microscopic examination.

Van Leeuwenhoek was the first to see protozoa under the microscope. He found microorganisms in the mouth and on the teeth and, for the first time, furnished exact descriptions of the shapes of bacterial clumps and chains as well as of individual bacilli. No one else was to see bacteria again for over a century. He also wrote about the cell nucleus and the structure of spermatozoa, gave the first accurate account of red blood corpuscles, delineated the conformation of the crystalline lens, and discovered the sarcolemma and the striped nature of skeletal muscle. His thorough examination of the capillary circulation, which Malpighi had recently touched on briefly without appreciating its significance, completed proof of the blood circulation proposed by Harvey sixty years earlier.

He carefully recorded his observations and sent over four hundred papers to the Royal Society and to the French Academy of Sciences. Most of these communications were in Latin and were first published in the *Philosophical Transactions of the Royal Society of London.* Subsequently, van Leeuwenhoek arranged the letters logically in groups and published them in numerous volumes, in both Latin and Dutch, between 1684 and 1722.

*Arcana Naturae Detecta* ("Nature's Secrets Uncovered") contains forty of the most interesting letters of this extremely active man, who was true to his hobby and little interested in anything but observing and describing, at which he was unexcelled. Van Leeuwenhoek is deservedly regarded as the father of protozoology and bacteriology. He died at the rather amazing age of ninety-one.

Anton van Leeuwenhoek. *Arcana Naturae Detecta.* Delft, 1695.

In this portion of one of Leeuwenhoek's plates are enlarged views of a worm, pupa, and cast-off shell, a female mosquito-like insect laying eggs, the greatly magnified head of a louse, a mite, and a mite's egg.

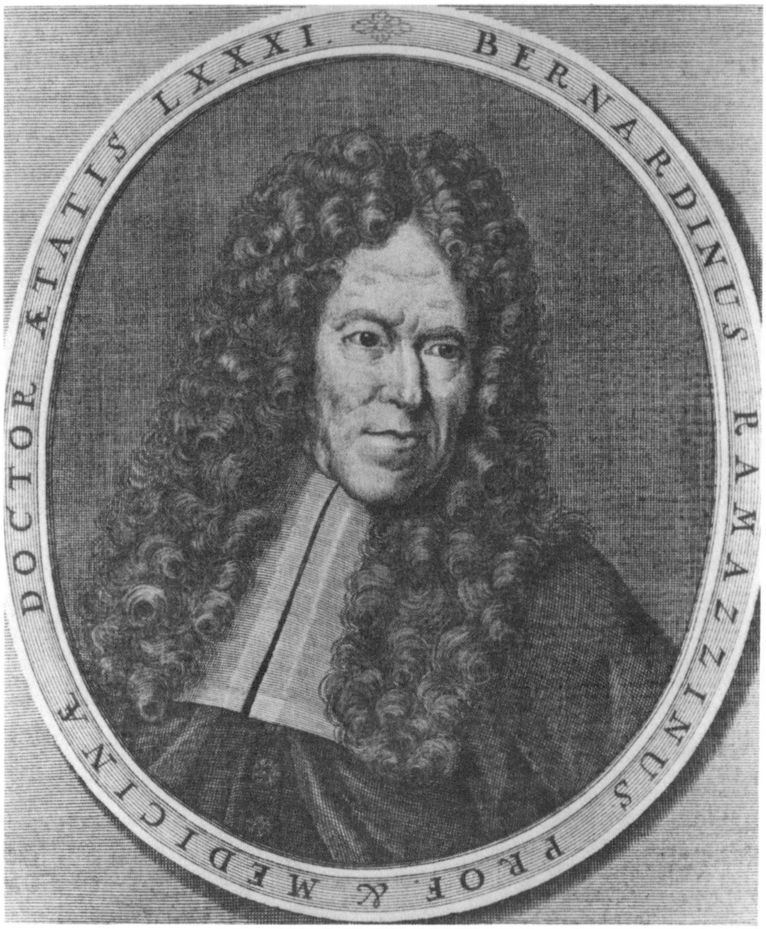
BERNARDINUS RAMAZZINUS PROF. & MEDICINÆ DOCTOR ÆTATIS LXXXI.

# Bernardino Ramazzini

## A TREATISE ON THE DISEASES OF TRADESMEN

Although Ramazzini (1633-1714) served as professor of medicine at Modena and subsequently at Padua, he is best remembered for his pioneer treatise on occupational disease. The book reflects an interest that Ramazzini acquired late in life; it was published in 1700, more than forty years after he had received his degree as doctor of medicine.

Ramazzini's concern with occupational diseases developed naturally from his studies of the environment as a cause of disease. The treatise covers the illnesses associated with forty to fifty different occupations, including general chapters on diseases of sedentary and standing workers and those of literary men. The first systematic survey of the subject, this book was reprinted at Utrecht in 1703, and an anonymous English translation appeared in 1705. At the age of eighty, Ramazzini revised the book; that expanded edition was published in 1713, the year before his death. He added new observations throughout, rearranging the second half of the volume and including a supplement of twelve new chapters on trades previously undescribed.

Among his more astute observations are his accounts of the "phthisis" acquired by stone-masons and miners (silicosis and pneumoconiosis), the eye problems of printers and gilders, the sciatica of tailors, and the lethargy of potters. Ramazzini pointed out that, in some lines of work, disorders can result from the strain of unusual physical demands or postures, such as those required of tailors; in other occupations, workers can develop disease from exposure to dangerous substances, such as lead or mercury. Ramazzini continues to be honored in Italy to this day by a medical journal that bears his name.

Ramazzini was also interested in epidemiology. From 1690 to 1695, he studied and then described a severe Italian epidemic of malarial fever. He became greatly concerned about this disease, which was endemic near undrained marshlands, and promoted the use of cinchona bark, as Thomas Sydenham (q.v.) was advocating, saying that cinchona did for medicine what gunpowder had done for war. He studied the effect of weather on recurrence of diseases and published his "barometric diary" in 1710, as Sydenham's follower John Locke had done in England in 1692.

Bernardino Ramazzini. *De Morbis Artificum Diatriba.* Modena, 1700.

"I choose to publish this Treatise of mine for the good of the Republick," Ramazzini wrote in his preface, "or at least for the Tradesmen . . . tho 'tis not very artfully writ."

TAB. II.

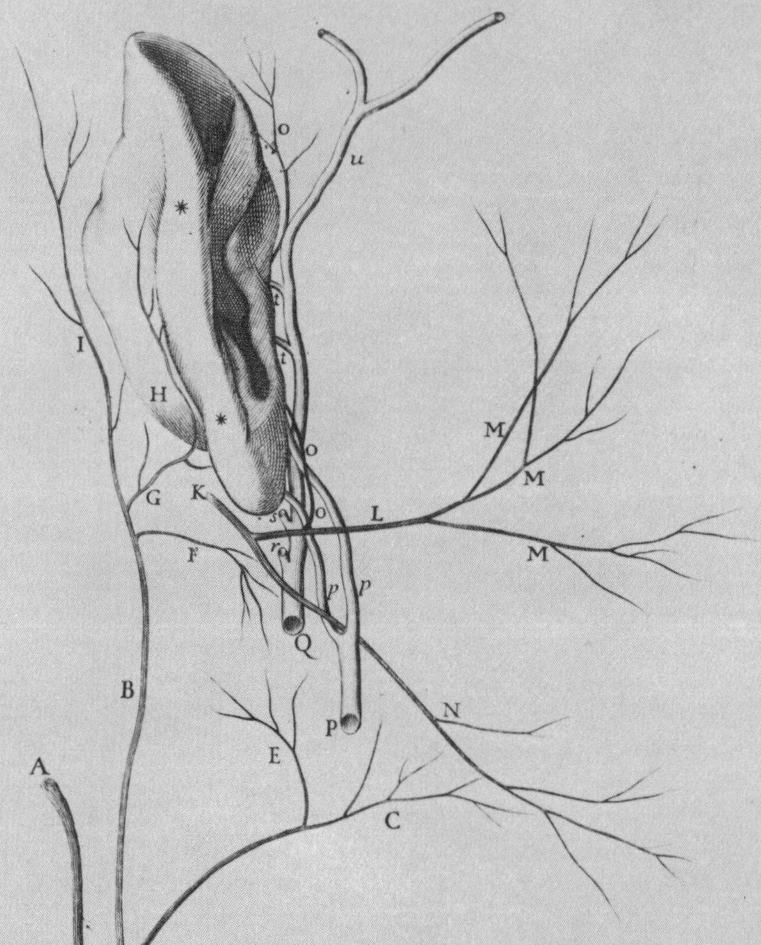

# Antonio Maria Valsalva

## TREATISE ON THE HUMAN EAR

Valsalva (1666-1723), of Bologna, who was one of Malpighi's students at Padua and the teacher of Morgagni, wrote the first full account of the minute anatomy of the ear in his *De Aure Humana Tractatus* ("Treatise on the Human Ear"), "in which the whole structure of the ear is described and illustrated with many new discoveries, and the uses of all its parts are investigated; in which is inserted a new description and delineation of the uvula and pharynx." He was the first to define the ear's three regions—outer, middle, and inner—and to explain their relative functions.

The "Treatise" is arranged in six chapters. The first three are anatomic and deal with the parts of the ear; the last three are physiologic and explain the functions of these parts. The auricle and auditory meatus, the tympanum and middle ear, and the labyrinth and inner ear are discussed. Chapter 2 includes Valsalva's report, promised on the title page, of the musculature of the uvula and pharynx; these are depicted on separate plates. The ten illustrations are good line engravings, of which the most striking are those of the nerves and blood vessels of the outer ear, the carotid artery, the semicircular canals, and the structure of the whole ear.

Valsalva described and named the eustachian tube, which connects the middle ear and the pharynx. His consideration of the eustachian tubes led to the "respiratory maneuver" named for him; if the tubes are patent and if the nose and mouth are closed, a forcible expiratory effort increases pressure on the tympanic membranes. Valsalva used this procedure to expel pus and foreign bodies from the middle ear. Since his time, the Valsalva maneuver has proved to be of value to the internist, the otologist, and the radiologist. In the section on the pharyngeal muscles, he detailed the dysphagia which has also been named for him. By the digital manipulation of "a kind of dislocation of the cartilaginous appendages of the hyoid bone," he relieved a woman who could not eat after a lump of beef had lodged in her throat.

Valsalva's collected works were edited with elaborate commentary by his more famous pupil, Morgagni. They include useful contributions to anatomy and surgery, of which the best remembered is his delineation of the sinuses of the aorta, still called "Valsalva's sinuses."

Antonio Maria Valsalva. *De Aure Humana Tractatus. . . .* Bologna, 1704.

Valsalva's line engraving shows the blood vessels of the outer ear. His classic work was accepted as a standard reference for many years and reflected his passionate interest in anatomic dissection.

# JO: MARIÆ LANCISII

Intimi Cubicularij, & Archiatri Pontificij

DE

# SUBITANEIS MORTIBUS

*LIBRI DUO.*

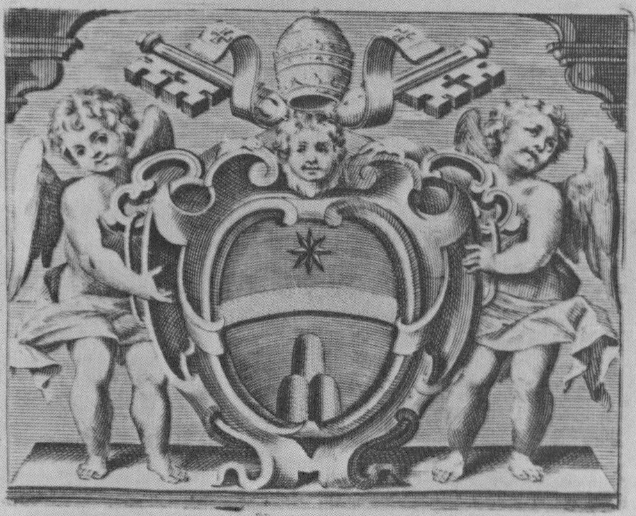

ROMÆ, Typis Io: Francisci Buagni. MDCCVII.

*SVPERIORVM PERMISSV.*

# Giovanni Maria Lancisi

## ON SUDDEN DEATH

Lancisi (1654-1720), regarded as the greatest Italian clinician of his time, was asked by Pope Clement XI to analyze and report on the pathogenesis of death in Rome. Lancisi responded with the treatise *De Subitaneis Mortibus* ("On Sudden Death"), published in 1707. In the first half of the book he dealt with sudden death in general, attributing it to three causes—"suffocation from intemperance," syncope, and apoplexy. More important, however, were the sections on heart disease, because here Lancisi laid the foundations of cardiac pathology. He described such conditions as cardiac syphilis, which had not previously been identified, and provided a classification of heart disease. Hypertrophy and dilatation of the heart were presented as manifestations of cardiac disease, and the existence of valvular vegetations was discussed for the first time. Lancisi's observations on heart disease were based on cases he had seen in his practice in Rome and include reports of autopsies in five fatal cases.

Lancisi died in 1720, but his later researches on the heart, with an important treatise on aneurysm, were published in 1728 by his former assistant, Francesco Soldati. In that book, the frequency of aneurysms of the heart was noted. Lancisi pointed out that the walls of some aneurysms are thin, whereas those of others are thick. Their causes, he stated, are diverse and include heredity, syphilis, asthma, palpitation, excesses, and violent emotions.

Lancisi had been much interested in epidemiology and possessed a clear insight into contagion not shared by his contemporaries. His book on the "Poisonous Effluvia of the Marshes" (1717), which described the Italian epidemic of malaria that had occurred in 1715, suggested that mosquitoes might be responsible for the spread of the disease.

Lancisi's considerable scholarship was further recognized when Clement XI asked him to edit the anatomic plates which Eustachio (q.v.) had executed in 1552 but which had been lost for 162 years. The rediscovered plates were published with Lancisi's notes in 1714.

Today the Biblioteca Lancisiana in Rome, founded by Lancisi in 1711 and considered one of the great historical medical libraries of Europe, houses the fine personal library that Lancisi dedicated to the use of the public.

Giovanni Maria Lancisi. *De Subitaneis Mortibus, Libri Duo.* Rome, 1707.

The papal tiara on the title page proclaims that this treatise was written at the request of Pope Clement XI.

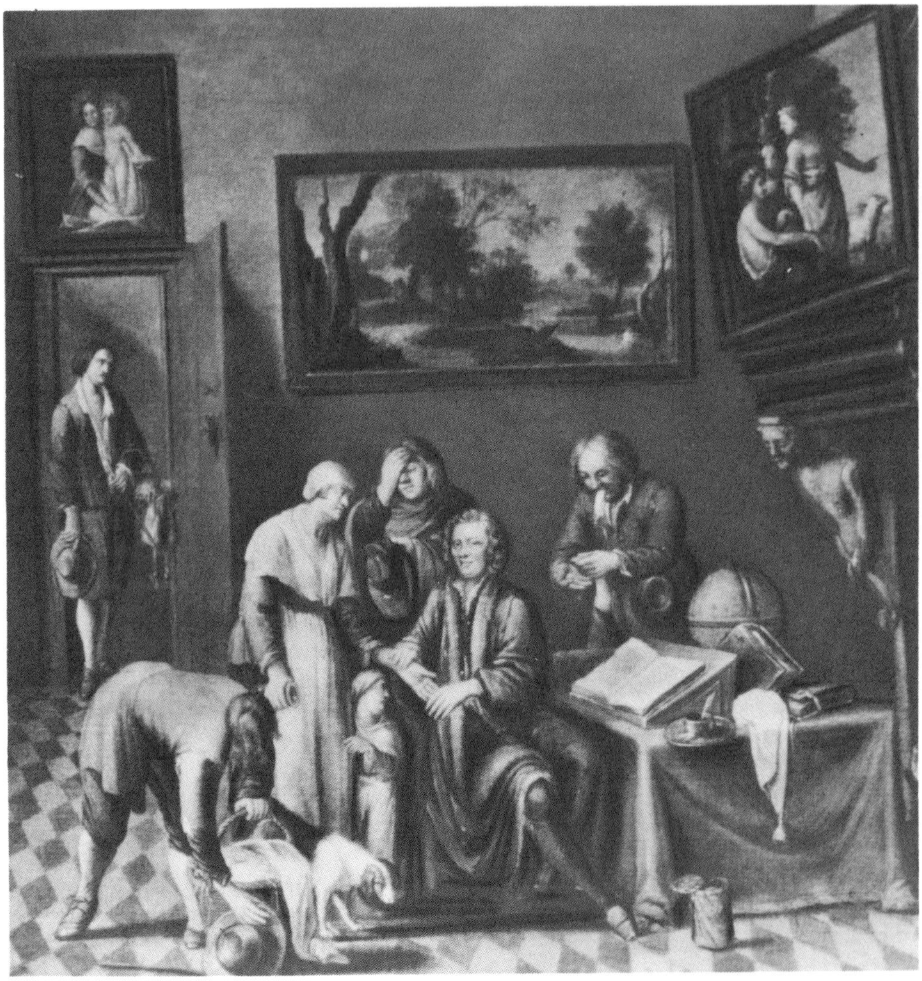

# Hermann Boerhaave

## INSTITUTES OF MEDICINE

No major medical discoveries are attributed to Boerhaave, but in his time he was Europe's leading physician, and his *Institutiones Medicae*, one of the first textbooks on physiology, was used in every medical school. It went through many editions and was translated even into Arabic and Turkish.

Boerhaave (1668-1738) exerted tremendous influence on medicine and related disciplines; he was an inspired teacher of clinical medicine, an experimental chemist, a botanist, and a consultant whose competence was recognized throughout Europe. He is credited with systematizing and synthesizing medical knowledge.

Boerhaave became a doctor of philosophy at the age of twenty-two and a doctor of physic at twenty-five. In 1701, when he was thirty-three, he was appointed lecturer in medicine at Leyden. Seven years later, his lectures were published in *Institutiones Medicae*; in the preface, Boerhaave described the text as "a little book which draws the lines within which my annual work with you is confined." It is divided into four sections: physiology, pathology, hygiene, and therapeutics. The title was used as the accepted name for courses on physiology in medical schools until well into the nineteenth century. Although he was not a great writer, his book was successful because of its simplicity, clarity, and eclectic wisdom. His warm personality and oratoric gifts made his lectures extremely popular. The many students who flocked to Leyden soon spread his teachings over Europe and America.

Boerhaave revived the instruction methods of Hippocrates; he took his students to the bedside of the patient and, by skillful questioning, drew from them the information needed for diagnosing the disease. Although he had only twelve hospital beds at his disposal, he utilized them to the fullest; under his guidance, Leyden became the site of one of Europe's most prestigious medical schools. Boerhaave also taught a private course on the theory of medical practice. The lectures from this course were published in *Aphorismi* in 1709.

Boerhaave was a cultured man with broad interests. He was an accomplished musician; he republished many ancient, Renaissance, and contemporary texts; he spoke five languages and could read in seven. Nobility and royalty from many countries visited him, but he said the poor were his best patients, "for God paid for them." He turned down tempting offers of professorships from several leading universities to continue teaching at Leyden. It was said he was so popular that church bells once signaled his recovery from gout.

Hermann Boerhaave. *Institutiones Medicae In usus annuae Exercitationis Domesticos Digestae*. Leyden, 1708.

Artist's conception
of a typical scene in Boerhaave's country home
outside Leyden, where he received and treated patients.
He was said to have treated more than
a hundred patients a day.

XXXIII

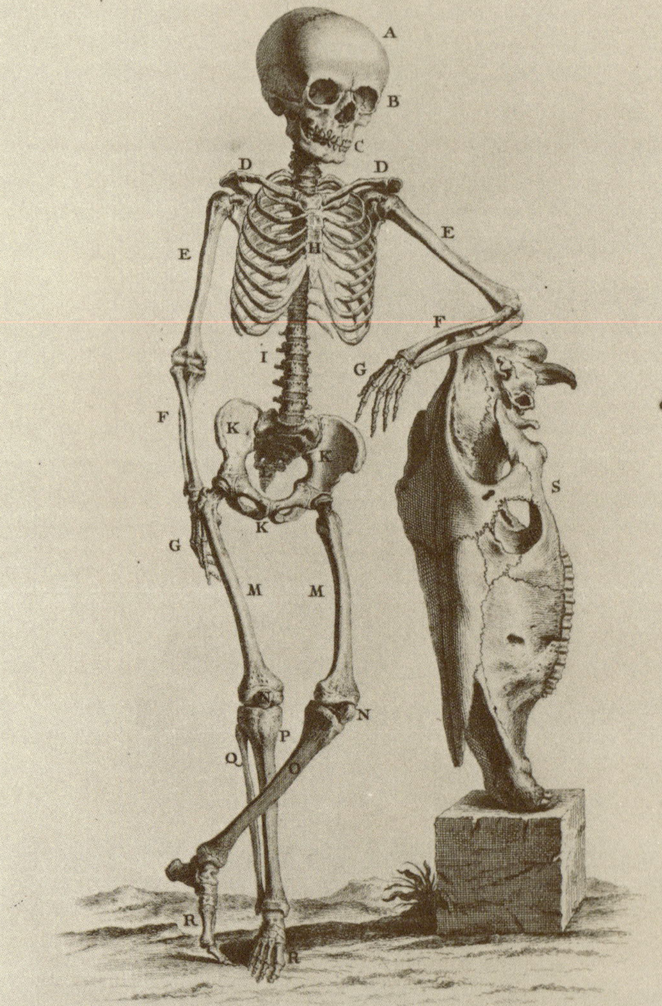

# William Cheselden

## THE ANATOMY OF THE BONES

Cheselden (1688-1752) became surgeon to St. Thomas's Hospital in 1718 and was an outstanding teacher of anatomy in London during the first half of the eighteenth century. *Osteographia,* his third book, is a monumental study of "all the bones of the human body displayed in their natural size." It contains fifty-six large plates of the human bones, with forty-four comparative anatomy vignettes, chiefly animal skeletons. Although the latter were intended as mere ornamental supplements, they constitute the first accurate delineations of some of the species shown. The book was clearly inspired by the skeleton plates in Vesalius's *Fabrica,* but Cheselden pointed out that Vesalius's illustrations were sometimes imprecise in detail. Cheselden used the camera obscura to assist van der Gucht with the drawings.

Cheselden's first book, on anatomy, was published in 1713 when he was only twenty-five, but it held the field against rival texts until the end of the century. In fact, the thirteenth edition was published in 1792. The book was intended for surgical students and was concerned almost entirely with the anatomy of the superficial parts and the extremities. The viscera, then not very accessible to the surgeon, are described rather summarily.

His second book, published in 1723, concerned the newly introduced "high," or suprapubic, operation for stone in the bladder. Because this involved Cheselden in a priority dispute with the brothers James and John Douglas, in which he was wildly abused and accused of plagiarism, he evolved the lateral operation. In 1728, he restored the sight of a blind boy by iridotomy with a needle to form an artificial pupil. This remarkable achievement, in addition to its surgical merit, provoked much discussion of the philosophic and psychologic implications of visual perception.

In addition to his surgical skills, Cheselden was a patron of boxing, an architect, and a draftsman. In the days before anesthesia, when speed of operation was a necessary attribute for all surgeons, he was notable among his peers for being able to perform a lithotomy within fifty-four seconds. His standing in eighteenth-century England can be inferred from Pope's lines:

> "I'll do what Mead and Cheselden advise,
> To keep these limbs and to preserve those eyes."

William Cheselden. *Osteographia, or the Anatomy of the Bones.* London, 1733.

The skeleton of a "boy nine years of age, leaning on the skull of an horse," an artistic pose showing their comparative sizes.

# AN ACCOUNT OF SOME Hydraulick and Hydroſtatical EXPERIMENTS made on the Blood and Blood-Veſſels of ANIMALS.

## EXPERIMENT I.

1. IN *December* I cauſed a Mare to be tied down alive on her Back, ſhe was fourteen Hands high, and about fourteen Years of Age, had a *Fiſtula* on her Withers, was neither very lean, nor yet luſty: Having laid open the left crural Artery about three Inches from her Belly, I inſerted into it a braſs Pipe whoſe Bore was one ſixth of an Inch in Diameter; and to that, by means of another braſs Pipe which was fitly adapted to it, I fixed a glaſs Tube, of nearly the ſame Diameter, which was nine Feet in Length: Then untying the Ligature on the Artery, the Blood roſe in the

# Stephen Hales

## STATICAL ESSAYS: CONTAINING HAEMASTATICKS

It is an oddity in the history of medicine that Stephen Hales (1677-1761), who introduced quantitative methods into the study of the circulation of the blood, was a doctor not of medicine but of divinity. After taking holy orders, the Reverend Dr. Hales served as curate at Teddington, a small parish in Middlesex, until his death. However, his labors as "perpetual curate" at St. Mary's-in-the-Meadows were overshadowed by his achievements in physiology and botany.

Hales began his study of the circulation by measuring the blood pressure of experimental animals, such as horses and sheep; his manometer was a long glass tube, connected to the animal's carotid artery by means of the windpipe of a goose. The blood pressure was measured directly from the height of the blood in the glass column.

Hales measured the volume of the ventricle by making a cast of the cavity with wax; multiplying this volume by the pulse rate gave the cardiac output. He computed the circulation rate and the velocity of the blood in capillaries, veins, and arteries. With simple but ingenious experiments, he explored peripheral vascular resistance and the complex interplay of pressure, flow, and resistance. His work was the first real advance in circulatory physiology since Harvey's pioneer observations.

Hales was equally adept at botanic experiments, devising new techniques to measure the movement of sap in plants and trees. The results of these experiments were published in *Vegetable Staticks* (1727). In 1733, after more than twenty years of experimentation, he consolidated the reports of his botanic experiments with those on the hemodynamics of the central and peripheral circulation *(Haemastaticks)* in two volumes of *Statical Essays.*

In later years, Hales became involved with the social aspects of medicine. His concern over poor ventilation in slave ships and prisons led him to devise a roof ventilator that could be operated by hand or by a windmill. He campaigned for temperance and was influential in the passage of the Gin Act of 1736. At the age of seventy, Parson Hales delivered the annual Croonian lecture to the Royal College of Physicians, but it dealt with theology, not physiology.

Stephen Hales. *Statical Essays: Containing Haemastaticks; or, An Account of some Hydraulick and Hydrostatical Experiments made on the Blood and Blood-Vessels of Animals.* Vol. II. London, 1733.

The classic simplicity of Hales's research is seen in this sample page of his book.

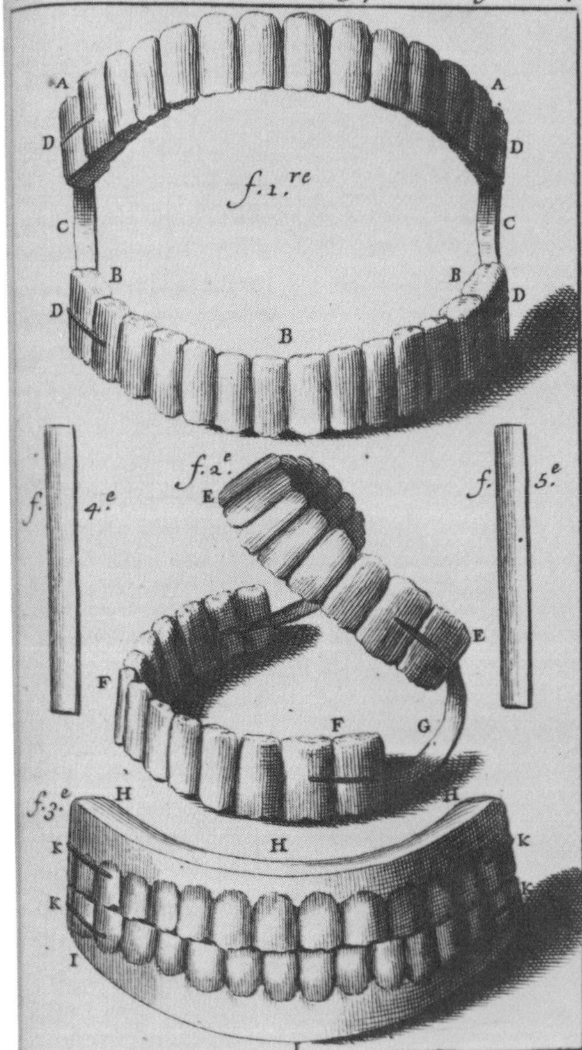
f. 1.re
A
A
D
D
C
C
B
B
B
D
D
f. 2.e
E
E
F
F
G
H
H
f. 4.e
f. 5.e
f. 3.e
H
K
K
K
K
I

# Pierre Fauchard

## THE SURGEON DENTIST

Pierre Fauchard (1678-1761) was a self-educated French *dentiste,* who invented that descriptive term for his profession. He was the first to use an orthodontal operation in the treatment of malocclusion and published this comprehensive scientific account of the care and treatment of the teeth when he was fifty. Because he had no academic standing, he obtained the support of the official surgeons of Paris and printed their signed "approbations" at the beginning of his work, which they praised as "methodical, intelligent and clear." Although small in format, the books are remarkably thorough and well illustrated. The first volume, of more than five hundred pages, contains thirty-seven chapters on the development, diseases, and care of the teeth and is illustrated with eight plates. In it appears the first account of pyorrhea alveolaris, now known as Riggs' disease. The second volume, somewhat shorter, deals with operative dentistry and artificial teeth and describes the dentist's armamentarium; thirty-two plates display instruments and dentures.

Fauchard improved removable dentures, carving bone or ivory to the shape required to fit the mouth. He also used artificial crowns, attaching them to the pulp cavity with a dowel or pin. Cavities were filled with gold, lead, or tin after the carious matter had been removed. Oil of cinnamon was applied to relieve pain. Fauchard is usually credited with having overthrown the belief that decay in teeth is caused by small worms.

The work is particularly interesting for its case histories and its detailed descriptions of instruments and appliances. In its own time, it was most influential in raising dental surgery from a rough trade to professional standing. An enlarged second edition was published in 1746.

The full title of *Le Chirurgien Dentiste* in translation reads: "The Surgeon Dentist or Treatise of the Teeth, in which are taught the methods of keeping them clean and healthy, beautifying them, repairing their loss, and treating their diseases and those of the gums and the accidents which can happen to the other parts near the teeth. With observations and reflections on several singular cases. The work is enriched with forty copperplate engravings."

Pierre Fauchard. *Le Chirurgien Dentiste, ou Traité des Dents.* 2 vols. Paris, 1728.

Some eighteenth-century dentures from the pioneer contribution of Pierre Fauchard.

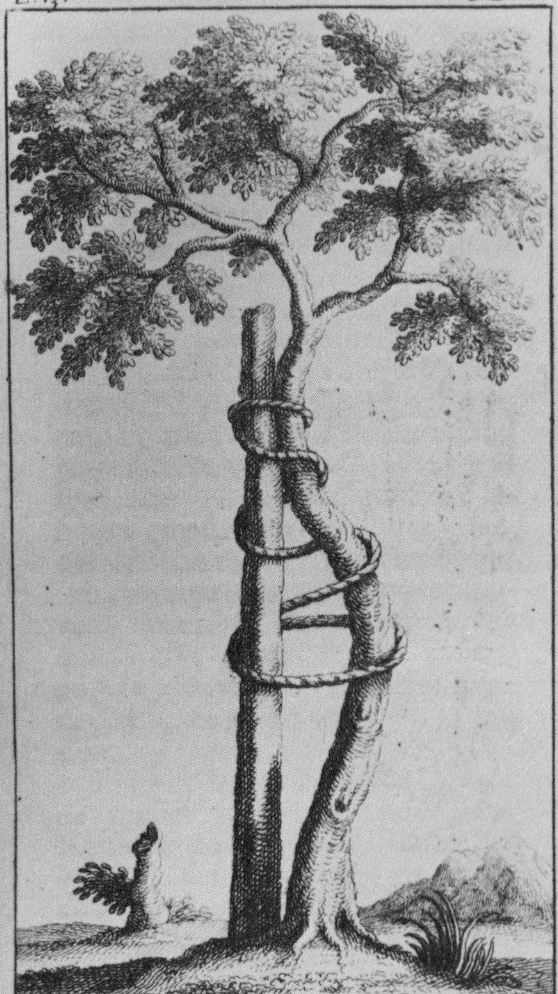

# Nicolas Andry

## ORTHOPEDICS

Nicolas Andry de Boisregard (1658-1742) was a professor of medicine at the University of Paris. At the age of eighty-three, he published an account of his experience in "the art of preventing and correcting deformities of the body in children," for which he coined the name "*L'Orthopédie*." "I have formed it," he wrote, "of two words, namely *orthos* (straight) and *paidos* (child)." Although he did not actually found the specialty of orthopedics (fractures were being treated by surgeons), he developed the concept of prevention.

At the beginning of his book, he stressed the importance of moderate exercise in the cure of deformities. On the whole, he treated deformities by improving posture and employing mechanical aids and sensible clothing. Children in Andry's day, especially those of the upper classes, were dressed in clothes that were extremely ill-suited for play. Tight waists and close-fitting breeches, corsets, and layers of petticoats made little boys and girls a pleasing spectacle in the drawing room but were thoroughly uncomfortable and severely limited the range of motion of their joints. Despite Andry's commonsense writing on the undesirable effects of such garments, physicians generally did not endorse his criticisms until near the end of the century.

The work on orthopedics is divided into four sections dealing, in turn, with a general anatomic survey of the exterior of the body; the prevention and correction of deformities, particularly by means of proper carriage of the body; the treatment of deformities in the extremities, head, and face, including the gums and teeth; and the treatment of mutism and voice defects.

A man before his time, Andry had also postulated in 1701 that air, water, fermenting wine, vinegar, cider, beer, and milk contained microörganisms. He went on to suggest that such organisms might also be found within the lesions of smallpox and other diseased tissues and that mercury's ability to kill them had enabled this element to cure syphilis. The idea was not well received by his medical colleagues and, in fact, became the subject of ridicule. His first descriptions of trigeminal neuralgia, however, were accepted from the start.

Andry's work made a great impact, because no comparable text had been written. An English translation was published promptly, in 1743. Sadly, Andry's many new approaches were not universally applied for nearly one hundred years, although surgeons did much good work in the meantime on a few deformities, such as clubfoot and diseases of the spine and joints.

Nicolas Andry. *L'Orthopédie ou l'Art de prévenir et de corriger dans les Enfans, les difformités du corps*. 2 vols. Paris, 1741.

Andry used a simple analogy from nature to illustrate his text on the correction of bone deformities in children.

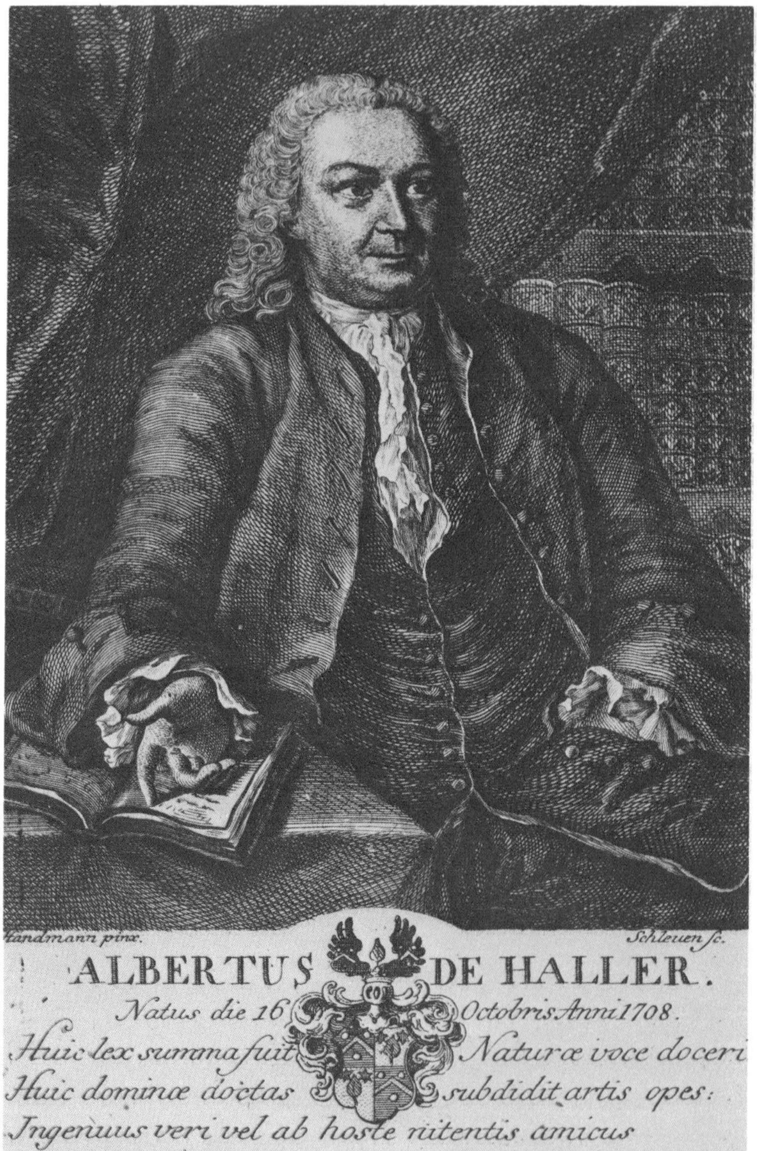
Handmann pinx.
Schleuen sc.
ALBERTUS DE HALLER.
Natus die 16 Octobris Anni 1708.
Huic lex summa fuit Naturæ voce doceri
Huic dominæ doctas subdidit artis opes:
Ingenuus veri vel ab hoste nitentis amicus
Censor et erroris candidus ipse sui
P. G. Werlhof

# Albrecht von Haller

## FIRST LINES OF PHYSIOLOGY

Albrecht von Haller (1708-1777) was professor of anatomy, medicine, surgery, and botany at the University of Göttingen in Hanover for seventeen years. Well known as an anatomist, botanist, and poet as well as writer, editor, and bibliographer, this remarkable man continued in public and academic service as well as with his research for a further twenty-four years after retiring to his native Switzerland, where he died at the age of sixty-nine.

The quantity of his writings and a record of the books he studied suggest that he must have read and written through every moment of his waking life. Yet he was a diligent dissector, traveler, collector, teacher, and administrator and kept up voluminous correspondence in several languages. He made original observations in the fields of anatomy and botany, wrote monographs in Latin, French, and German, and edited volumes of classical and contemporary medical writings.

His most lasting gift to medicine was that of establishing experimental physiology as the basis for advances in medical knowledge. His most notable experiment was the demonstration that contractility is the property of muscle and sensibility the property of nervous tissue. He is sometimes considered the founder of modern neurology.

A summary of his lectures, *Primae Lineae Physiologiae,* was published in 1747. It was soon translated from Latin into English and other languages and later was revised and expanded several times by the author. The second edition (1751) is one hundred pages longer than the first, but the same arrangement of the contents was kept. Von Haller's style is clear and lively. As briefly as possible and in a continuous descriptive style rather than a tabulation, he gives many facts, precisely detailed and concisely explained.

This introductory book was followed, between 1757 and 1766, by the eight volumes of his "Elements of the Physiology of the Human Body," which the French physiologist François Magendie, in 1827, called "that cursed book in which everything can be found." John F. Fulton, who like von Haller was both physiologist and bibliographer, characterized it as "a vast and well-systematized storehouse of physiological knowledge, replete with citation and an incredible number of accurate references to literature."

The "First Lines" is a small book, closely printed, comprising 857 numbered paragraphs and arranged in thirty-five chapters. Even today it provides a sound and intelligent guide for a beginner in physiology.

Albrecht von Haller. *Primae Lineae Physiologiae in Usum Praelectionum academicarum.* Göttingen, 1747.

This portrait (date unknown) appropriately places von Haller in the setting of a library. A prolific writer and editor, he produced several hundred monographs and books.

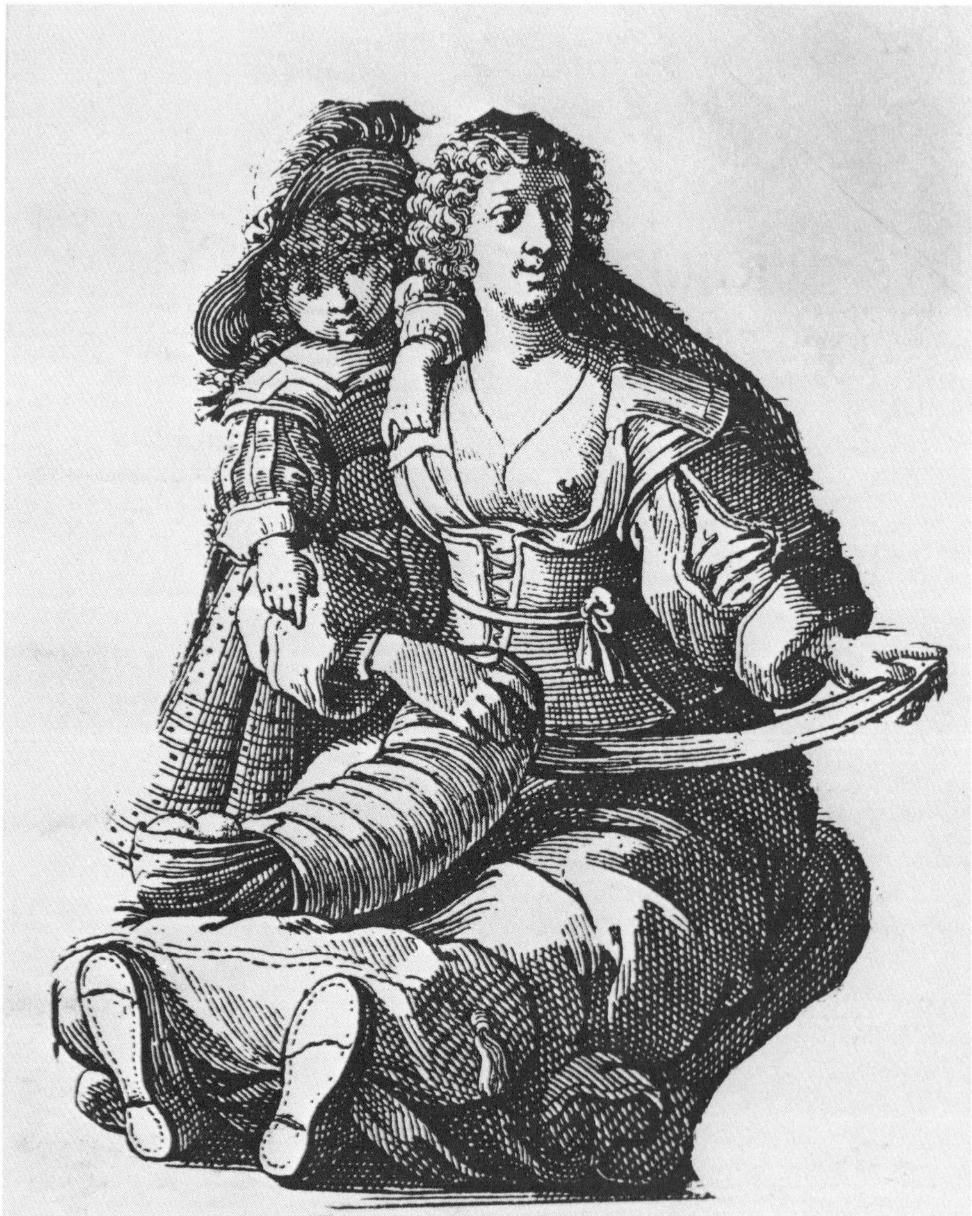

# William Cadogan

## NURSING AND THE MANAGEMENT OF CHILDREN

Infant mortality in eighteenth-century London was as high as 50 percent. The majority of the inhabitants were poor, and children were often unwanted and subjected to neglect, whether they were born in or out of wedlock. One of the first attempts to correct this situation and provide a home for abandoned waifs was the establishment of the Foundling Hospital, which was opened in 1745.

Cadogan (1711-1797), an Oxford graduate who had served aboard a hospital ship as a naval surgeon with John Hunter (q.v.) during the war with Spain, was physician to the Bristol Infirmary when he published this essay addressed to "One of the Governors of the Foundling Hospital." It was accepted by the committee of the hospital, which authorized its publication in 1752. Thereafter, Cadogan was appointed physician to the hospital and moved to London from his practice in Bristol.

In his opening sentences, Cadogan railed against the practices of mothers of the day: "You perceive, Sir, by the Hints I have already dropp'd, what I am going to complain of is, that children in general are over-cloath'd and over-fed, and fed and cloath'd improperly. To these Causes I impute almost all their Diseases. But to be a little more explicit. The first great Mistake is, that they think a new-born Infant cannot be kept too warm; from this Prejudice they load and bind it with Flannels, Wrappers, Swaths, Stays, &c.... which all together are almost equal to its own Weight....But what is worse than this, at the End of the Month, if things go on apparently well, this Hot-bed Plant is sent out into the Country, to be rear'd in a leaky House, that lets in Wind and Rain from every Quarter. Is it any Wonder the Child never thrives afterwards?" Cadogan stressed the paramount importance of breast feeding, which was most necessary when the cleanliness of artificial feedings was suspect and the mixing of cow's milk, sugar, and water in the correct proportions to simulate human milk was not yet understood.

The book, though little more than a pamphlet, ran to at least twelve editions. For many years it was considered the most important pediatric text. In its day, it was an important innovative step in practical child care.

In 1771, Cadogan published *A Dissertation on the Gout and All Chronic Diseases,* of which ten reprintings were called for in two years. A sufferer from the disease himself, he recommended temperance for reducing the frequency of attacks. Although it was widely read, Cadogan's advice was unpopular and received with much derision.

William Cadogan. *An Essay upon Nursing, and the Management of Children, From their Birth to Three Years of Age.* London, 1748.

An engraving by Abraham Bosse illustrates one of the conditions Cadogan undertook to change. The wrapping of a new baby in swaddling clothes, he maintained, lessened its chances for good health.

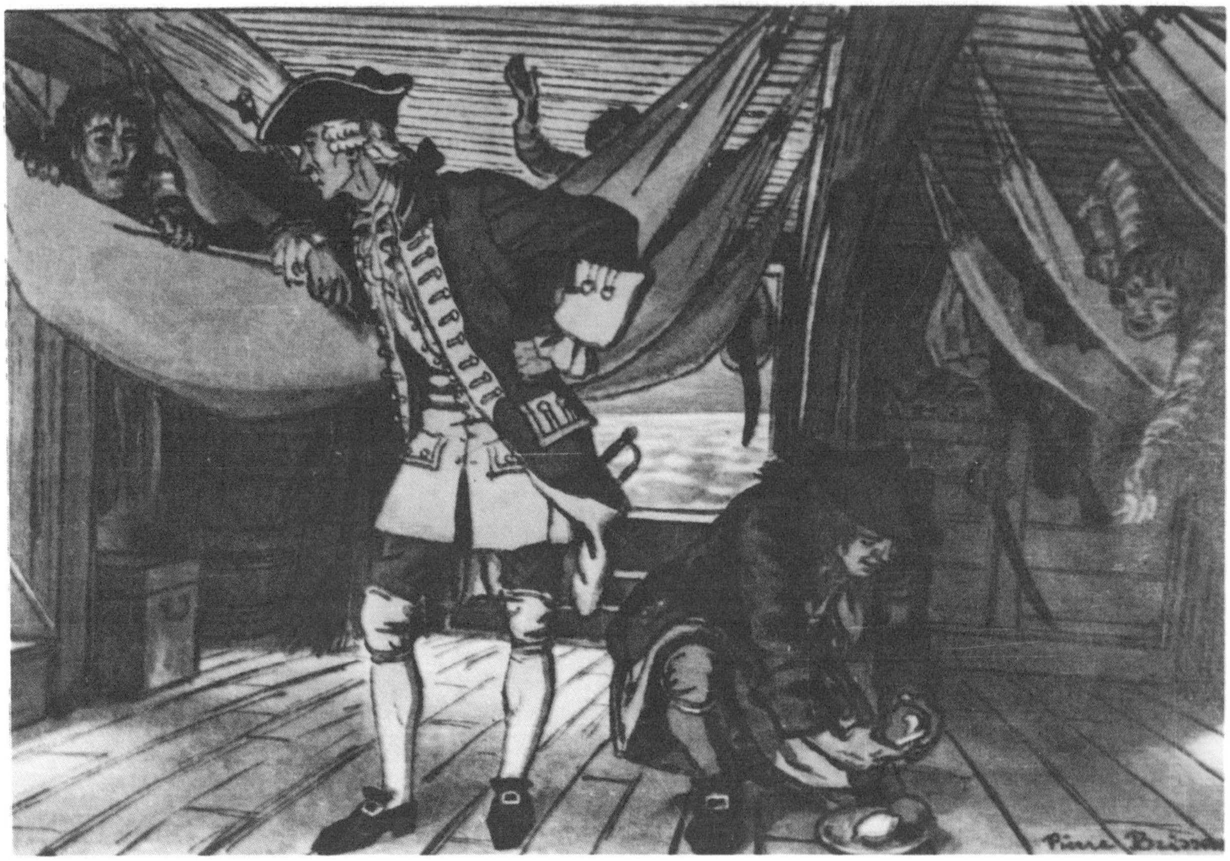

# James Lind

## A TREATISE OF THE SCURVY

James Lind (1716-1794), a Scottish-trained surgeon, began his reforms in naval hygiene with this treatise on scurvy. The work was not entirely original, because the clinical nature of the disease and the preventive properties of fresh fruits and vegetables had been explored by Lind's predecessors. Nevertheless, his practical suggestions for including antiscorbutic foods in sailors' daily menus during long sea voyages exerted a tremendous influence. His statements about the cause and cure of scurvy were not confirmed and elucidated until the early twentieth century, when the effects of vitamin C deficiency were precisely defined.

While serving at sea as a surgeon's mate in 1747, Lind carried out a controlled experiment on the diet of the sailors. Perhaps the first clinical trial, the study showed that citrus juice could prevent and cure scurvy. Six years later, after he had received a medical degree from the University of Edinburgh, Lind published this book. It presented a critical account of current opinion, demonstrating that the disease is not congenital, hereditary, or infectious; a description of the disease, its cause, prevention, and cure; and a digest of everything written previously about scurvy.

The treatise describes Lind's experiment. Each of six pairs of patients was given one of the following dietary supplements: cider, "elixir vitriol," vinegar, seawater, oranges and lemons, and "an electuary of garlic, mustard seed, radish, Peru balsam, and gum myrrh" with garlic water. All other conditions were kept constant. In comparing the results, Lind found "sudden and visible effects from the use of the oranges and lemons." The tender sprouting tops of green wheat also served to protect men against scurvy, he noted.

Moreover, Lind observed that cartilaginous prominences, especially those of the ribs and the knees, were the parts most noticeably affected by scurvy. These effects were seen as pain and swelling during the course of the disease and by abnormalities at autopsy. More than one hundred and fifty years later, it was shown that ascorbic acid is necessary to maintain the production and integrity of collagen.

Lind's classic, well-controlled clinical trial offered firm support to previous recommendations that citrus juice be given to prevent scurvy. Convinced by Lind's work, Captain James Cook included citrus juice in the diet of the sailors on his South Sea voyage of 1772-1775 and reported its unprecedented success to the Royal Society in 1776. In spite of this support, the use of citrus juice was not officially adopted by the British navy until forty years after the publication of Lind's treatise.

Lind also fought for the establishment of hospital ships, cleanliness and ventilation in sick bays, and other measures for which he has been called the "father of nautical hygiene."

James Lind. *A Treatise of the Scurvy.* Edinburgh, 1753.

In this reproduction of a colored drawing, Lind observes British sailors being treated with citrus fruits (oranges and limes) to cure scurvy. The nickname "limey" for sailors can be traced to Lind's discovery.

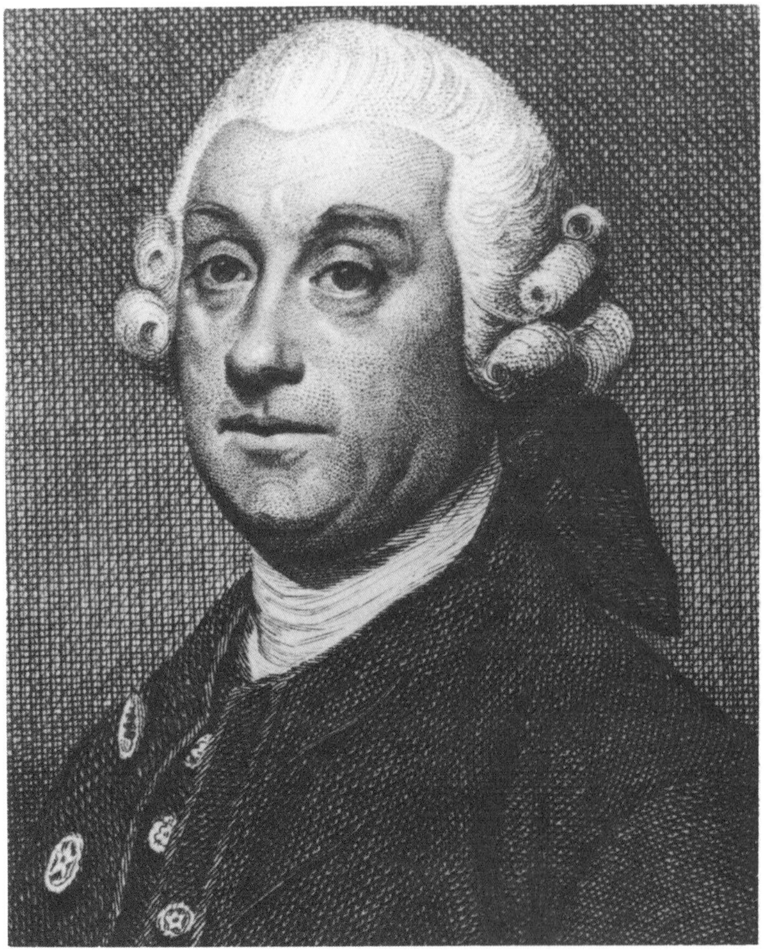

# Percivall Pott

## A TREATISE ON RUPTURES

Pott (1714-1788), one of the most prominent surgeons and teachers of surgery in London during the third quarter of the eighteenth century, published the first description of congenital hernia in this survey of the varieties of hernia and their treatment. He always wrote in clear, natural English, directly from his own experience, and recorded that he had "two intentions" in writing about ruptures: "To lay before the young practitioner a plain practical account of the three most frequent species of ruptures, and from my own experience to remove the prejudice against the profession with regard to this disease which the repeated assertions of advertising quacks have raised." He called the trusses provided by such quacks "melancholy proofs of ignorance."

Noting the advances that surgery had made in the previous years, he suggested that the time had come for the public to trust surgeons to deal adequately with ruptures. In this book, he classified hernias not by site but by condition: "Those suitable for immediate reduction, those irreducible from their size, ancient date or adhesions, those reducible but the reduction difficult and attended with pain and trouble, and those reducible only by surgical operations."

Although he described his methods in cases in which surgery was practical, he dismissed the possibility of "a radical cure" and criticized the use of cautery or caustic as "fallacious, uncertain, and therefore disused by good surgeons." Pott revised his book on hernias three times for later editions.

Pott's name is associated with a number of pathologic conditions. He described the chimney sweep's carcinoma of the scrotum and recognized it as an occupational disease (1775), the first such example. He has also become immortalized by his account of the kyphosis, known as Pott's disease, which results from tuberculosis of the spine (1779), and by the ankle fracture involving the lower fibula and the medial malleolus (1765).

He lived in the era when surgeons finally broke with the barbers and helped make that break. It is interesting that a compound fracture of his own leg led to a long convalescence and gave him the time to write this, his first book.

Pott, a short but elegant gentleman and scholar, was a busy London surgeon whose practice included the aristocracy of the age. He was a kind, humane person, greatly admired and respected by his contemporaries.

Percivall Pott. *A Treatise on Ruptures*. London, 1756.

Portrait of the famous surgeon.
As surgeon to the illustrious of London society, Pott was called on to treat, among others, the actor David Garrick and lexicographer Samuel Johnson.

As the practice of Inoculation always divided people into parties, ſome contending warmly for it, and others as ſtrongly againſt it; the latter aſſerting that the advantages pretended were imaginary, and that the Surgeons, from views of intereſt, conceal'd or diminiſh'd the true number of deaths occaſion'd by Inoculation, and magnify'd the number of thoſe who died of the *Small-pox* in the common way: It was reſolved by the Magiſtrates of the town, to cauſe a ſtrict and impartial enquiry to be made by the Conſtables of each ward, who were to give in their returns upon oath; and that the enquiry might be made more ſtrictly and impartially, ſome of the partiſans for and againſt the practice were join'd as aſſiſtants to the officers, and accompany'd them in their progreſs through the wards from houſe to houſe. Their ſeveral returns being received, and ſumm'd up together, the numbers turn'd out as follows,

| Had the Small-pox in the common way, | | Of theſe died | | Received the diſtemper by Inoculation, | | Of theſe died | |
|---|---|---|---|---|---|---|---|
| Whites | Blacks | Whites | Blacks | Whites | Blacks | Whites | Blacks |
| 5059 | 485 | 452 | 62 | 1974 | 139 | 23 | 7 |

It appeared by this account that the deaths of perſons inoculated, were more in proportion at this time than had been formerly obſerved, being ſomething more than one in a hundred. The favourers of Inoculation however would not allow that this was owing to any error in the former accounts, but rather to the Inoculating at this time many unfit ſubjects, partly through the impatience of people who would not wait the neceſſary preparation, leſt they ſhould take it in the common way; and partly from the importunity of parents prevailing with the Surgeons againſt their judgment and advice to inoculate weak children, labouring under other diſorders; becauſe the parents could not immediately remove them out of the way of the diſtemper, and thought they would at leaſt ſtand a better chance by being inoculated, than in taking the infection, as they would probably do, in the common way. The Surgeons and Phy-

ſicians

# Benjamin Franklin

## INOCULATION FOR THE SMALL-POX

Although not a physician, the remarkable Benjamin Franklin (1706-1790) made many valuable contributions to medicine. He was a founder and the first president of the Pennsylvania Hospital, of which he wrote a history. He invented the bifocal lens and a flexible catheter and wrote on the use of electricity for the treatment of paralysis. This treatment was named for him (franklinization). He also studied and wrote about lead poisoning, night blindness, sleep, the "heat" of blood, the infectious nature of colds, infection from cadavers, the infant death rate, and medical education. His *Dialogue with Gout* (1759) is of special interest because he himself suffered from this disease.

Public health was one of Franklin's many interests, but at first he opposed smallpox inoculation, which at that time was indeed dangerous. Later, when his youngest son died of the disease, he regretted his opposition and became an advocate. Variolation, the practice of inoculating humans with dried, unmodified matter to prevent contagious smallpox, had been introduced into western Europe from Turkey about 1720. In England it was strongly advocated by Dr. Richard Mead, the leading London physician. However, it was not until the 1750's, when severe epidemics of smallpox recurred, that variolation became general. While he was in England between 1757 and 1762 as agent for the Pennsylvania Assembly, Franklin gathered statistics from both English and American sources to present a strong argument in favor of variolation. He published these in his pamphlet, together with "Plain Instructions" for inoculation. The latter were written at his request by a London physician who has been variously identified as Edward Archer or William Heberden. The page of Franklin's text reproduced here reminds us that the present-day problems of designing and evaluating clinical investigations are nothing new.

Improved methods of variolation were introduced in the 1760's, but the preliminary treatment was severe, the results were unpredictable, and a permanent reservoir of smallpox carriers was created. Search for a safer preventive measure therefore went on; the search culminated in Jenner's vaccination, announced in 1798.

The short pamphlet in the Lilly Library is an important contribution to the movement that finally led to eradication of this dread disease.

Benjamin Franklin. *Some Account Of the Success of Inoculation for the Small-Pox in England and America. Together with Plain Instructions, By which any Person may be enabled to perform the Operation, and conduct the Patient through the Distemper.* London, 1759.

In Franklin's time, smallpox vaccination was a highly controversial and a somewhat dangerous procedure, as evidenced in this page of his pamphlet.

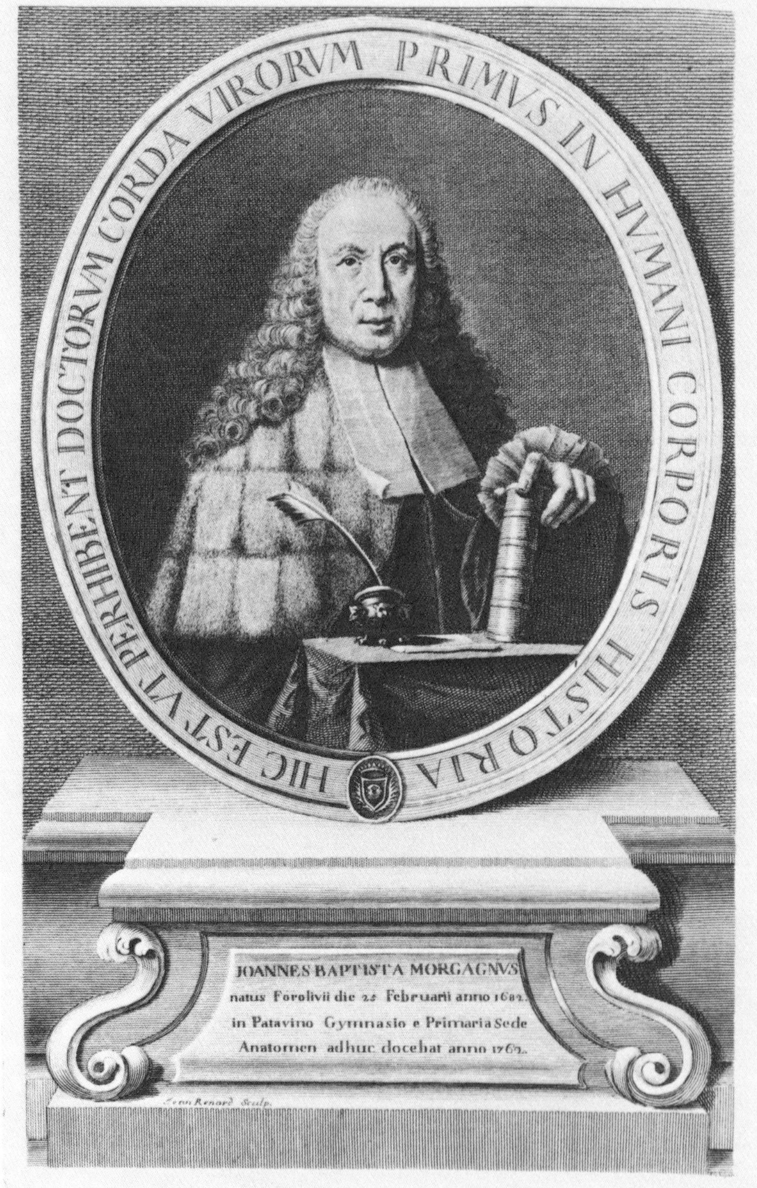
HIC EST VT PERHIBENT DOCTORVM CORDA VIRORVM PRIMVS IN HVMANI CORPORIS HISTORIA
JOANNES BAPTISTA MORGAGNVS
natus Forolivii die 25 Februarii anno 1682.
in Patavino Gymnasio e Primaria Sede
Anatomen adhuc docebat anno 1762.
Renard Sculp.

# Giovanni Battista Morgagni

## ON THE SEATS AND CAUSES OF DISEASE

Morgagni (1682-1771), professor at Padua for sixty years, was a renowned man of medicine in Europe in the mid-eighteenth century. In fame and achievement, he was rivaled only by Boerhaave at the beginning of his career and by von Haller in his later years. Because Venice was at that time the most frequented city in Europe and the university town of Padua was nearby, Morgagni was accessible for consultation to a great number of patients. His earlier anatomic work appeared in the six series of letters of his *Adversaria Anatomica* between 1706 and 1719. During the 1720's, he published another series of letters commenting on the ancient Roman medical texts. He also edited the works of his master, Valsalva, with an elaborate commentary (published in 1740) running to more than a thousand pages, six times longer than the Valsalva material.

Morgagni's "Five Books on the Seats and Causes of Diseases Investigated by Anatomy, Comprising Almost Innumerable Dissections and Observations Now First Published for the Benefit of Physicians, Surgeons, and Anatomists" is considered one of the great books in the history of medicine. Issued in Venice when he was seventy-nine, it appeared in two volumes and ran to some 850 tall pages with double columns of print. As though to guarantee acceptance throughout the learned world, each of the five "books" is dedicated to a prominent physician or surgeon in a different city.

Morgagni's hundreds of case histories are correlated with necropsy reports in such a simple and attractive style that his vast collection remains one of the most readable of all medical books. The reports are replete with astute observations, and, in many cases, Morgagni described conditions that were not generally recognized until decades later. Especially noteworthy are discussions of cardiac valves (aortic insufficiency, mitral stenosis), syphilitic aneurysm, pneumonia, and tuberculosis of the kidney. A number of eponyms have kept his name familiar to future generations; certain crypts, foramens, tubercles, sinuses, valves, columns, and other structures are associated with Morgagni.

This monumental work may be said to establish the organ concept of disease and to make pathologic anatomy a major medical discipline. By coincidence, the book was published the same year as Auenbrugger's (q.v.) major contribution on percussion. The age of observation had arrived.

Giovanni Battista Morgagni. *De Sedibus, et Causis Morborum per Anatomen Indagatis, Libri Quinque....* 2 vols. Venice, 1761.

"This is the man, as learned judges have named him, who is first among men in the study of the human body."

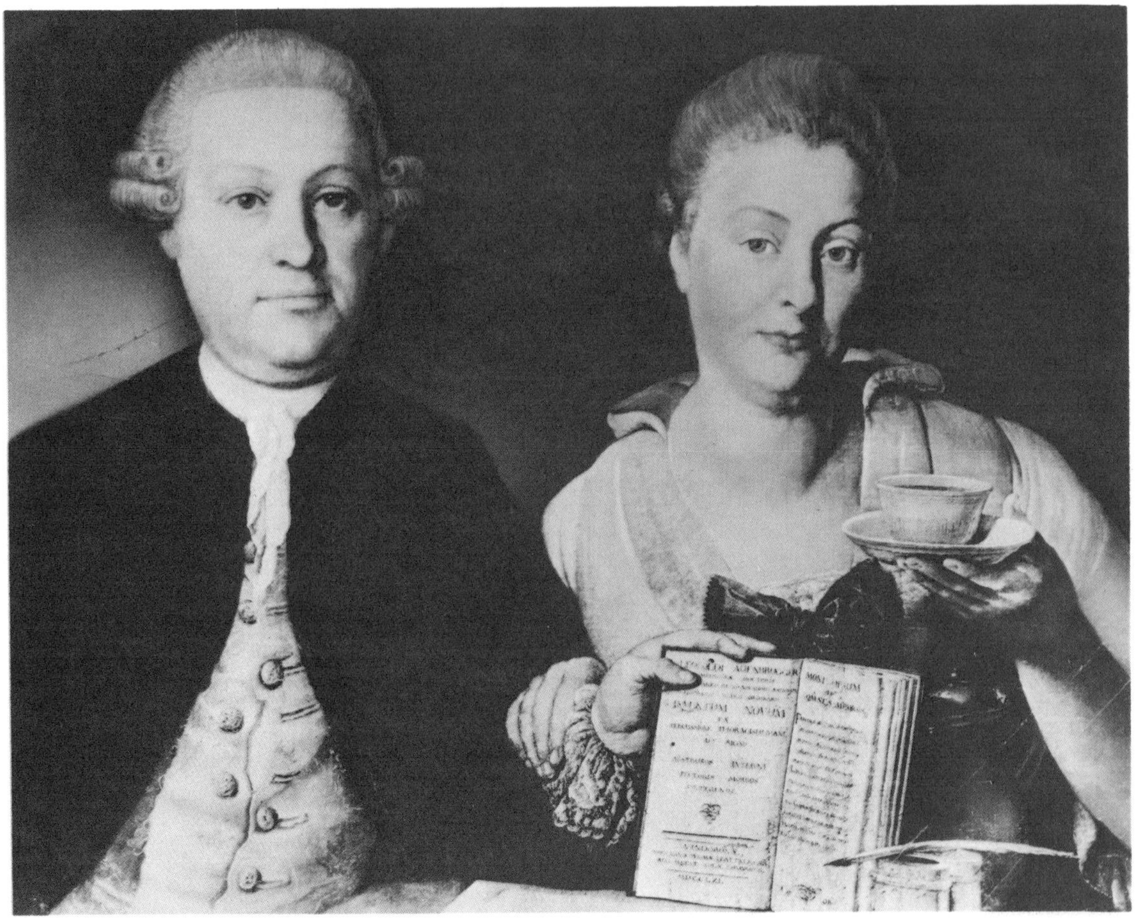

# Leopold Auenbrugger

## NEW DISCOVERY ON PERCUSSION OF THE CHEST

Auenbrugger (1722-1809) used his "New Discovery of Detecting from Percussion of the Human Chest Obscure Diseases within the Breast" while he was physician to the Spanish Hospital in Vienna. He had carefully verified his findings by dissection before committing them to paper. The book begins with general chapters on chest diseases, then describes the special uses of his method, and includes fourteen case histories.

Auenbrugger was gifted with a musical ear and distinguished the "drum" sound emitted by the healthy chest from the higher "tympanitic" sound, the indistinct sound, or the dull "flesh" sound of a diseased chest. By tapping over fluids which had been injected into the chests of cadavers, he established the percussion note characteristic of pleural effusion. Applying the technique in his practice, he was able to prove his diagnosis by thoracentesis. Although he gave notice "to all doctors" that percussion "deserves first place after examining the pulse and respiration," his method was not adopted by van Swieten—the leading Viennese physician—his former teacher, nor by de Haen, physician to the Vienna Clinic. De Haen's successor, Maximilian Stoll, took it up but died prematurely, and the procedure was dropped. Auenbrugger had also expressed the wish that his method might prove "a solace of the wretched and an increase of their art for true cultivators of medicine." The book was translated into French in 1770, but the translation also was ignored.

Although not widely followed, the new method of percussion was taught in several German university medical schools and was adopted by some prominent physicians. Corvisart (q.v.), Napoleon's physician, learned of it from Stoll's writings and mentioned his own success with it in his book; he followed this by editing Auenbrugger's original text in a new French translation (1808). Nearly fifty years after Auenbrugger's publication, Corvisart's advocacy firmly established percussion as a necessary procedure for every physician.

Auenbrugger retired from his hospital in 1762, had a distinguished career in private practice, and was ennobled in 1784 for his medical achievement. In 1783, he published a psychologic study of the urge to commit suicide, citing this urge as a real disease.

As a distinguished member of the Viennese court, Auenbrugger delighted Empress Maria Theresa by writing a libretto for Salieri's operetta, *The Chimney Sweep*. Unassuming and sedate, he did not appear concerned that his new method of diagnosis remained almost unnoticed until a year before his death.

Leopold Auenbrugger. *Inventum novum ex Percussione Thoracis humani ut signo abstrusos interni Pectoris Morbos.* Vienna, 1761.

In this portrait with his wife,
Auenbrugger proudly holds a copy of his *magnum opus*.
It was some fifty years before his concept
of percussion was generally accepted.

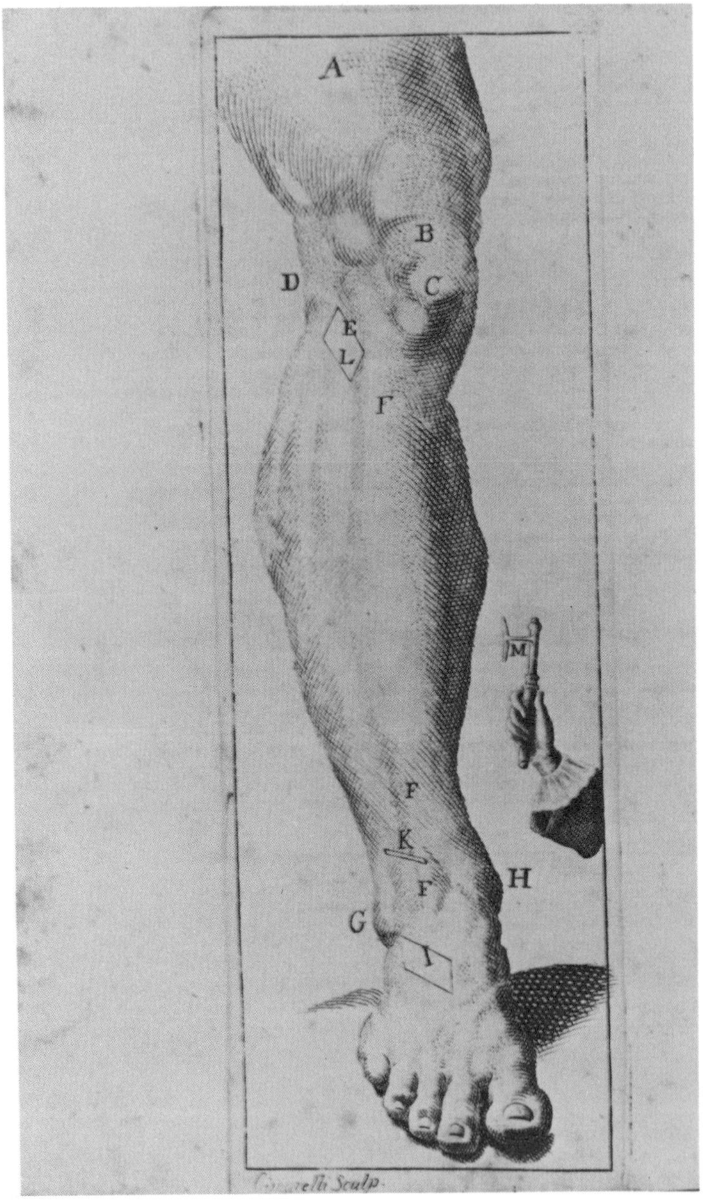

Cipparelli Sculp.

# Domenico Cotugno

## TREATISE ON SCIATICA

Throughout his career, Cotugno (1736-1822), or Cotunnius, was physician at the Hospital for Incurables in Naples, the most important city in Italy at that time. He had traveled as a young man in northern Italy and studied under Morgagni at Padua; in middle age he visited Austria and Germany in attendance on his king. During the first half of his life, he was active in research on anatomy and its bearing on physiologic problems. He was also a scholarly connoisseur of books and amassed a fine library.

At the age of twenty-five, he followed Valsalva's discovery of aural structure with a study of the fluids of the inner ear, *De Aquaeductibus Auris Humanae Internae* (Naples, 1761), in which he described the parts of the inner ear, established the existence of the labyrinthine fluid, and offered a theory of resonance to explain the process of hearing. He is also known for his careful account of the pathologic findings in the intestines of persons who had died of typhoid fever and for his demonstration that albuminuria can be detected by boiling the urine.

*De Ischiade Nervosa Commentarius,* in fifty-seven chapters, was published when he was twenty-eight. It differentiated between two kinds of "sciatica," neurologic and arthritic, by showing that the sciatic nerve is involved with the former. Cotugno covered in great detail the symptoms and etiology of sciatica and also outlined his methods of treating it. In the course of this account, he gave the first extensive description of the cerebrospinal fluid, which had been mentioned by Valsalva (q.v.) in 1692. Cotugno revised the book for three subsequent editions, and it was also translated into English (1785) and German (1792).

Cotugno anticipated Richard Bright by more than fifty years in his description of nephrosis, wrote a useful book on smallpox (1769), and advocated the public control of tuberculosis. He lived to the age of eighty-six.

Domenico Cotugno [Dominicus Cotunnius]. *De Ischiade Nervosa Commentarius.* Naples, 1764.

In this illustration, Cotugno indicated the points at which heat (blisters) should be applied for treatment of sciatica.

PLATE III

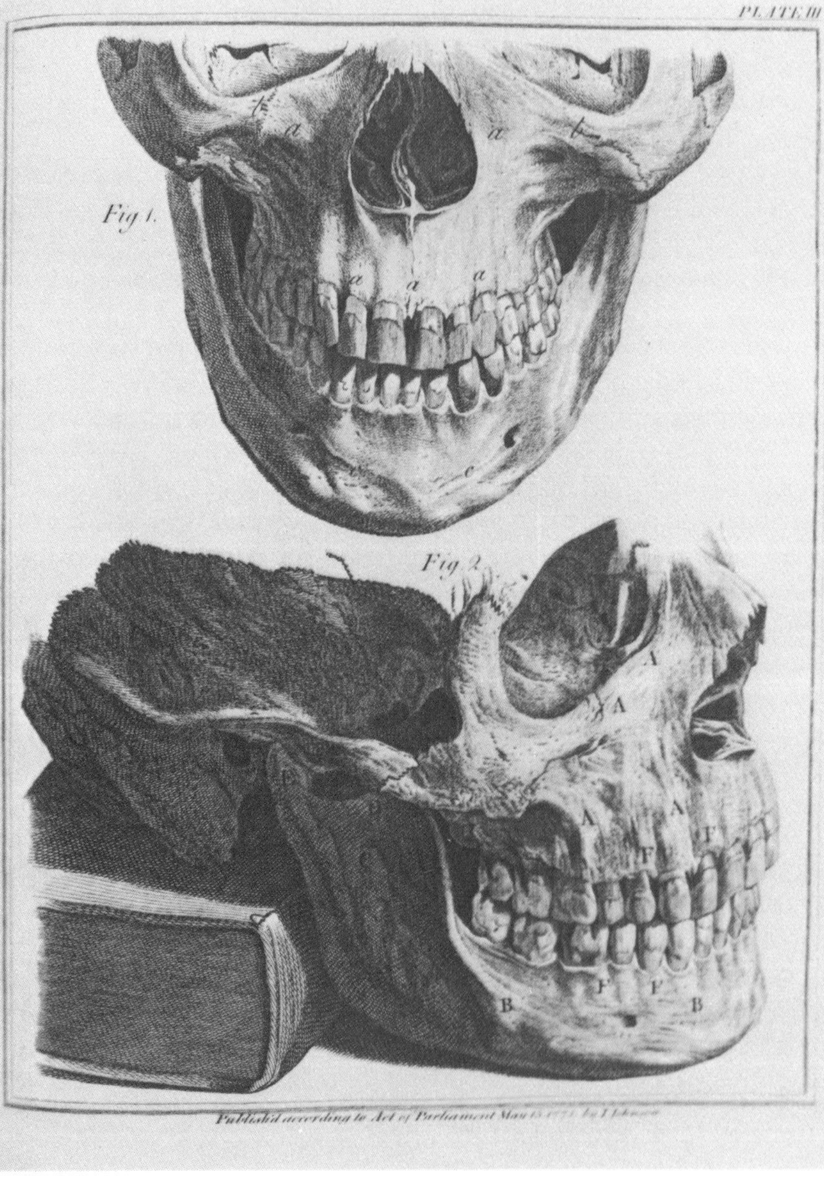


*Publish'd according to Act of Parliament May 15 1771 by J Johnson*

# John Hunter

## THE NATURAL HISTORY OF THE HUMAN TEETH

John Hunter (1728-1793) was brought from Scotland to London as a rough, uncouth twenty-year-old to learn dissection at his brother William's school of anatomy. John showed such a striking aptitude for the new activity that, within a year, he was demonstrating the art of dissection. Although he never had a traditional medical education, he began to study surgery at the age of twenty-three under William Cheselden (q.v.).

John Hunter's superb background in comparative anatomy and pathology and his ability to relate structure to function made him one of England's greatest surgeons and perhaps the founder of experimental surgery. Among his innovations was a technique for treating aneurysms without amputation by use of a single ligature to tie off the artery in the healthy tissue. He is said to have elevated surgery from an art to a science by showing that the proper route to the operating room led through the laboratory.

In a busy life devoted to research, teaching, and the practice of surgery, Hunter found time to study the structure, development, and diseases of the teeth and to collect and arrange a series of dental specimens. Hunter's two treatises on the teeth rank him as one of the founders of modern scientific dentistry.

In the first book (1771), Hunter classified the teeth in the system still used today and was the first to state definitely that the human teeth "are never more than thirty-two." He traced their development in the fetus and the child and established their structure of pulp, bone, and enamel. At the end of the book are descriptions of devices to correct malocclusion and even suggestions for a method of transplantation.

The second volume (1778) dealt with pathology. Hunter discussed the diseases of the teeth, the alveolar processes, and the gums; abscesses; and nerve pains in the jaws. He concluded that tooth decay starts on the surface of the tooth and not in the interior.

Like his brother William, John founded a famous museum. Housing more than 13,000 specimens demonstrating comparative anatomy and the physiologic processes in animals and man, it was also a menagerie that contained numerous live mammals. After his death, the great Hunterian Museum became the property of the Royal College of Surgeons. It was partially destroyed by Nazi bombs in 1941.

John Hunter was a student of Percivall Pott, a teacher of Edward Jenner, and, with William Heberden, a consultant on an illness of Benjamin Franklin. Originally buried in St. Martin's-in-the-Fields, his body was moved to Westminster Abbey sixty-six years after his death.

John Hunter. *The Natural History of the Human Teeth*. London, 1771. Bound with *A Practical Treatise on the Diseases of the Teeth*. London, 1778.

Artist Jan Riemsdijk, working from Hunter's specimens, provided sixteen full-page drawings for this first scientific study of the human teeth.

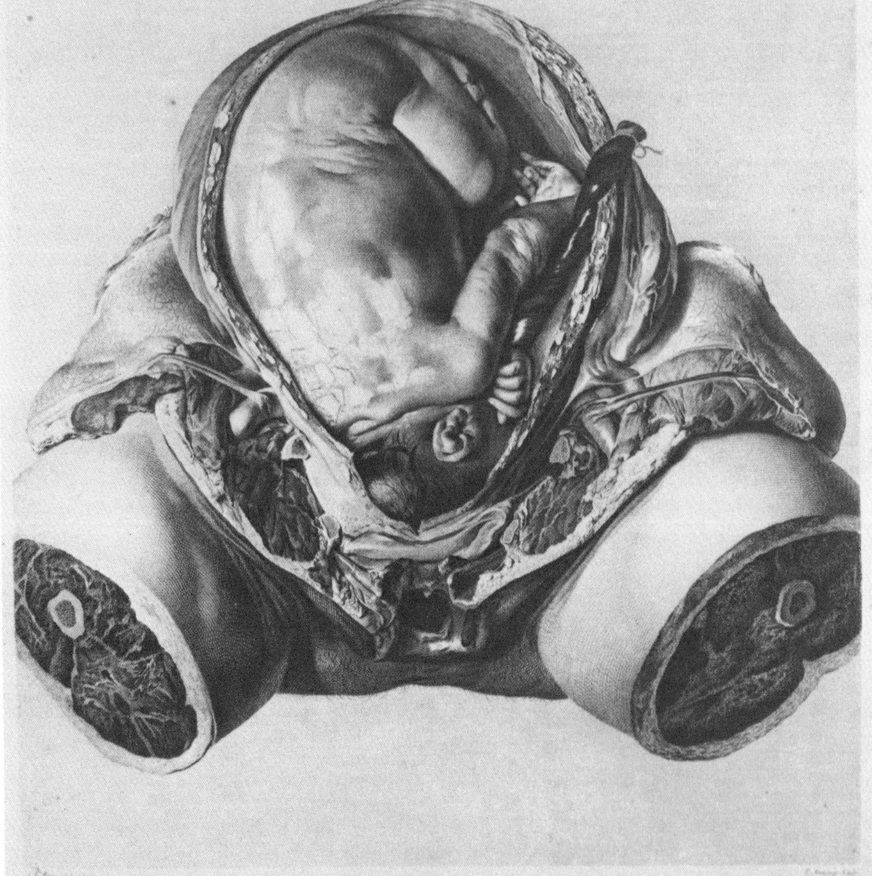

TAB. VI. Fœtus in utero, prout a natura positus, rescissis omnino parte uteri anteriori, ac Placenta ei adhaerente.

Pub. Nov. 1 1775 by D. Hunter.

# William Hunter

## THE ANATOMY OF THE HUMAN GRAVID UTERUS

As London's foremost obstetrician, William Hunter (1718-1783) attended Queen Charlotte at the birth of each of her sixteen children. Hunter was an inspired teacher; his school of anatomy attracted men who became famous anatomists and surgeons. Among the latter was his brother John, who was ten years his junior. William Hunter's home housed not only the school of anatomy but also a museum for his collections—books and manuscripts, paintings, coins, medals, and anatomic and pathologic specimens. These collections were later bequeathed to the University of Glasgow, where Hunter had studied for five years.

Hunter spent almost twenty-five years preparing *The Anatomy of the Human Gravid Uterus*, the most magnificent obstetric atlas ever published. He engaged the best artists to draw and engrave the thirty-four illustrations, and it was printed by John Baskerville, the finest printer of the age, at the peak of his career. The life-size line engravings, many measuring 54 by 46 centimeters, achieve effects of depth and contrast without losing sharpness of detail and present a wide range of normal and pathologic conditions of the womb and fetus. Each page of text is printed in two columns, one in Latin and the other in English.

William and his brother John explored the anatomy of the placenta and described the separate circulatory systems of the mother and the fetus. The brothers later quarreled over who should receive recognition for this work and separated professionally about three years before William's death.

William Hunter was the first to describe retroversion of the uterus (1770). Outside the field of obstetrics, he is remembered for the first description of arteriovenous aneurysm and for clarifying the anatomy and physiology of the lymphatics. He was professor of anatomy in the Royal Academy and a Fellow of the Royal and Antiquarian societies.

Hunter never married. A hardworking, disciplined man who lived simply and frugally, he was troubled by severe attacks of gout, a disease that also affected other members of his family. He died in 1783 at the age of sixty-four.

William Hunter. *Anatomia Uteri Humani Gravidi tabulis illustrata*. Birmingham, 1774.

The infant *in utero* has never been more magnificently depicted than in this engraving. The original full-page illustration is life-size.

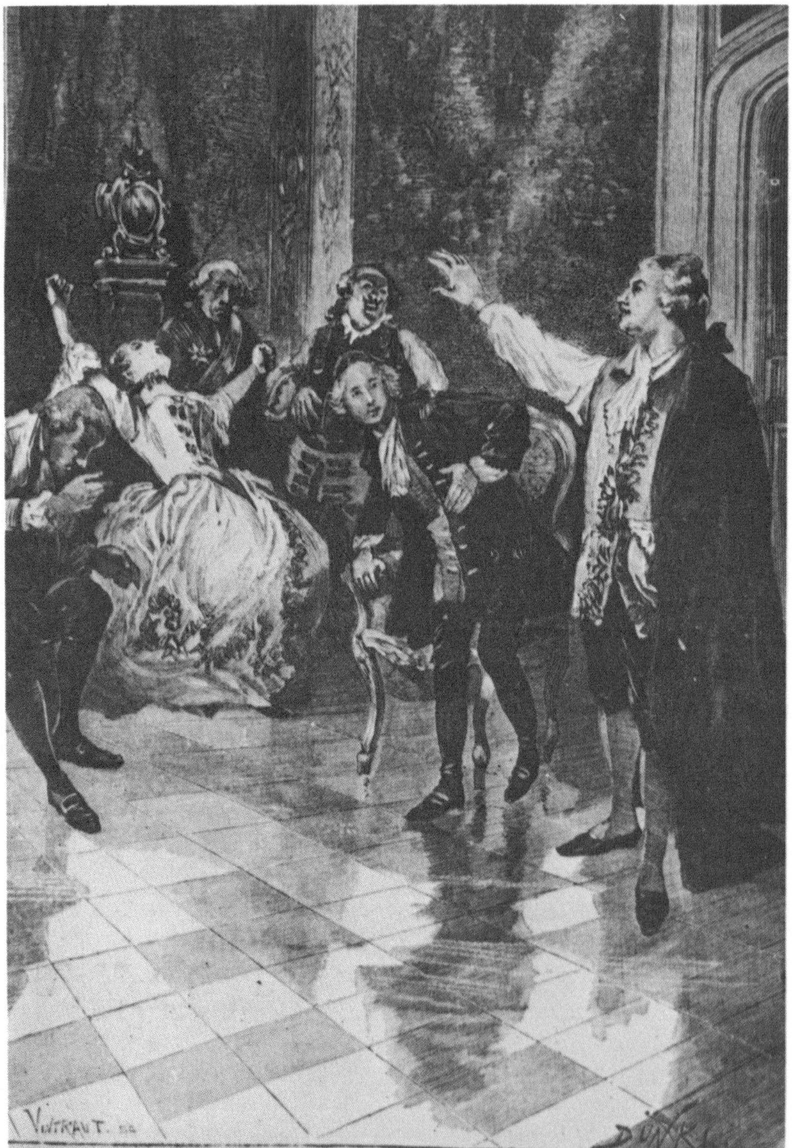

UNE SÉANCE DE MAGNÉTISME DE MESMER, DANS SON HOTEL DE LA PLACE VENDÔME (PAGE 131)

II.

# Franz Anton Mesmer

## ANIMAL MAGNETISM

Mesmer's magnetotherapy, though without scientific foundation, evoked such excitement in the late eighteenth century that his name has endured since then in the term "mesmerism." A native of Switzerland, Mesmer (1734-1815) studied medicine in Vienna under van Swieten and de Haen. His graduating thesis proposed the theory that heavenly bodies act upon living beings by means of a subtle fluid he called "animal magnetism."

Mesmer came to believe in the therapeutic efficacy of iron magnets placed on the patient's body or passed over it. During 1773 and 1774, while practicing as a physician in Vienna, he claimed that he had "cured" some hysterical patients. He had done this, he explained, by utilizing the flux and reflux of magnetic currents in the body under the influence of hypnotic suggestion. In experimenting with magnets, he conceived the idea that similar power is possessed by the human hand. Anton Stoerck, the chief physician in Vienna, refused to believe Mesmer's claims, and in 1777 Mesmer was ordered to discontinue this form of treatment and leave the city. He moved to Paris in 1778 and there erected a temple to the god of health, where, with a background of soft music, the purple-clad Mesmer would hold hypnotic seances, waving a magnetized wand. Although the afflicted thronged to this temple and his activities became a sensation, a commission was finally appointed to investigate the phenomenon. Among the examiners were Benjamin Franklin and Antoine Lavoisier. The commission decided that magnetism was due to the imagination, Mesmer's claims were denounced, and the clinic was suppressed in 1784.

In self-justification, Mesmer published the book *Mémoire sur la découverte du magnétisme animal* in 1779. After an "Advice to the Public" in his own favor, Mesmer records the case histories of the patients he had treated successfully in Vienna, with some account of his controversies. Twenty-seven theoretical "Propositions" follow and provide a pseudoscientific basis for his treatment. These include statements that there is "a universal fluid susceptible of receiving, propagating, and communicating the impression of movement," although "up to the present its laws are unknown," that there are a "flux and reflux" of this fluid in animal bodies, and that "I call this property of the animal body, which is analogous to the properties of the magnet, Animal Magnetism."

Mesmer's work had minimum medical value in itself, but it seems clear in retrospect that he was curing psychosomatic ailments by suggestion. Ultimately, "mesmerism" stimulated research on nerve impulses and influenced the rise of psychotherapy.

Franz Anton Mesmer. *Mémoire sur la découverte du magnétisme animal*. Geneva and Paris, 1779.

Mesmer's "cures" may have been effected more by hysteria than by science. This scene, from a lithograph by Figuier, suggests that the seances were fraught with drama.

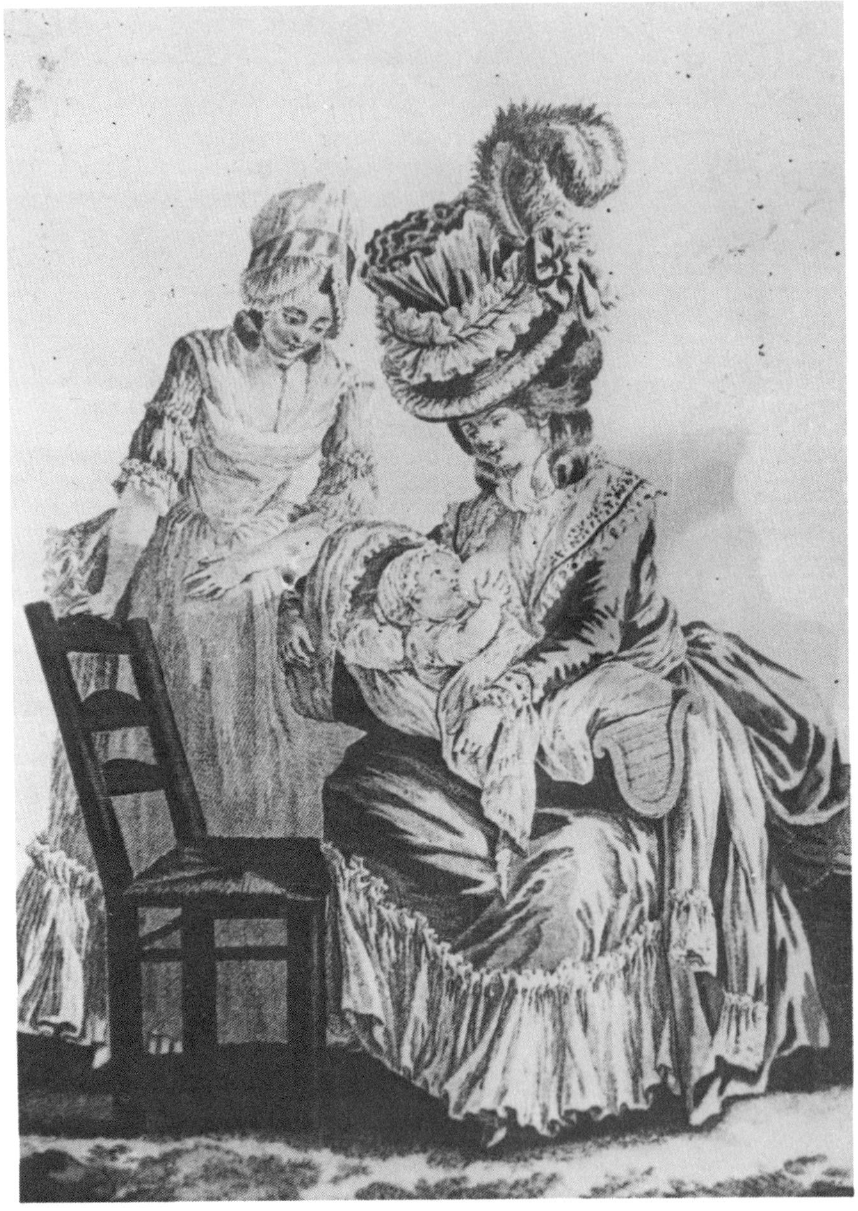

# Michael Underwood

## THE DISEASES OF CHILDREN

Michael Underwood (1737-1820) published *A Treatise on the Diseases of Children* in 1784, one year after another physician-author, George Armstrong, had issued the last version of his *Essay* on the same subject. Underwood was accused of plagiarizing, although the work of contemporary authors discussing the same subject could easily overlap. Underwood was better qualified than Armstrong but less original. He had trained in Paris and at St. George's Hospital in London and had practiced as a surgeon for a quarter of a century. After obtaining a license in obstetrics, he practiced as a "man-midwife" for the rest of his long life. He died at the age of eighty-four. It was Underwood who was called to attend the Princess of Wales at the birth of Princess Charlotte, the first legitimate grandchild of George III. Through his book on the diseases of children, which he kept carefully up to date in successive editions, Underwood became the most influential pediatrician of his time.

The volume is small, about 10 by 17 centimeters. This first edition followed the arrangement of Armstrong's book in describing ailments caused by intestinal toxemia, then disorders of teething, and, finally, exanthematous fevers, rickets, and whooping cough. Underwood was more thorough than Armstrong, however; his useful chapter on "Thrush," for instance, fills ten pages. The "Directions for Management of Infants from the Birth" again follow Armstrong's method but add enlightened instructions as to psychologic aspects, the "passions of the mind," including control of "the tempers of wet-nurses." Underwood was also a pioneer in the development of artificial infant feedings that were nutritionally sound and came close to duplicating the food values found in mother's milk. He recommended boiled cow's milk diluted with barley water.

Later editions were three times as long as the first and were divided into volumes covering "The Province of the Physician," "The Province of the Surgeon," and the duties of the nurse. Underwood indicated that "The Work is calculated not only for Medical People, but for the Direction of the Intelligent Parent." He also added new observations; in the second edition (1789), he first defined poliomyelitis as a distinct disease, and in the fourth (1799), he wrote the earliest account of congenital heart disease in children. He himself prepared seven editions, and three more followed his death; the tenth appeared in 1846, sixty-two years after the first. There were seven American editions between 1793 and 1842 and several French and German translations. The influence of this book must have been profound.

Michael Underwood. *A Treatise on the Diseases of Children, With Directions For the Management of Infants From the Birth; Especially Such as are brought up by Hand.* London, 1784.

This French engraving undoubtedly was designed to help popularize breast feeding among the affluent, many of whom preferred to rely on wet nurses or on artificial feedings of possibly questionable nutritional value.

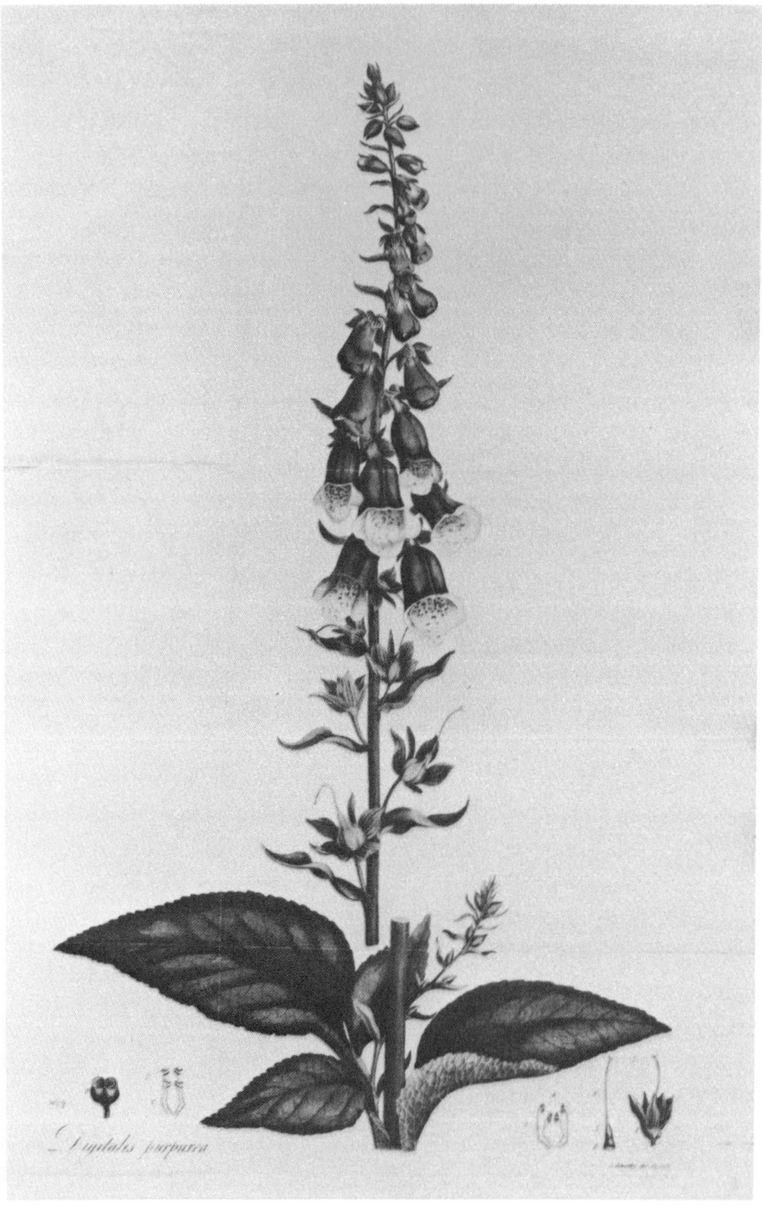

*Digitalis purpurea*

# William Withering

## AN ACCOUNT OF THE FOXGLOVE

William Withering (1741-1799) discovered the efficacy of digitalis in the treatment of cardiac edema by analyzing a folk remedy and observing that the active ingredient was found in the common foxglove plant *(Digitalis purpurea)*, which had been used in other herbal remedies for asthma. The drug was known to physicians but had been given indiscriminately; Withering not only pointed out the cases in which it could be prescribed with advantage but also determined the correct dosage.

Withering graduated from the University of Edinburgh in 1766. He began his career in the English Midlands, practicing as a physician first in Stafford and then, from 1775 to 1792, in Birmingham. There he was appointed one of the physicians to the General Hospital when it opened in 1779. Three years earlier he had published *Botanical Arrangement of All the Vegetables*, a monograph on British flora, which was widely studied; it was arranged according to the new Linnaean system, was often revised, and became a standard reference during the following hundred years. He also wrote an influential study of scarlet-fever epidemics in 1779. After 1784, Withering was attacked by tuberculosis and gradually withdrew from his very successful practice to devote more time to botany and chemistry.

When Withering first used digitalis in 1775, he noticed that "lives were hazarded by its unguarded exhibition" or that, on the other hand, "a medicine of efficacy was rejected as dangerous and unmanageable." By the time he published his *Account*, he had had ten years' experience with the drug and could offer "rules and precautions" for its preparation and administration. The main part of the text, some ninety pages, presents 156 cases from his private practice, followed by reports on eight hospital patients. The next section contains histories of similar cases sent to him by correspondents. The remaining pages convey "practical remarks" on the preparation, dosage, and effects of the medicine, suggest rules and cautions, and, finally, discuss dropsy.

Withering introduced digitalis as a diuretic in the treatment of dropsy. He recognized that certain individuals responded best to the drug, and his descriptions show that these were cardiac patients. However, it was more than forty years before Richard Bright differentiated cardiac dropsy from renal dropsy. Withering pointed out to colleagues, when they reported failures with the drug, that they were not following his rules but were giving excessive doses in unsuitable cases. His careful analysis made this powerful medicine safe for the treatment of heart diseases.

William Withering. *An Account of the Foxglove, and Some of its Medical Uses: with Practical Remarks on Dropsy, and other Diseases.* Birmingham, 1785.

The sole illustration in Withering's book is this exquisite foldout plate of the foxglove *(Digitalis purpurea)*, which appears uncolored in some copies of the book, delicately tinted in others.

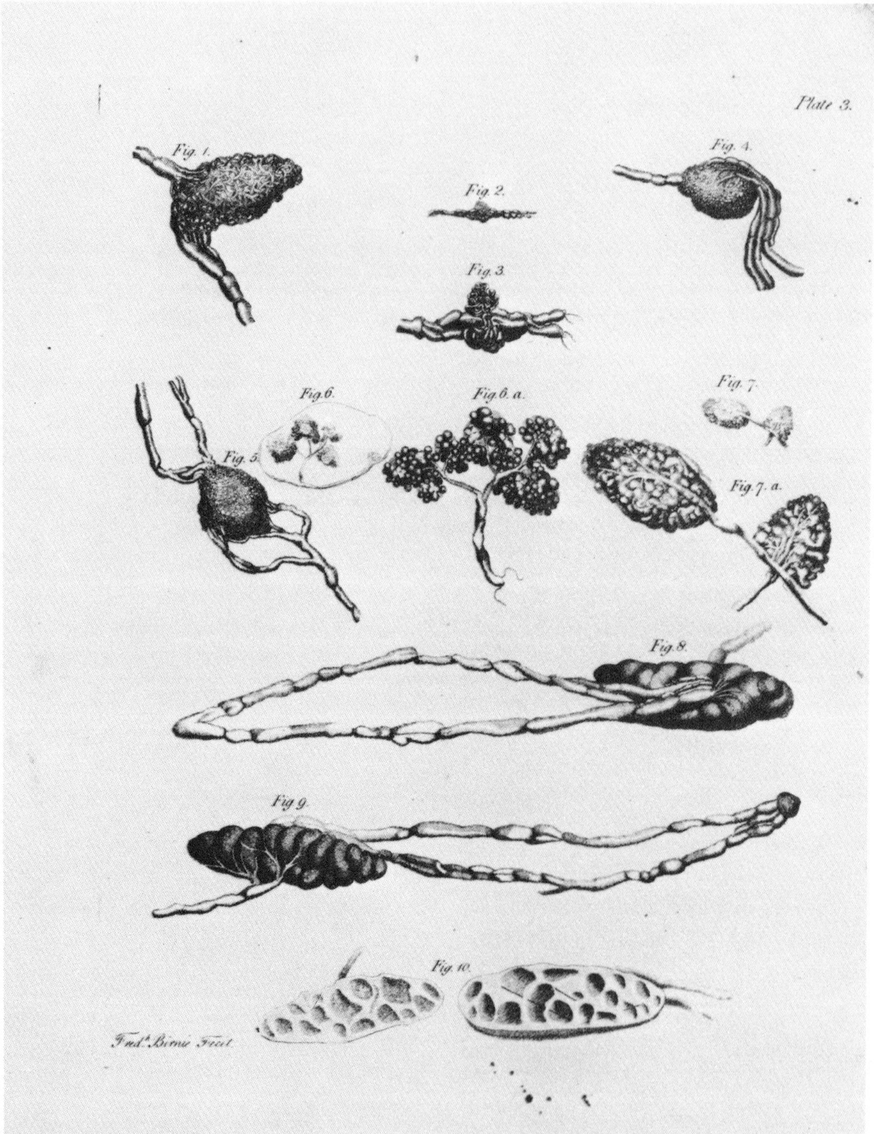
Plate 3.
Fig. 1.
Fig. 2.
Fig. 3.
Fig. 4.
Fig. 5.
Fig. 6.
Fig. 6. a.
Fig. 7.
Fig. 7. a.
Fig. 8.
Fig. 9.
Fig. 10.

# William Cruikshank

## THE ANATOMY OF THE ABSORBING VESSELS

Cruikshank (1745-1800) concluded the investigation of the lymphatics, which had occupied anatomists since the middle of the seventeenth century. He was associated with William Hunter's anatomy school, where the problem had been explored by John Hunter, William Hewson, and John Sheldon. All of them had published valuable reports, but it was Cruikshank's book that gave the definitive account of the human lymphatic system.

Part 1 of the book is a digest of earlier writings on the "Absorbing Vessels and their Glands in those animals in general in which they have yet been found," and Part 2 is the anatomic description of the human lymphatic system. Of this, he wrote, "...fluids absorbed by the lacteals are transmitted to the lymphatics and through them, at last, conveyed to the blood...proof that lymphatics are absorbents, is, that whenever fluids are extravasated on surfaces, or into cavities, or whenever such fluids preternaturally distend their reservoirs, the lymphatics belonging to these surfaces and cavities are found full of the same fluid."

Although he originally had intended to become a Presbyterian minister, Cruikshank spent four years as an apprentice in surgery and pharmacy after he graduated in theology and the arts from the universities of Edinburgh and Glasgow. In 1771, he moved from his native Scotland to London, where he became an assistant and later a partner in William Hunter's famous school of anatomy. There, in addition to dissecting and lecturing, he undertook his experimental research in embryology, neurology, and physiology, including studies of the "insensible perspiration," in which he showed that the skin gives off carbon dioxide.

After William Hunter's death in 1783, Cruikshank carried on the anatomy school in partnership with Hunter's nephew, Matthew Baillie. Cruikshank also became well known in London as a surgeon, numbering Dr. Samuel Johnson and Admiral Nelson among his patients. For his many achievements in research, he was elected a Fellow of the Royal Society shortly before his death.

William Cumberland Cruikshank. *The Anatomy of the Absorbing Vessels of the Human Body.* London, 1786.

The first edition of Cruikshank's book contained three memorable line engravings by J. Thornthwaite and Frederick Birnie, of which this is one. Two more plates were added in a later edition (1790).

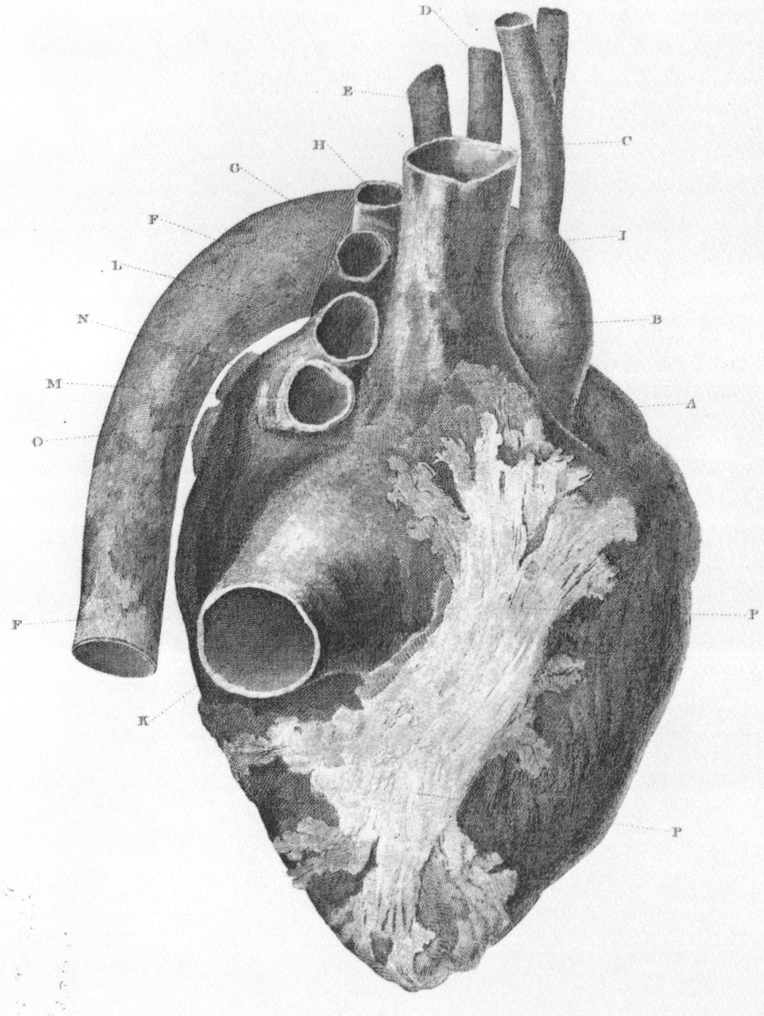
D
E
C
H
G
F
I
L
B
N
M
A
O
F
P
K
P

# Matthew Baillie

## MORBID ANATOMY

Matthew Baillie's *Morbid Anatomy*, published when he was thirty-two, offered a new approach to the understanding of disease by systematically describing the morbid appearance of each organ at autopsy and correlating these findings with a full case history. It was perhaps the first example of the modern concept of pathology.

In contrast to previous authors who had recorded organic lesions underlying the outward evidences of diseases, Baillie (1761-1823) classified such lesions according to types—softenings, hardenings, thickenings, ulcers, tumors, aneurysms, and so on. He confined his surgery to the thoracic and abdominal organs and the brain and wrote unusually well about diseases of the heart, lungs, liver, and kidneys. Baillie kept to objective description and avoided hypothetical correlations, although clinical symptoms were added in his second edition. He noticed that organic lesions may occur without clinical symptoms and that apparently similar symptoms may represent different lesions.

Baillie combined his own observations with those of his two distinguished uncles, William and John Hunter. He was educated for the ministry but later turned to medicine. He inherited William Hunter's famous anatomy school and museum in London in 1783 and directed the school for nearly twenty years. In 1787, he was appointed physician to St. George's Hospital, where John Hunter was one of the senior surgeons. Baillie became responsible for his uncle's very remarkable biomedical museum after John Hunter's death in 1793. From the age of forty, he was absorbed in his successful and extensive practice as a physician.

Baillie has been credited with the first accounts of several diseases, including cirrhosis, emphysema, and dermoid cysts of the ovary. These descriptions were original and also were presented concisely and clearly. He wrote, for instance, "[Ulcers of the stomach]...frequently...have a peculiar appearance. Many of them are hardly surrounded with any inflammation...nor is there any particular diseased alteration in the structure of the stomach in the neighbourhood. They appear very much as if some little time before a part had been cut out from the stomach with a knife, and the edges had healed, so as to present an uniform smooth boundary round the excavation which had been made."

Baillie later provided a volume of pathologic illustrations, the best that had yet been published. His textbook proved to be most popular and reached its fifth edition before Baillie's death in 1823.

Matthew Baillie. *The Morbid Anatomy of some of the most important parts of the Human Body*. London, 1793.

Baillie's plates illustrating *The Morbid Anatomy* were published separately six years after the book appeared. This one shows a rarely found ossification on the surface of the heart.

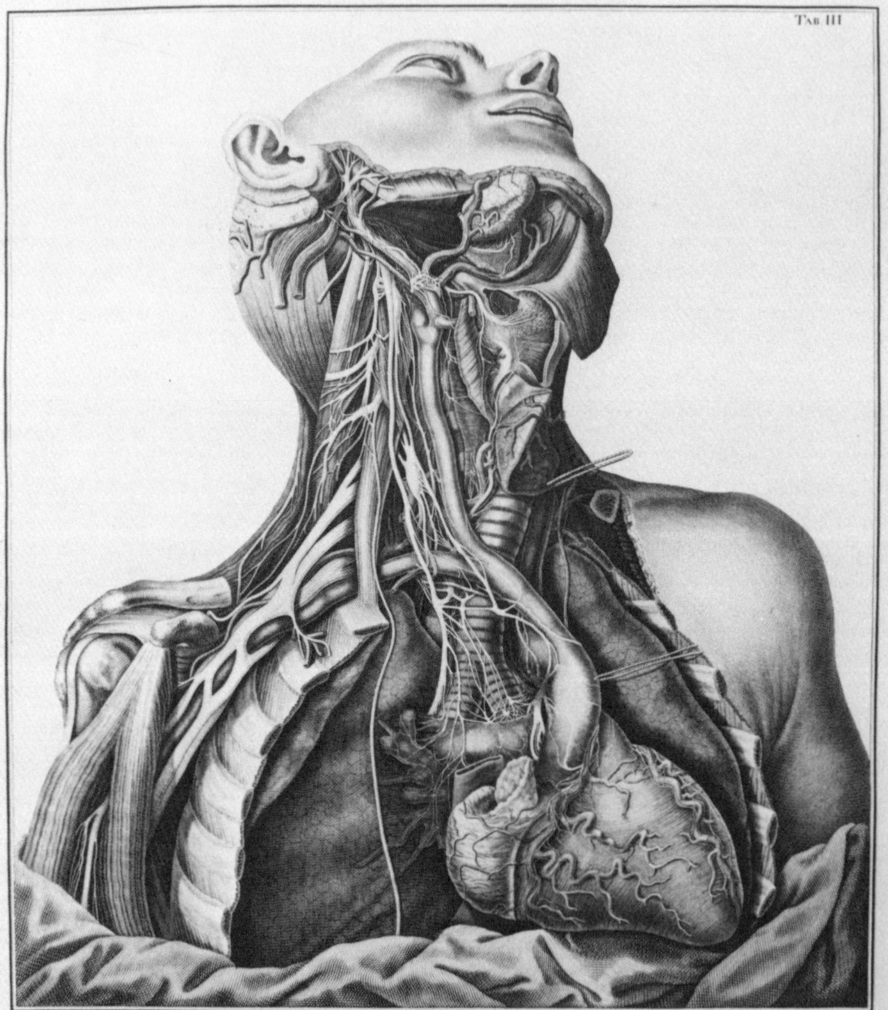


ANT. SCARPA del. F. Anderloni sculp.

# Antonio Scarpa

## NEUROLOGIC PLATES

Antonio Scarpa (1752-1832), born in Venice, was the most brilliant pupil of Morgagni, the great anatomist and clinical pathologist at Padua. Scarpa received his medical degree at the age of eighteen and, at twenty, was appointed professor of anatomy at Modena. Here he immediately published, with his own superb illustrations, a book on his discovery of the membranous labyrinth in the ear. When he was thirty-one, he moved to the more important chair of anatomy at Pavia, which he held for twenty years. In 1787, in addition, he assumed the chair of surgery and held it until 1812. He was equally distinguished as research worker, surgeon, and teacher; wrote well in Latin and Italian; and drew his own illustrations with skill.

Perhaps his greatest achievement was his large atlas of "Neurologic Plates," illustrating the cardiac, cerebral, glossopharyngeal, and pharyngeal nerves. This was published in Latin in 1794. The text includes a general essay on neurology, with accurate criticism of illustrations published by earlier anatomists, such as Willis, Vieussens, and von Haller. The essay is followed by descriptions of his own plates, providing brief, precise comments on the nerves illustrated, with mention of previous accounts. The seven engravings are so large that some organs are pictured life-size. Engraved by Faustino Anderloni from Scarpa's drawings, the plates are both accurate and brilliant in light and shade. The book offered the first detailed representation and description of the nerves of the heart.

The author is best remembered for Scarpa's triangle, an area bordered by the inguinal ligament and superficial thigh muscles. It was first delineated in his report on an operation for popliteal aneurysm.

Scarpa's anatomic investigations spanned a period of nearly sixty years and included comparative studies of the auditory and olfactory apparatus and the deep structure of bone. His surgical work covered masterly and influential research on the diseases of the eye, congenital clubfoot, aneurysms, hernia, and arterial disease. On each subject, Scarpa offered new knowledge with practical application for the surgeon and clear, well-defined illustrations.

Scarpa became director of the Medical Institute at Pavia and continued his research and writing until a year before his death at eighty-one. His work as surgeon and anatomist was carried on in the best tradition of the Italian school.

Antonio Scarpa. *Tabulae Neurologicae ad illustrandam Historiam Anatomicam Cardiacorum Nervorum, Noni Nervorum Cerebri, Glossopharyngaei, et Pharyngaei ex Octavo Cerebri*. Pavia, 1794.

Anderloni's engraving from Scarpa's drawing shows a view of the nerves to the heart. This brilliant illustration is life-size.

| | | died. |
|---|---|---|
| Brought forward | | 1768 |
| October | 1 | 74 |
| | 2 | 66 |
| | 3 | 78 |
| | 4 | 58 |
| | 5 | 71 |
| | 6 | 76 |
| | 7 | 82 |
| | 8 | 90 |
| | 9 | 102 |
| | 10 | 93 |
| | 11 | 119 |
| | 12 | 111 |
| | 13 | 104 |
| | 14 | 81 |
| | 15 | 80 |
| | 16 | 70 |
| | 17 | 80 |
| | 18 | 59 |
| | 19 | 65 |
| | 20 | 55 |
| | | 3318 |

| | | died. |
|---|---|---|
| Brought forward | | 3318 |
| October | 21 | 59 |
| | 22 | 82 |
| | 23 | 54 |
| | 24 | 38 |
| | 25 | 35 |
| | 26 | 23 |
| | 27 | 13 |
| | 28 | 24 |
| | 29 | 17 |
| | 30 | 16 |
| | 31 | 21 |
| November | 1 | 13 |
| | 2 | 21 |
| | 3 | 15 |
| | 4 | 15 |
| | 5 | 14 |
| | 6 | 11 |
| | 7 | 15 |
| | 8 | 8 |
| | 9 | 6 |
| Total, | | 3881* |

From this table it appears that the principal mortality was in the ſecond week of October. A general expectation had obtained, that cold weather was as fatal to the contagion of this fever as

* In the above accounts there is a deficiency of returns from ſeveral grave-yards of 163.

heavy



heavy rains. The uſual time for its arrival had come, but the weather was ſtill not only moderate, but warm. In this awful ſituation, the ſtouteſt hearts began to fail. Hope ſickened, and deſpair ſucceeded diſtreſs in almoſt every countenance. On the *fifteenth* of October it pleaſed God to alter the ſtate of the air. The clouds at laſt dropped health in ſhowers of rain, which continued during the whole day, and which were ſucceeded for ſeveral nights afterwards by cold and froſt. The effects of this change in the weather, appeared firſt in the ſudden diminution of the ſick, for the deaths continued for a week afterwards to be numerous, but they were of perſons who had been confined before, or on the day in which the change had taken place in the weather.

The appearance of this rain was like a dove with an olive branch in its mouth, to the whole city. Public notice was given of its beneficial effects in a letter ſubſcribed by the mayor, of Philadelphia, who acted as preſident of the committee, to the mayor of New York. I ſhall inſert the whole of this letter. It contains, beſides the above information, a record of the liberality of that city, to the diſtreſſed inhabitants of Philadelphia.

K 2 "SIR,

# Benjamin Rush

## YELLOW FEVER IN PHILADELPHIA IN 1793

Rush's account of the great epidemic of "West Indian Yellow Fever," which killed nearly four thousand people in Philadelphia between August and November, 1793, is a fascinating medical, social, and personal record. He described the course of the disease in many individual patients whom he attended; he discussed the causes of the disease's rise and decline; and he recounted the controversies among physicians concerning the correct methods of combating the spread of the epidemic and of treating the sick. Rush (1745-1813) printed the texts of notices issued by the city government and the College of Physicians, with letters he and other physicians had written to the papers, and he set forth the psychologic as well as the physical ravages of the disease as he himself experienced them and observed them in his own family. By proclaiming his belief that yellow fever was the result of filth in the city and not an importation, he aroused the anger of many citizens of Philadelphia. Now his book is considered a classic in epidemiology.

Another important contribution to medical literature was his *Medical Inquiries and Observations, upon the Diseases of the Mind* (1812), the first American text on psychiatry, which had a profound effect on practitioners for several generations.

A religious man strongly committed to a concern for the public welfare, he limited his materia medica to just a few drugs and, in order to strip medicine of some of its mystery, refused to write prescriptions in Latin.

Rush poured his tireless energy into countless activities. He was a professor of medicine at the new University of Pennsylvania, a signer of the Declaration of Independence, and surgeon general (but later resigned) for one department of the Continental army. Furthermore, he was active in the reform movements to abolish slavery and capital punishment and to establish public schools and free medical dispensaries. He discredited fraudulent cancer cures and, perhaps most significant, insisted that insanity was a disease. He was one of the founders of Dickinson College and of the school now known as Franklin and Marshall College and, for the last fourteen years of his life, was Treasurer of the United States Mint.

Benjamin Rush. *An Account of the Bilious remitting Yellow Fever, As It Appeared in the City of Philadelphia, in the Year 1793.* Philadelphia, 1794.

Flashes of a poetic style relieve the grimness of Rush's account of the yellow-fever epidemic in Philadelphia.

# MEDICAL REPORTS,

ON THE

## EFFECTS OF WATER,

COLD AND WARM,

AS A REMEDY IN

## *FEVER, AND FEBRILE DISEASES;*

WHETHER APPLIED TO THE SURFACE OF THE BODY, OR USED AS A DRINK:

WITH

*OBSERVATIONS ON THE NATURE OF FEVER;*

AND ON THE EFFECTS OF

OPIUM, ALCOHOL, AND INANITION.

---

BY JAMES CURRIE, M.D. F.R.S.

Fellow of the Royal College of Physicians, Edinburgh, and Physician to the Liverpool Infirmary.

---

*Intentiones operationum, quas proposuimus (ut arbitramur) verissimae sunt, remedia intentionibus fida. * * Rem ipsam experimentum et comprobavit et promovebit. * * Opera consilii cujusque prudentioris, sunt effectu admiranda, ordine quoque egregia, modis faciendi tanquam vulgaria.*

BACON. Historia vitae et mortis.

---

LIVERPOOL,

PRINTED BY J. M'CREERY,

FOR CADELL AND DAVIES, LONDON.

1797.

# James Currie

## THE EFFECTS OF WATER AS A REMEDY IN FEVER

James Currie (1756-1805) emigrated from Scotland to Virginia as a young man in 1775, hoping to make his fortune. At the opening of the Revolution, he published a loyalist manifesto, made a hazardous escape to Britain, and began medical studies at Edinburgh in 1777. He practiced in Liverpool with great success from 1780 until shortly before his death at the age of forty-nine.

Currie was interested in literature and politics as well as medicine. He attacked the slave trade at a time when Liverpool was its shipping center, wrote against the repressive policy of the British government during the war with republican France, and campaigned for better care for French prisoners of war, which earned him notoriety as an unpatriotic revolutionary. For the benefit of Robert Burns's family, he edited the first collection of his poems, but in so doing he annoyed the poet's idolaters.

From the time of his student days, Currie advocated sponging and bathing with cold water for treating fever; in his book of 1797, he gave the first precise directions for such procedures and showed the need to measure body temperature during the process. William Wright, after long practice in Jamaica, had published a paper in 1786 describing cold-water baths as successful therapy for fever, and, a year after Currie's book appeared, Robert Jackson, a British army surgeon, reported similar success with typhus and yellow fever. However, neither of these writers considered measuring body temperature repeatedly to determine when a cold bath would do the most good.

The term "fever" was still employed in the late eighteenth century to characterize specific disease, especially typhus, although physicians knew that fever was a symptom of many different conditions. This ambiguity lingered in Currie's writing. His book began with a recital of Wright's 1786 report. He then described his own experience at Liverpool with "cold affusions" followed by sea bathing. He explained "the manner in which the affusion of cold water ought to be used"; namely, "from six to nine in the evening, or at any time of the day when there is no sense of chilliness, when the heat of the surface is steadily above what is natural, and when there is no general or profuse sensible perspiration." To measure body temperature, Currie first tried "a small mercurial thermometer of great sensibility after a form invented by Mr. Hunter and used in his experiments on animals," but he soon modified this to an "instrument with a small bulb and curved at the end, introduced under the tongue."

James Currie. *Medical Reports, on the Effects of Water, Cold and Warm, as a Remedy in Fever, and Febrile Diseases....* Liverpool, 1797.

Currie prescribed cold-water baths to reduce fever. According to the title-page quotation, he apparently believed with Roger Bacon that "experience has not only proved but will also advance the matter itself."

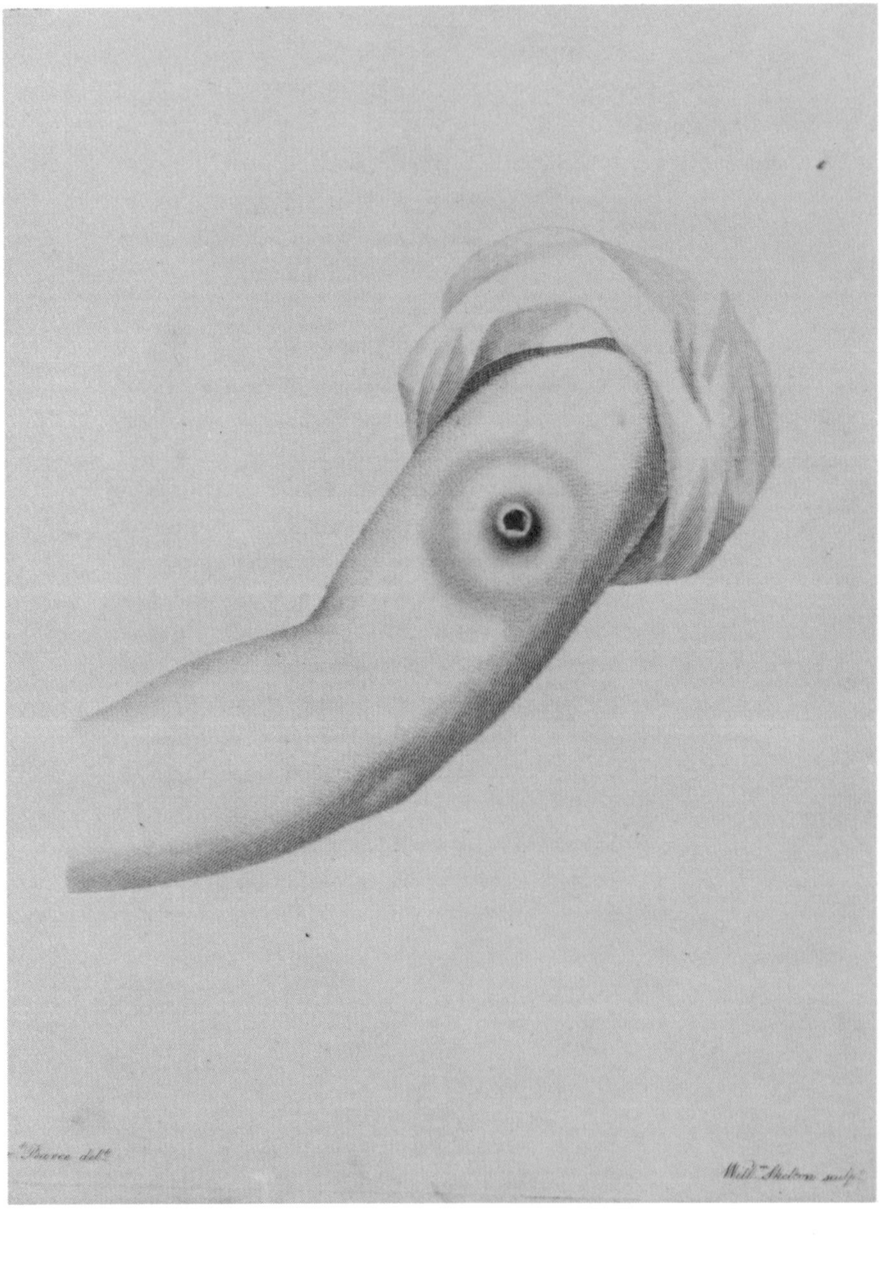
Pearce del.
Willm Skelton sculp.

# Edward Jenner

## AN INQUIRY INTO THE COW POX

Jenner (1749-1823) was nearly fifty when he published this slim book that brought a new understanding of the prevention of disease and had a profound influence on the future growth of medicine. For many years, Jenner had been a country practitioner and was respected by his local colleagues for his interest in heart disease and his skill in treating it. However, he was more widely known as a naturalist and was a Fellow of the Royal Society. Because he practiced for half the year at the fashionable spa of Cheltenham, influential London physicians referred their important patients to him there.

It had long been claimed by farmers and dairymaids that a person who had had an attack of cowpox would be immune against smallpox. Jenner was perhaps the first to give this matter serious study. He contended that inoculation with cowpox matter was a practical method of prophylaxis, simpler and safer than inoculation with the attenuated smallpox pus introduced in England in the 1720's.

In his book Jenner advanced three points. First, he maintained that the protective "virus," which was found in horses, became safe for human inoculation only after it had been transmitted to cows. This confused theory he quietly dropped after longer experience. The next point was that only the "true virus" gave protection and that "matter from other pustulous sores" was ineffective. Lastly, he stated that vaccination gave permanent protection. He modified this opinion later and recommended revaccination in times of smallpox epidemics.

Jenner supported these three contentions with twenty-three case histories in his book. The critical ones were those of Sarah Nelmes, the milkmaid from whose hand Jenner first took the cowpox virus, and a boy named James Phipps. In May, 1796, Jenner inoculated the eight-year-old James with "vaccinia," or cowpox material, and then with virulent smallpox pus to which, as Jenner anticipated, James did not react.

Other histories included those of a boy who was inoculated in 1798 with matter taken directly from the cow and of another inoculated with material from the arm of the first youth. From this second subject, inoculations were transferred to "several children and adults" and thence to "several others," all of whom were protected from smallpox, as demonstrated by direct challenge. (Incidentally, the author recorded the first observed case of anaphylaxis.)

Jenner's book was issued three months after this successful venture, in June, 1798. There are four good plates in the book, three engravings of arms and one picture of the hand of Sarah Nelmes, showing the position and development of the cowpox pustules.

For the remaining twenty-four years of his life, Jenner campaigned actively for vaccination, writing pamphlets and articles and carrying on a worldwide correspondence. He lived to see vaccination generally accepted and successful in abolishing smallpox.

Edward Jenner. *An Inquiry into The Causes and Effects of the Variolae Vaccinae, A Disease Discovered in Some of the Western Counties of England, Particularly Gloucestershire, and known by the Name of The Cow Pox.* London, 1798.

"The efflorescent blush around the part punctured in the boy's arm was so truly characteristic of that which appears on variolus inoculation, that I have given a representation of it."

# PROGRESS OF THE NEW INOCULATION IN AMERICA.

TWO years ago, I published a tract, entitled, "*A Prospect of exterminating the Small pox; being the history of the Variola Vaccina or Kine-pox, as it appeared in England; with an account of a series of inoculations performed in Massachusetts.*"

It was said in that pamphlet, that, on receiving the vaccine virus from England,* I commenced the experiment, July 8th, 1800, on my own children, four of whom, with three of my domestics, passed regularly through the distemper; and that they soon after went into the licensed small-pox hospital in this neighbourhood, and all seven of them were inoculated by Dr. Aspinwall with the matter of the small-pox, without the least trait of infection. This decisive experiment encouraged others to follow the example set by my own family, so that by the first of September I had inoculated about fifty persons, of different ages, sexes and conditions.

By this time the public attention was thoroughly excited, and, judging by the very numerous letters I received from all parts of New England, requesting further information, as well

* From Dr. Haygarth of Bath; procured for him by Mr. Creaser, Surgeon, in that city.

# Benjamin Waterhouse

## A PROSPECT OF EXTERMINATING THE SMALL-POX

Benjamin Waterhouse (1754-1846) introduced vaccination against smallpox into the United States by demonstrating its effectiveness on his own children and describing the experiment in his pamphlets on extermination of the disease.

Waterhouse's interest in vaccination was aroused in 1798, when an English physician friend wrote to him about cowpox inoculation and then sent him a copy of Edward Jenner's work on the effects of variola vaccine. Convinced that Jenner's work was valid, Waterhouse obtained cowpox matter from England in 1800 and vaccinated his five-year-old son. Satisfied with the boy's response, he vaccinated his other children and servants. A servant boy was then exposed to the disease in a smallpox hospital near Boston and proved to be immune.

After receiving fresh supplies of cowpox matter from England in the early spring of 1801, Waterhouse continued the vaccinations and then reported on his work in a supplement to his first pamphlet. The supplement, on "the progress of the new inoculation in America," was much longer than the original publication.

Among Waterhouse's other projects was the writing of a popular book in which he warned young people against the evils of tobacco and alcohol. Eight editions of this book were published, including one each in French and German. Waterhouse also lectured on natural history, botany, and mineralogy, first at Rhode Island College and then at Harvard University. In 1782, on his return from seven years' study in England and Europe, he suggested the formation of a humane society and, three years later, helped draw up plans for such an organization in Massachusetts.

Waterhouse became the first professor of the theory and practice of physic in Harvard's newly established department of medicine in 1783. In 1810 he learned of a plan to move the medical school from Cambridge to nearby Boston. So vigorously did he oppose the idea that in 1812 he was forced to resign his professorship, a position he had held for twenty-nine years. The following year, he was appointed medical superintendent of all military posts in New England. While serving in this position, he is believed to have edited (or even written) a romantic narrative, *A Journal of a Young Man of Massachusetts* (1816). His last literary work was the editing, at the age of eighty, of John B. Wyeth's *Oregon,* published as a deterrent to western immigration.

Benjamin Waterhouse. *A Prospect of Exterminating the Small-Pox.* . . . 2 parts. Boston, 1800 and 1802.

The introductory page of Volume II of Waterhouse's book, which also contains letters to the author from Edward Jenner and Thomas Jefferson, then President of the United States.

Pl. IIme 

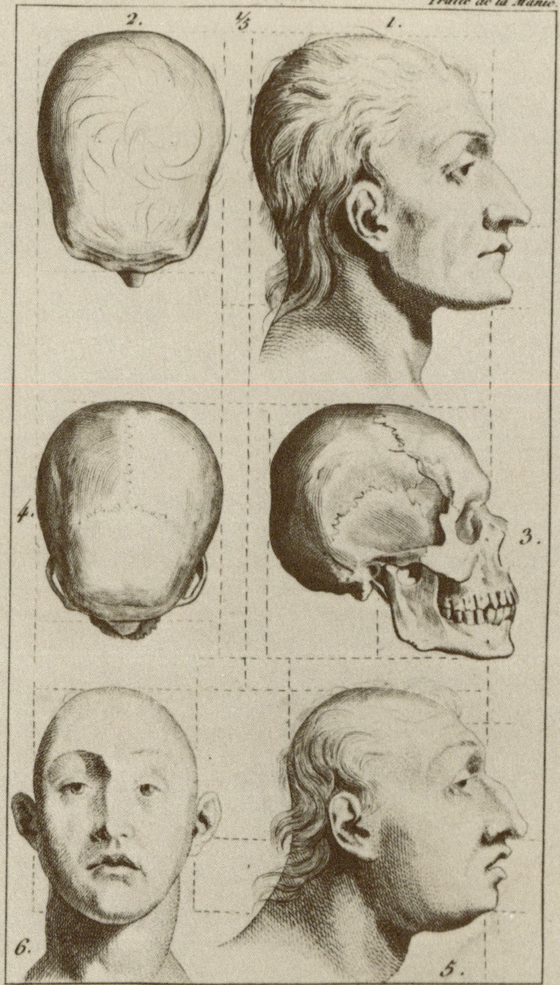

# Philippe Pinel

## TREATISE ON MENTAL DISEASE

On the twenty-fourth of May, 1798, in one of the most dramatic moments in the history of medicine, Pinel (1745-1826) had the manacles and chains removed from forty-nine of his male psychiatric patients at Bicêtre, a hospital near Paris. Two years later, he was called to La Salpêtrière, the famous hospital where the insane female patients were kept. Pinel had them placed in the care of sympathetic physicians and treated with compassion while doing away with other maltreatment, such as bloodletting, which had been employed previously for the purpose of repression. He prescribed quieting drugs for some and occupational therapy for others. Because of these innovations, he is considered the founder of "open-door" psychiatry.

Pinel's "Treatise on Mental Disease" combines a psychologic study with a social program for the humane care and rehabilitation of the insane. His teaching was a product of the Enlightenment that accompanied the French Revolution and was based on long experience in a mental hospital. He included, on a foldout page of his book, a table listing pertinent data about patients he had cured. Although the date of publication is 1801, Pinel refers on page 3 to an unpublished report on the insane that had been submitted in 1791 or 1792 to the Société de Médecine. Perhaps the treatise represents that report, the publication of which may have been delayed until 1801 by the French Revolution.

Pinel first discussed periodic, or remittent, mania and its "moral treatment." Next he described his anatomic research on cranial deformities (illustrated). He then analyzed the "distinct kinds of alienation," classifying them as melancholia, mania without and with delirium, dementia ("the abolition of thoughts"), and idiotism ("the obliteration of the intellect and the affective faculties"). That nomenclature is obsolete, but current classifications are strikingly similar, e.g., depression, psychopathic personality, manic psychosis, schizophrenia, and mental deficiency. Although it was based on clinical observation, the book was written in the deductive philosophic manner of the time, for the pathology of the brain was not understood.

Pinel's original contribution is in the final chapters; there reform in the management of his mental hospital is described, with occupational therapy as the "fundamental law." The book ends with his principles for medical treatment and care in convalescence.

He refused an appointment as personal physician to Emperor Napoleon, possibly because he preferred to continue practicing, teaching, and studying.

Philippe Pinel. *Traité médico-philosophique sur l'aliénation mentale, ou la manie.* Paris, An IX [1801].

This engraving from Pinel's book shows a deformed skull and the corresponding external conformation of the head.

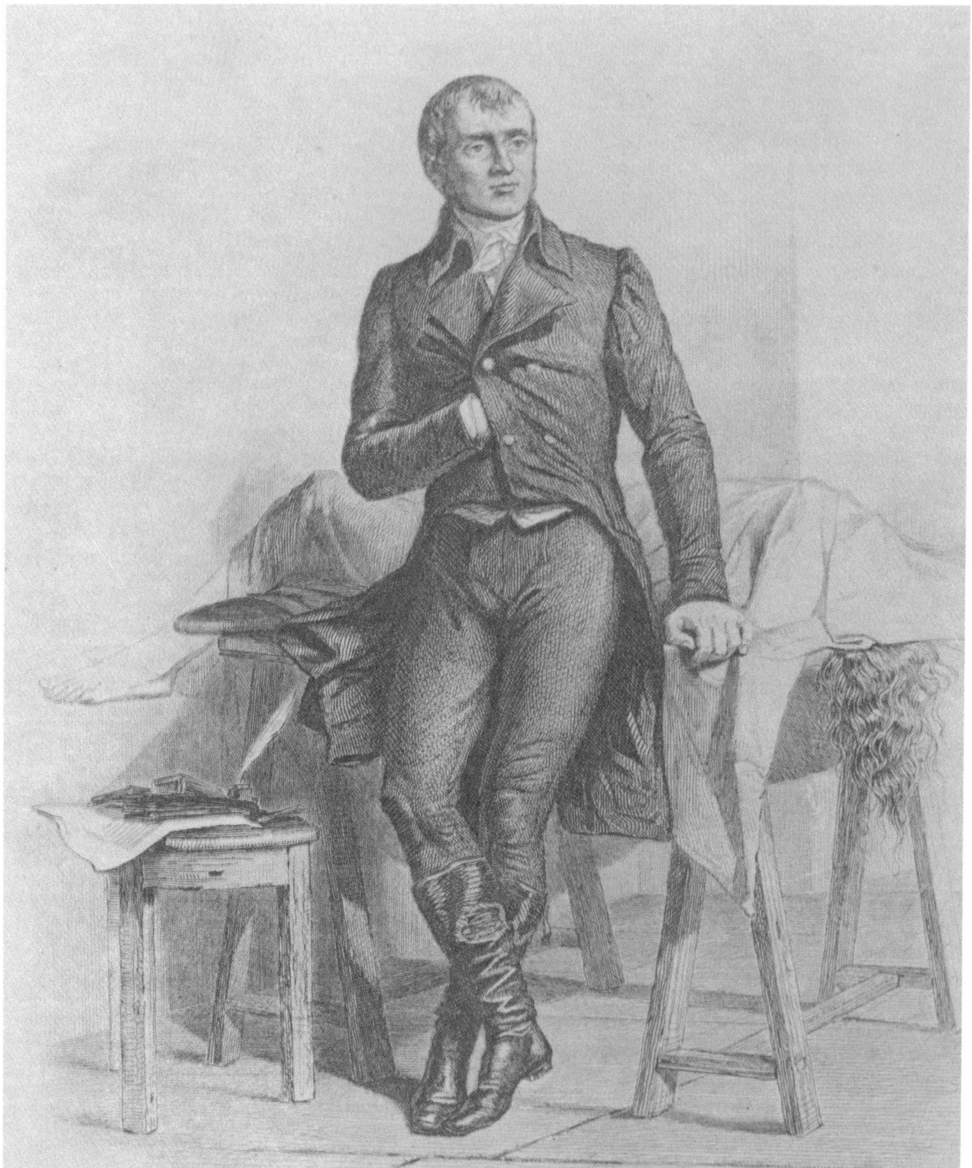

# Marie-François-Xavier Bichat

## GENERAL ANATOMY

Bichat (1771-1802) changed the course of pathologic anatomy by transferring interest from organs to tissues and by establishing histology as the basis for investigating structure and function. "The different organs have membranes and tissues in common," he wrote, "and the seat of disease is in the constituent tissues and not in the individual organs."

He began his clinical work at Lyons but moved to Paris when he was twenty-three to attend Pierre Desault's surgical clinic. When Desault died in 1795, Bichat edited his writings on membranes and on the relationships of organs and continued research along these lines. His large-scale *Anatomie générale* ("General Anatomy") covered the pathology of the tissues, system by system, and was followed by an even longer "Treatise of Descriptive Anatomy," of which Bichat had completed three volumes (of a projected five) before he died in 1802 at the age of thirty-one.

His early death, probably from an infection acquired while dissecting, prompted Corvisart, the emperor's personal physician, to write to Napoleon: "Bichat has just fallen on a battlefield which numbers more than one victim. No one has done so much and so well in so short a time." Because, like the emperor, he had accomplished a great deal in only a few years, he became known as the "Napoleon of medicine." The emperor ordered that a bust of Bichat be placed in the Hôtel-Dieu.

Working essentially without benefit of a microscope (then still unperfected), Bichat identified some twenty-one different types of tissues and showed that tissues from different organs are similar and subject to the same diseases. Modern histology may be said to have been founded by this young physician. He made animal experiments as well as clinical observations in his search for the "vital properties of each tissue" but defined his thoughts in the negative statement, "Life is the sum of the forces that resist death."

Bichat laid the foundation for a biologic attitude to medical problems and influenced such successors as Laënnec and Bernard in France, Bell and Brodie in England, and Virchow and von Kölliker in Germany.

Marie-François-Xavier Bichat. *Anatomie Générale, appliquée à la Physiologie et à la Médecine.* 2 vols. Paris, An IX [1801].

This portrait of Bichat offers evidence that he was sometimes called "the Napoleon of medicine." The cadaver for dissection and the writing materials symbolize two important aspects of his work.

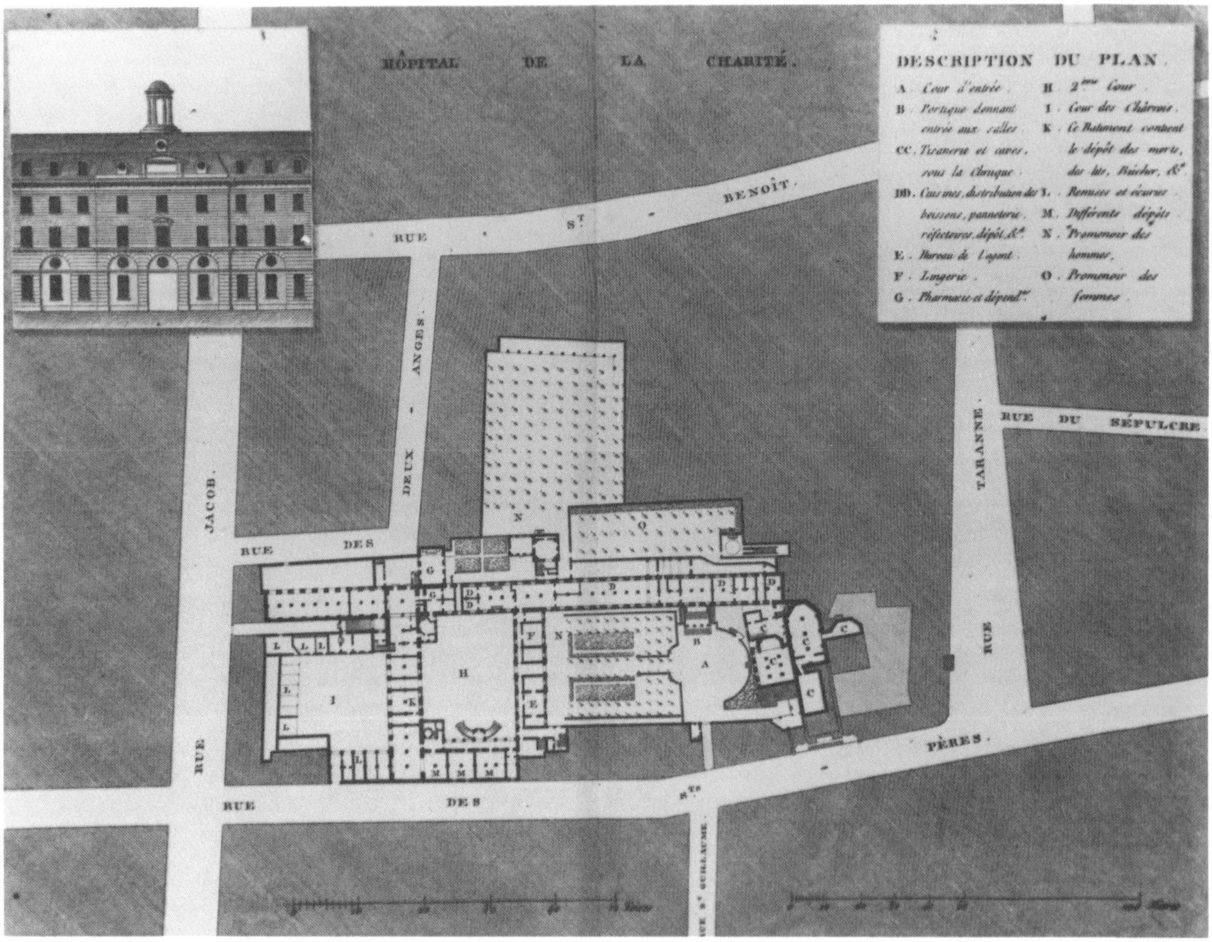
HÔPITAL DE LA CHARITÉ.
DESCRIPTION DU PLAN.
A. Cour d'entrée.
B. Portique donnant entrée aux salles.
CC. Tisanerie et caves, sous la Clinique.
DD. Cuisines, distribution des boissons, panneterie, réfectoires, dépôt, &c.
E. Bureau de l'agent.
F. Lingerie.
G. Pharmacie et dépend.ces
H. 2ème Cour.
I. Cour des Chârons.
K. Ce Batiment contient le dépôt des morts, des lits, Bûcher, &c.
L. Remises et écuries.
M. Différents dépôts.
N. Promenoir des hommes.
O. Promenoir des femmes.
RUE ST. BENOIT.
RUE DES DEUX ANGES.
RUE JACOB.
RUE TARANNE.
RUE DU SÉPULCRE.
RUE DES STS. PÈRES.

# Jean-Nicolas Corvisart

## ESSAY ON DISEASES AND ORGANIC LESIONS OF THE HEART

Corvisart (1755-1821) published this significant book while he was the leading physician in Paris. He had graduated under the old regime, became professor of clinical medicine under the Republic, and was appointed physician to Napoleon when the emperor assumed control of France.

The book contains a storehouse of deductions from a vast experience and is based on Corvisart's teaching course at the Charité, which became a center of clinical instruction largely because Corvisart taught there. He differentiated heart from lung disorders and first adequately classified the symptoms of heart disease. He dealt in turn with the pathology of the pericardial sac, the muscular substance and the fibrous tissue of the heart, its organic diseases, and aneurysm of the aorta. He was the first to describe carditis. Each section is illustrated by case histories from his own practice, with an appendix of other physicians' reports. These clinical chapters fill three-quarters of the text. The fourth quarter contains "Corollaries," a general discussion of causes, signs, symptoms, progress, and treatment. Corvisart recorded many conditions that would be "discovered" again by later investigators. His book was translated into English and thus had a profound effect on medical thinking in many countries. Throughout his career, he combined the most acute clinical observations with knowledge of anatomy and pathology. This correlation was a notable advance in education.

Corvisart was also alert to other men's work. He translated Maximilian Stoll's book on fever from German and published a commentary on Boerhaave's "Aphorisms." An unusual contribution to medicine was his translation of Auenbrugger's book, which brought percussion into practice after fifty years of neglect and led directly to Laënnec's great work. "I know very well," Corvisart wrote, "how little reputation is allotted to translators and commentators, and I might easily have elevated myself to the rank of an author, if I had elaborated anew the doctrine of Auenbrugger and published an independent work on percussion. In this way, however, I should have sacrificed the name of Auenbrugger to my own vanity, a thing which I am unwilling to do. It is he, and the beautiful invention which of right belongs to him, that I desire to recall to life."

In fact, it was Corvisart's careful manner of examining the chest, including percussion, which first attracted the emperor's attention to him at a time when Napoleon was suffering from a respiratory infection. Corvisart retired from practice following the emperor's abdication and died a few months after his famous patient.

Jean-Nicolas Corvisart. *Essai sur les Maladies et les Lésions organiques du Coeur et des Gros Vaisseaux.* Paris, 1806.

Corvisart's classes at the old hospital, La Charité, in Paris attracted many of the most earnest medical students from both sides of the Atlantic.

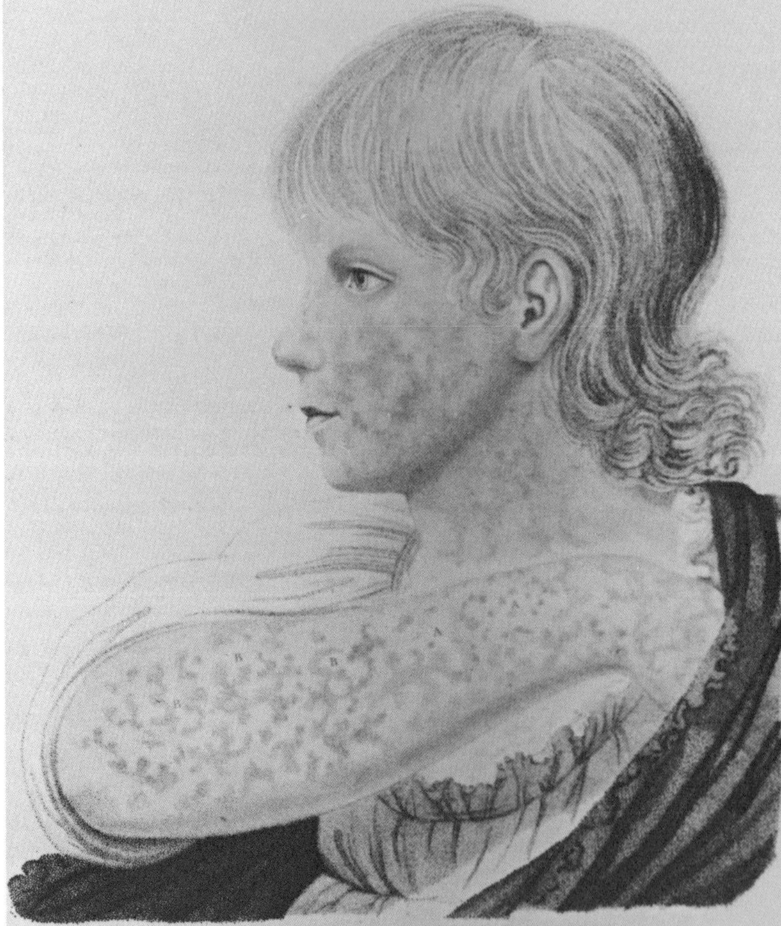

*Rubeola sine catarrho*

London, Pub. Nov.r 1, 180[illegible], by J. Johnson, St. Pauls Church Yard

# Robert Willan

## ON CUTANEOUS DISEASES

Willan (1757-1812), one of the founders of modern dermatology, was perhaps the first to classify cutaneous diseases in a logical system. He named eight categories according to the appearance of the skin: papular, squamous, exanthematous, bullous, vesicular, pustular, tubercular, and macular. The nomenclature was compiled from Greek, Latin, and Arabic terms. This classification, presented to the Medical Society of London, won him the Fothergillian gold medal in 1790. It was generally adopted in English-speaking countries and is largely in use at the present time.

Willan intended this book to be the first volume in a definitive series on dermatology, but it was the only volume the author managed to complete before his death at the age of fifty-five. The contents, originally published serially, covered only part of the classification proposed in the introduction. His student, Thomas Bateman, continued the description in a work published in 1817, which also contains a series of Willan's engravings.

He made many original observations, describing for the first time or providing the first clear differentiation of such disease entities as impetigo, lupus, psoriasis (sometimes known as Willan's syndrome), scleroderma, ichthyosis, sycosis, and pemphigus.

Willan was an early supporter of Edward Jenner, whose announcement of vaccination was published in the summer of 1798, about the same time as the first part of Willan's *On Cutaneous Diseases.* Jenner had drawn Willan's attention to the "entanglement" of cowpox herpes, the effect of one virus on another in the same host. Willan himself published a treatise entitled *On Vaccine Inoculation* in 1806, which strongly advocated compulsory vaccination.

He was an accomplished scholar in Latin and Greek, and perhaps that is why certain relatively unfamiliar terms are still used in dermatology. He was also greatly concerned with the sick and indigent and worked to improve the public health of his time.

Although Willan's purely descriptive pathology was superseded by the more profound "morbid anatomy" introduced in his lifetime by Matthew Baillie (q.v.), his book remains one of the foundation stones of modern dermatologic knowledge.

Robert Willan. *On Cutaneous Diseases.* Vol. I. London, [1796]-1808.

The new art of colored stipple engraving enabled Willan to provide detailed portraits of patients so lifelike that they could be used as diagnostic guides by physicians.

ACTUALITÉS 2

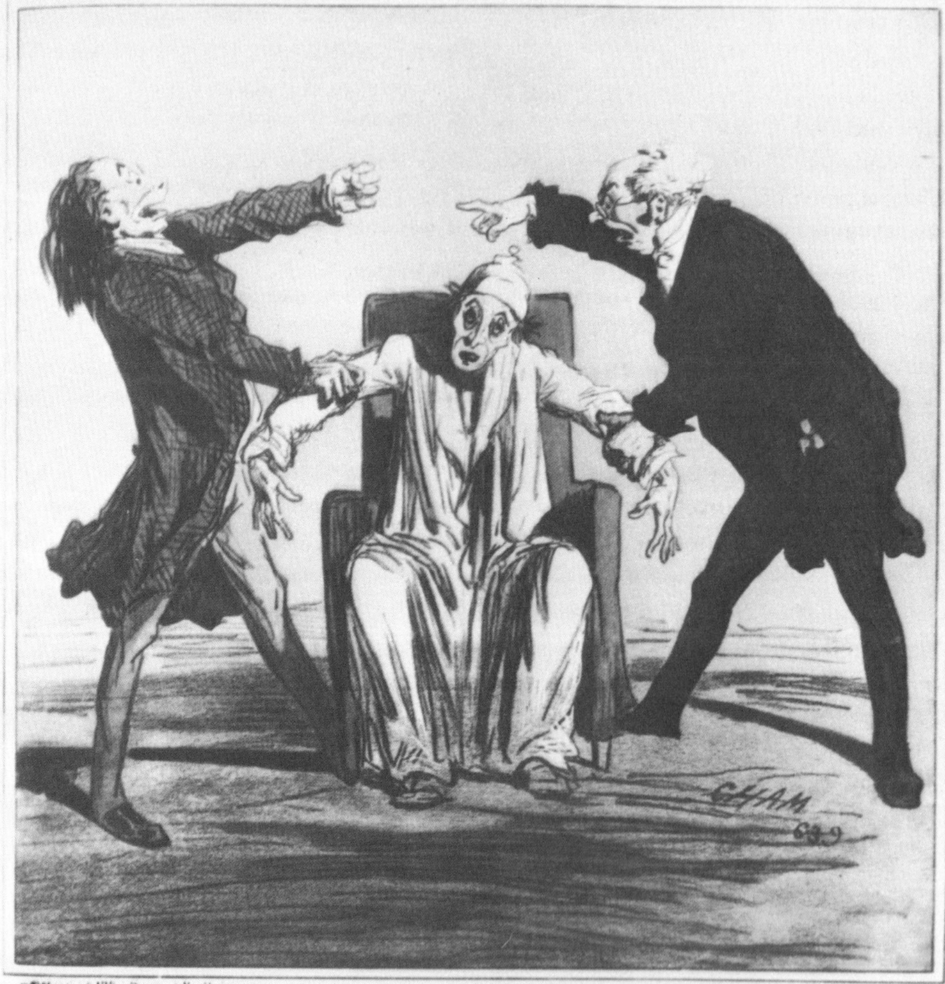


- Homœopate!....vous êtes un drôle......monsieur ne mourra que de ma main
- Allopate !....vous êtes un polisson !!......monsieur ne périra que par moi .....
- Ma foi, je m'en moque de leur querelle, je vois que pour moi le résultat sera toujours le même

# Samuel Hahnemann

## A SYSTEM OF RATIONAL THERAPEUTICS

The reaction of a German physician against the abusive polypharmacy and the bleeding, purging, and vomiting of early nineteenth-century treatment initiated a counterrevolution in the form of homeopathy.

Hahnemann (1755-1843) practiced successfully in Dresden and Leipzig for only a short time before rejecting the current medical practices. During a period of brooding and study, he wondered why quinine cured the paroxysms of malaria. Upon taking the drug, he was promptly seized by a reaction similar to that of malaria patients; after his wife and five children also reacted this way, he decided that quinine cured malaria by producing counterfeit disease. He evolved the concept of *similia similibus curantur* (like should be cured by like) after several years of experimentation. According to this principle, a patient should be given a specific drug that would reproduce in a healthy individual the symptoms, or the clinical picture, of the disease under treatment. Hahnemann introduced the new system publicly in 1796. His method stressed careful history-taking and the use of very small doses of single drugs in preference to overdosage with many. In the context of the practice of the day, it was a welcome improvement in therapeutics.

His most important book, on "rational treatment" (1810), had a considerable impact on medical practice. It naturally aroused the enmity of the apothecaries, who forced him to leave Leipzig in 1821.

He became rich and famous in time and, at the age of seventy-nine, married a wealthy woman who was forty-five years his junior. The couple moved to Paris, where Hahnemann developed a highly successful practice among the aristocracy. He continued to work until his death at the age of eighty-eight.

The concept of homeopathy spread rapidly in Europe and in the United States, where medical schools were established to teach this system. However, the introduction of pure chemicals and controlled animal experiments led to the establishment of more rational therapeutics and the rise of modern pharmacology.

Samuel Hahnemann. *Organon der rationellen Heilkunde.* Dresden, 1810.

The quarrel between followers of homeopathy and allopathy, unlike most medical controversies, was taken up by the popular press, which used satire such as this cartoon to point out the real loser—the patient.

Plate VIII.

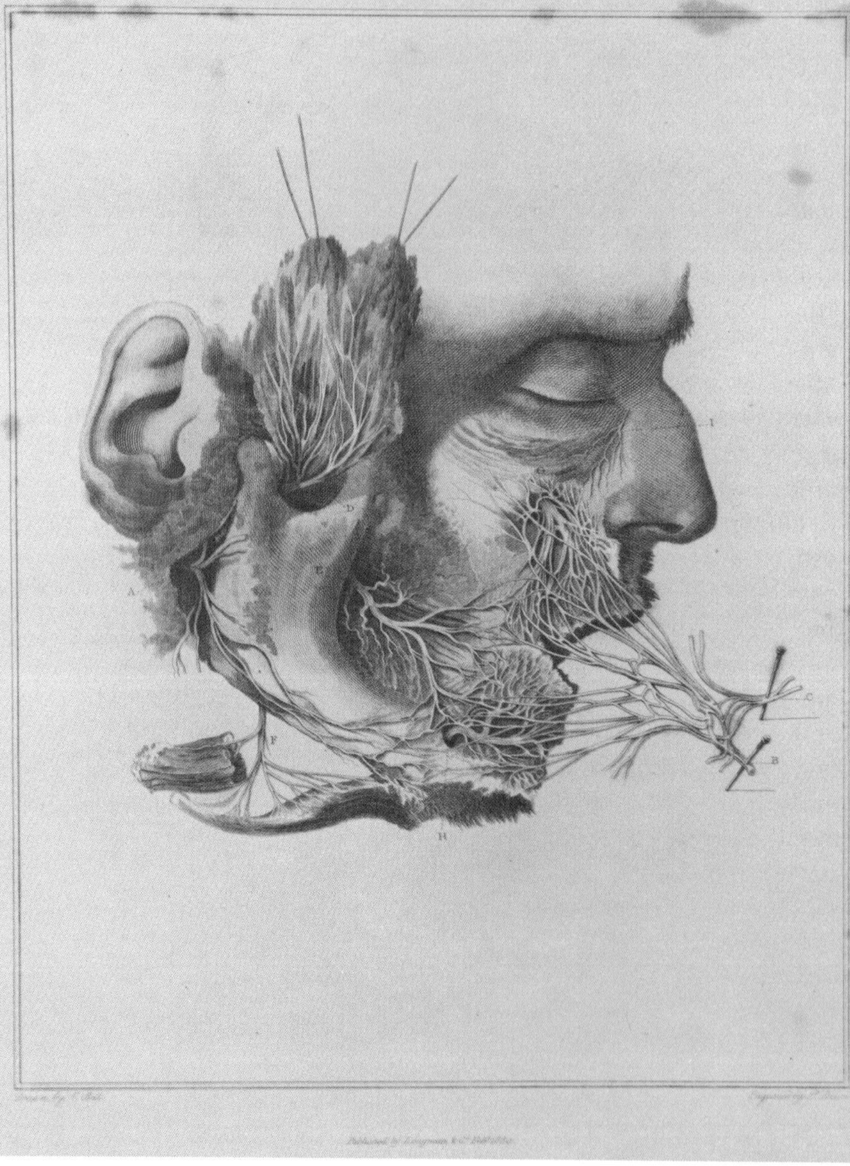

# Sir Charles Bell

## A NEW ANATOMY OF THE BRAIN

In 1809, Charles Bell (1774-1842) wrote to his brother, George Joseph, "Could you get a little tiny book printed for me, of twenty pages of the smallest 8vo?" When the booklet appeared in 1811, it was a bit longer than Bell had anticipated—thirty-six pages—but it was a milestone in neurology, because it contained the first reference in medical literature to the functions of the spinal nerve roots.

Only one hundred copies of the pamphlet were printed, and Bell distributed these to his friends for comment. In the pamphlet, Bell maintained that different parts of the brain serve different functions. He had cut certain spinal-nerve roots in experimental animals and showed by the changes in their behavior that the nerves were anatomically "united for convenience of distribution, but distinct in office." Such functional specificity, he deduced, was derived from the part of the brain with which the nerve was connected.

"On laying bare the roots of the spinal nerves," he wrote, "I found that I could cut across the posterior fasciculus of nerves which took its origin from the posterior portion of the spinal marrow without convulsing the muscles of the back, but that, on touching the anterior fasciculus with the point of the knife, the muscles of the back were immediately convulsed." However, Bell failed to grasp the significance of this observation and classed all nerves as sensory, calling the posterior roots "sensible" and the anterior roots "insensible." In a similar experiment eleven years later, Magendie provided clear proof that the anterior roots are motor, and Bell then accepted his findings.

Bell was trained in Edinburgh but spent the busiest years of his active and productive life in London, where he was known as a surgeon, an anatomist, a teacher, and a writer. A two-volume *System of Operative Surgery* brought him fame and success. He later joined the school founded by John and William Hunter (q.v.). His talent for sketching and drawing was useful to him in illustrating his medical works. He published additional papers on the nervous system and subsequently collected them in *The Nervous System* (1830). Bell was knighted in 1829 for his physiologic discoveries. He returned to his beloved Edinburgh in 1836 and held the chair of surgery at the University of Edinburgh until his death.

Bell is remembered chiefly for his later demonstration of the sensory and motor functions of the fifth cranial nerve, for his discovery of the long thoracic nerve that bears his name, and for his description of the facial paralysis, known as Bell's palsy, which results from facial-nerve neuropathy.

Charles Bell. *Idea of A New Anatomy of the Brain: submitted for the Observations of his Friends.* London, 1811.

Bell was an accomplished artist as well as surgeon. His drawing from a later work, *The Nervous System of the Human Body* (1830), shows a dissection of the branches of the facial nerve that is involved in Bell's palsy.

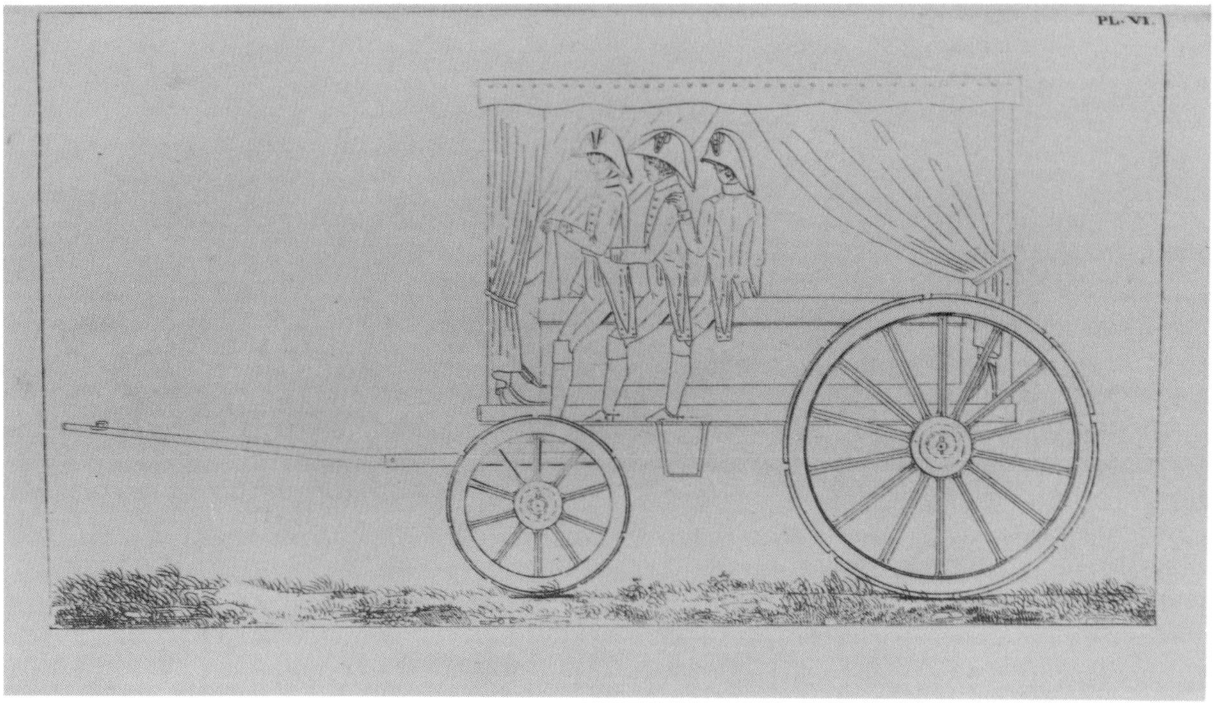
PL. VI.

# Dominique-Jean Larrey

## MEMOIRS OF A MILITARY SURGEON

Modern military medicine begins with Larrey (1766-1842), chief surgeon to Napoleon. This four-volume history of his battlefield experiences includes the whole epic of Napoleon's campaigns. Volume one begins with Larrey's work before the Revolution, when he sailed for Newfoundland as a naval surgeon. He had returned to Europe by the time war broke out in 1792 and was made surgeon major in the Army of the Rhine. In this capacity, Larrey initiated the practices that mark him as a man with imagination and organizational ability. Under his direction, triage and first aid were performed on the battlefield; the critically wounded were taken to military hospitals in light one-horse carriages called "flying ambulances" (illustrated). Until then, ambulances had "never arrived in less than twenty-four or thirty-six hours, so that most of the wounded died for want of assistance."

In 1794, Larrey was appointed chief surgeon of the army bound for Corsica. When he reported at Toulon for this assignment, Larrey met Bonaparte for the first time; Larrey was twenty-eight and Bonaparte, then commander of an artillery brigade, was twenty-five.

The books deal with the Egyptian campaign; the famous victory of Austerlitz in December of 1805, by which Napoleon consolidated his power over Europe; the Spanish campaign, which wasted the emperor's resources; and the disastrous Russian campaign of 1812. In the fourth volume, Larrey tells laconically how he turned back at the Berezina River to save a case of surgical instruments. He returned to the river to find one bridge remaining, filled with a frantic mob. Larrey was recognized and passed forward from shoulder to shoulder by the struggling soldiers. He reached the other side moments before the bridge was destroyed by artillery fire.

Larrey practiced debridement of wounds and was one of the first to amputate at the hip joint, an operation that he twice executed successfully under battlefield conditions. During the battle of Borodino, Larrey is said to have performed two hundred amputations in one day. In his book he discussed the therapeutic effects of maggots on wounds and was the first to describe trench foot.

He himself was wounded three times and was captured by the Prussians, only to be released because he had once saved the life of his captor's son.

Larrey's courage, skill, and humane care were admired not only by the soldiers but also by Napoleon, who left 100,000 francs to "Larrey, the most virtuous man I have ever known."

Curiously, it was not until the Civil War in the United States that Larrey's concepts were widely accepted and the wounded removed from the battlefield on the day they were injured.

Dominique-Jean Larrey. *Mémoires de chirurgie militaire, et campagnes.* 4 vols. Paris, 1812-1817.

The modern ambulance traces its origin to Larrey's one-horse carriage, which saved the lives of many of Napoleon's wounded soldiers.

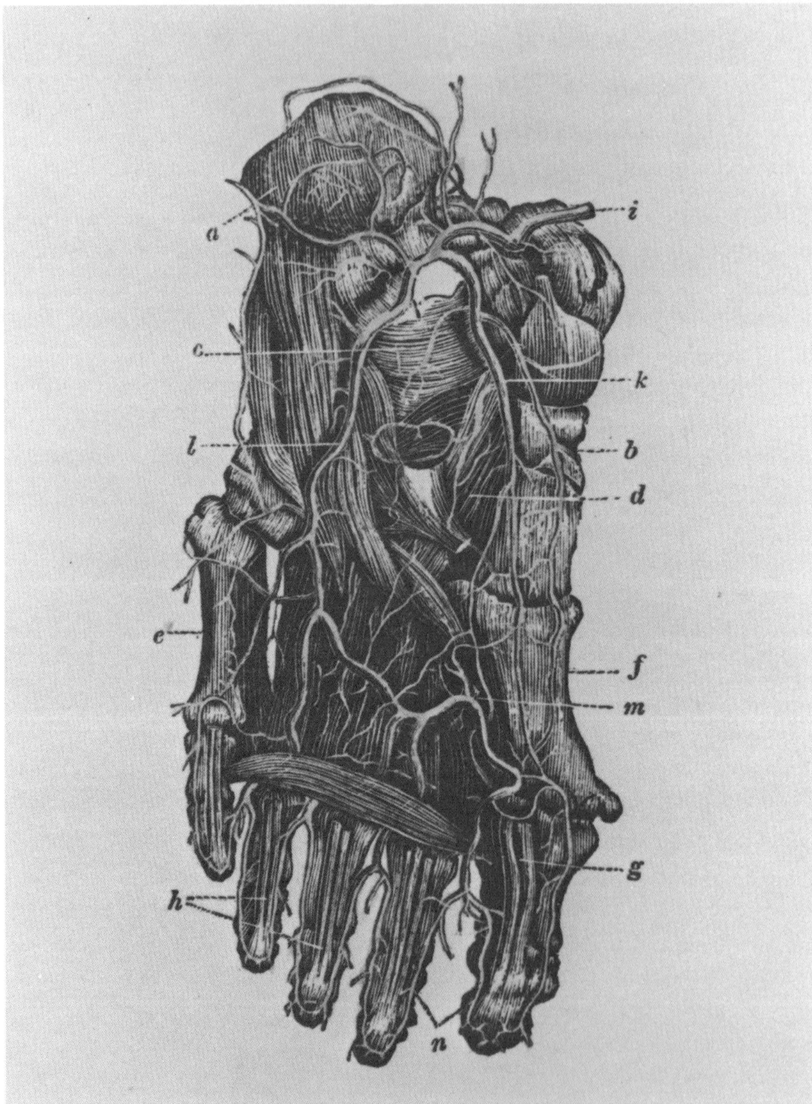

i
a
c
k
l
b
d
e
f
m
g
h
n

# John Collins Warren

## THE ARTERIES OF THE HUMAN BODY

John Collins Warren (1778-1856) was the son of John Warren, one of the founders of Harvard Medical School and a leading surgeon in Boston. The younger Warren was trained in London, Edinburgh, and Paris; at Guy's Hospital, he was a pupil of Astley Cooper, the greatest English surgeon among the successors of John Hunter. On coming home to America, Warren became his father's assistant in anatomic research and teaching and in his surgical practice. He was surgeon to the Massachusetts General Hospital from its opening in 1821, was associated with it for thirty-six years, and enjoyed wide recognition as the outstanding American surgeon of the first half of the nineteenth century.

In the course of his teaching, he realized the need for an anatomic atlas of the arteries. Accordingly, he had an accomplished medical artist, Josiah Foster Flagg, prepare copies of the artery plates from *Icones Anatomicae,* or "Images of Anatomy," which had been published by the renowned Albrecht von Haller between 1743 and 1756. Haller had improved upon his predecessors' work by giving accurate representation of actual dissections; these varied, as always in nature, from the ideal which earlier illustrators had tried to show.

Warren and Flagg did not work directly from the plates in Haller's book but used an anonymous manual for dissectors issued in London in 1808. This little English edition, with Haller's plates reduced in size, was published in St. Thomas's Street, London, and was probably intended for the students of the United School of St. Thomas's and Guy's Hospitals, where Warren had studied. Flagg, a dentist and pioneer in the development of porcelain false teeth, was in a class by himself as a medical artist. He engraved the fifteen plates on wood and printed them in two colors to show the arteries in red against the surrounding tissues in black. They were the first anatomic illustrations in color to be printed in the United States.

Warren revised the descriptions and added a general account of the arteries. This striking book is very rare; the Lilly Library copy is in its original covers.

Warren also published *Surgical Observations on Tumors* in 1837, a work famous in its day, but he is now chiefly remembered as the first surgeon to operate on a patient under total anesthesia. This was in 1846, when he was sixty-eight. After his death, the family tradition was continued by his son, grandson, and great-grandson, all of whom were surgeons in Boston.

John Collins Warren. *Anatomical Description of The Arteries of the Human Body, illustrated by several coloured Engravings, selected and reduced from the Icones of Haller, Exhibiting the Parts as they appear on Dissection. From the last London Edition. Corrected and Improved.* Boston, 1813.

Flagg's engravings for Warren's book showed the arteries in red with the supporting tissues in black. The artist's treatment gives a strong three-dimensional effect.

AN

# ESSAY

ON THE

# SHAKING PALSY.

## CHAPTER I.

### DEFINITION—HISTORY—ILLUSTRATIVE CASES.

SHAKING PALSY. *(Paralysis Agitans.)*

Involuntary tremulous motion, with lessened muscular power, in parts not in action and even when supported; with a propensity to bend the trunk forwards, and to pass from a walking to a running pace: the senses and intellects being uninjured.

THE term Shaking Palsy has been vaguely employed by medical writers in general. By some it has been used to designate or-

# James Parkinson

## THE SHAKING PALSY

The name of James Parkinson (1755-1824) was immortalized by his description of the mysterious nervous disorder he named "the shaking palsy." His small and modest pamphlet, published in 1817 when he was sixty-two, is remarkable because his conclusions were reached entirely by inference from external symptoms. He recorded ten cases, differentiating paralysis agitans from other forms of paralytic disease, but remained in "uncertainty and indecision" about the cause. He could neither indicate a cure nor suggest any useful treatment, because, he wrote, "internal medicines are scarcely warrantable.... all that art is capable of accomplishing is to check the further progress of the disease."

The little book has five chapters; the first defines the disease and illustrates it with six case histories. Chapter 2 contains descriptions of the two diagnostic symptoms—the "involuntary tremulous motions with lessened voluntary muscular power" and "a propensity to bend the trunk forwards and to pass from a walking to a running pace." Chapter 3 differentiates shaking palsy from anomalous convulsion, disordered nervous control, and passive tremblings. Chapter 4 suggests that the cause is some disease of the spinal marrow in the superior cervical vertebrae and the medulla oblongata. A case of convulsive palsy following suspected injury of the spinal marrow is contrasted with four more case histories of the shaking palsy. The last chapter proposes bleeding or blistering at the neck in the hope of checking the disease. It is noteworthy that the book does not mention the characteristic masklike facies.

Parkinson, a general practitioner in London, attended John Hunter's lectures on surgery (and recorded them in shorthand). He was the first to report in English on a case of appendicitis with perforation. He wrote another book on medical education, *The Hospital Pupil*, which was well received after its publication in 1800.

A political radical, he often engaged in agitations for reform, to the annoyance of those in government. He was an active pamphleteer, fighting for the disenfranchised, equitable taxes, legal protection of the poor, and other causes. He also contributed to chemistry, geology, and paleontology. His book on paralysis agitans remained the basic text on Parkinson's disease until quite recent times and is still a masterful example of clinical description.

James Parkinson. *An Essay on the Shaking Palsy*. London, 1817.

The first page of Parkinson's text.
Because neither "paralysis agitans" nor "shaking palsy" is now considered an accurate or scientific designation, the eponym "Parkinson's disease" or "parkinsonism" has come to be the most commonly used medical term.

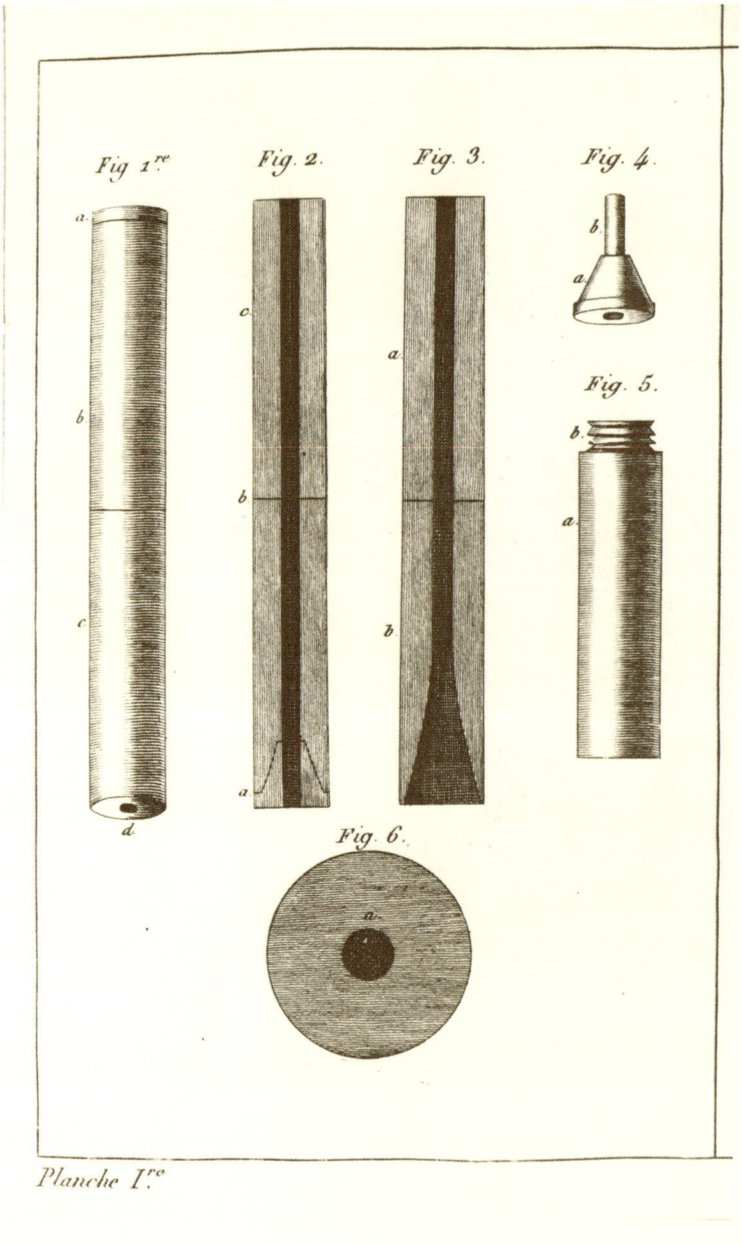


Planche Ire

# René-Théophile-Hyacinthe Laënnec

## STETHOSCOPIC AUSCULTATION

At the age of thirty-eight, Laënnec (1781-1826), a physician to the Hôpital Necker in Paris, provided the first adequate method for diagnosing diseases of the thorax. Matthew Baillie, the leading British physician of the time, wrote to him that his book was "the fullest and most able account of the diseased appearances of the Heart and Lungs which has yet been published." It enjoyed immediate international success, and in 1826, the year of his death, Laënnec brought out an expanded edition, giving more attention to pathology and treatment.

Auscultatory percussion, the evocation of sounds within the chest by tapping with the fingers, had been introduced by Auenbrugger nearly fifty years earlier but spread only slowly into practice until 1806, when Corvisart, Laënnec's teacher, began to advocate its use. Laënnec's innovation was the stethoscope, an instrument for "indirect auscultation" through amplification of the chest sounds.

In its four parts, the book deals with exploration of the voice and the diagnosis of phthisis; study of the respiratory organs, pneumonia, emphysema, pleurisy, and pneumothorax; the bronchial sounds; and investigation of the circulation, including analysis of heart sounds, diseases of the heart, and aneurysm of the aorta. The illustrations on four double plates show Laënnec's newly invented stethoscope, pathologic conditions of the lung, and deformity of the chest from chronic latent pleurisy.

Laënnec also wrote numerous works on other medical subjects, including treatises on peritonitis, the capsule of the liver, and pathologic anatomy, especially that type of liver cirrhosis which has been named for him. He added significantly to the knowledge of pathology with his method of correlating clinical observations with postmortem findings.

His abiding interest, however, was the diagnosis of diseases of the chest, a preoccupation quite possibly attributable to the fact that his mother had died of tuberculosis when he was a very small child. This heritage, along with a frail constitution and close association with pulmonary disease patients, led, ironically, to his own death from tuberculosis at the age of forty-five.

René-Théophile-Hyacinthe Laënnec. *De l'auscultation médiate....* Paris, 1819.

Laënnec's very first stethoscope was a roll of paper. Here is shown his refined version, a short wooden tube with a narrowing lumen, for use at one ear.

Pl. XVI.

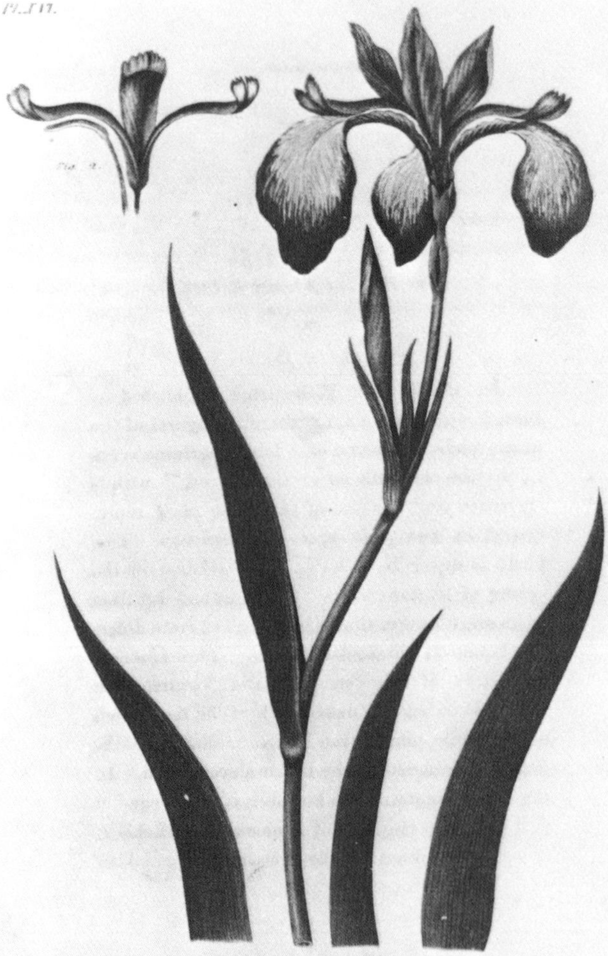

Fig. 2.

*Iris versicolor*

# Jacob Bigelow

## TREATISE ON THE MATERIA MEDICA

Jacob Bigelow (1787-1879), who lived to the age of ninety-two, practiced as a physician in Boston for sixty years. A professor of materia medica at Harvard from 1815 to 1855, he distinguished himself first as a botanist. He had studied under Benjamin Smith Barton, of Philadelphia, whose *Elements of Botany* (1803) was the first textbook on the subject published in the United States. Barton had proposed that Bigelow describe the flora of Virginia and Pennsylvania, but Bigelow, more methodical than cooperative, instead published the three-volume *American Medical Botany* (1817-1821). This comprehensive survey in six parts contained sixty plates colored by a special process he had invented. It was one of the first two American books issued with colored illustrations of plants. The other was that of William Barton, nephew of Benjamin Barton and also a professor of botany at Philadelphia, whose *Vegetable Materia Medica of the United States* came out at the same time (1817-1818).

Bigelow went on to promote compilation of a national pharmacopoeia. The Massachusetts Medical Society had printed its pharmacopoeia in 1808, the first state issue of such a work, but Bigelow had wider views. He joined in a convention of physicians and botanists who met in Washington, D. C., to assemble the first *Pharmacopoeia of the United States of America* and was instrumental in having it published in both Latin and English in 1820.

He continued his campaign by writing and publishing his *Treatise on the Materia Medica* in 1822, which he "intended as a sequel to the *Pharmacopoeia*" and as a convenient handbook of practice for the physician and the dispenser. The *Treatise* begins with an explanation of the classification of medicines according to their action. The main text is arranged in an alphabetical sequence of Latin headings, such as *Linimenta, Pilulae,* and *Tincturae*. He departed from custom by insisting on simplicity of nomenclature but provided a "Table of Synonymes" which compared the terminology of the American pharmacopoeia with that of similar works.

Thus, early in the development of the nation, Bigelow's vision insured that the whole United States would have a single unified materia medica. Bigelow's son, Henry Jacob Bigelow, became one of the great surgeons of his day, a pioneer in anesthesia and orthopedic surgery.

Jacob Bigelow. *A Treatise on the Materia Medica intended as a Sequel to the Pharmacopoeia of the United States.* Boston, 1822.

This iris, delicately tinted by a printing process of Bigelow's invention, is one of sixty plates from *American Medical Botany*. He recommended a tincture of *Iris versicolor* as a diuretic.

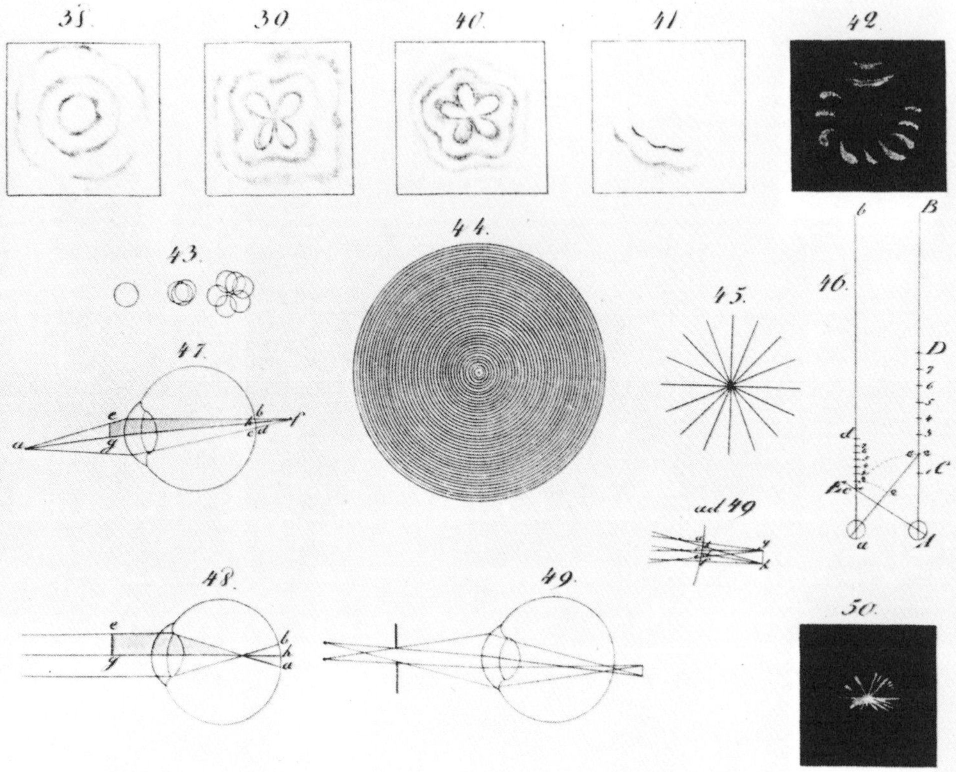
38.
39.
40.
41.
42.
43.
44.
45.
46.
47.
48.
49.
ad 49
50.
b
B
D
d
C
a
A

# Johann Evangelist Purkinje

## THE SUBJECTIVE ASPECT OF VISION

Purkinje (1787-1869) was graduated in 1819 from Charles University in Prague, Bohemia, then the third kingdom of the Austrian Empire, and was appointed to the chair of physiology at the University of Breslau in Saxony early in 1823. His graduation dissertation had concerned subjective visual phenomena, a topic he further explored in this three-part article published in 1825. Some of the findings reflect Purkinje's experiments on himself after he had taken belladonna.

Purkinje was a histologist and a physiologist. He was one of the most original of the young men in many countries who, by using up-to-date improved microscopes, were advancing rapidly in knowledge of living processes. He reported new observations on myopia, hypermetropia, and accommodation and on reflex eye movements, including nystagmus, while noting the impossibility of observing the inner eye in the living.

In 1850, Purkinje returned to his native country as professor of physiology at Prague, a position he retained until his death.

In preparing tissues for microscopic examination, Purkinje was the first to employ a properly focused light source of high intensity, a microtome, potassium bichromate, glacial acetic acid, and Canada balsam. Whereas microscopy had until then provided not much more than the means of magnifying tissue architecture, these contributions permitted the detailed study of the types of cells that characterize a tissue.

While studying the structure of the brain, Purkinje noted those ganglionic cells that are peculiar to the cerebellum and are now called "Purkinje cells." Likewise, he was the first to describe the "Purkinje fibers" of the heart. He introduced the word "protoplasm," invented investigative instruments such as moving recorders for the study of cardiac action, and gained an international reputation for his discoveries in cytology, embryology, and cardiology.

Some of his important works were overlooked for decades because they were in his native Czech. However, he himself was fluent in no less than twelve languages. Many of his significant discoveries were made in his home laboratory. Purkinje's wide-ranging interests included the inventing of a spirometer and a hearing aid, a detailed study of fingerprints, and investigation of gastric secretion. In his spare time, he founded a journal of natural history.

Johann Evangelist Purkinje. *Neue Beiträge zur Kenntniss des Sehens in subjectiver Hinsicht.* In *Magazin für die gesammte Heilkunde,* Vol. 20; edited by Dr. J. N. Rust. Berlin, 1825.

These drawings record the visual phenomena seen by Purkinje after he had taken digitalis. The fact that they appear in his graduation dissertation shows that, even in his day, students sometimes experimented with drugs.

Tab. 3.

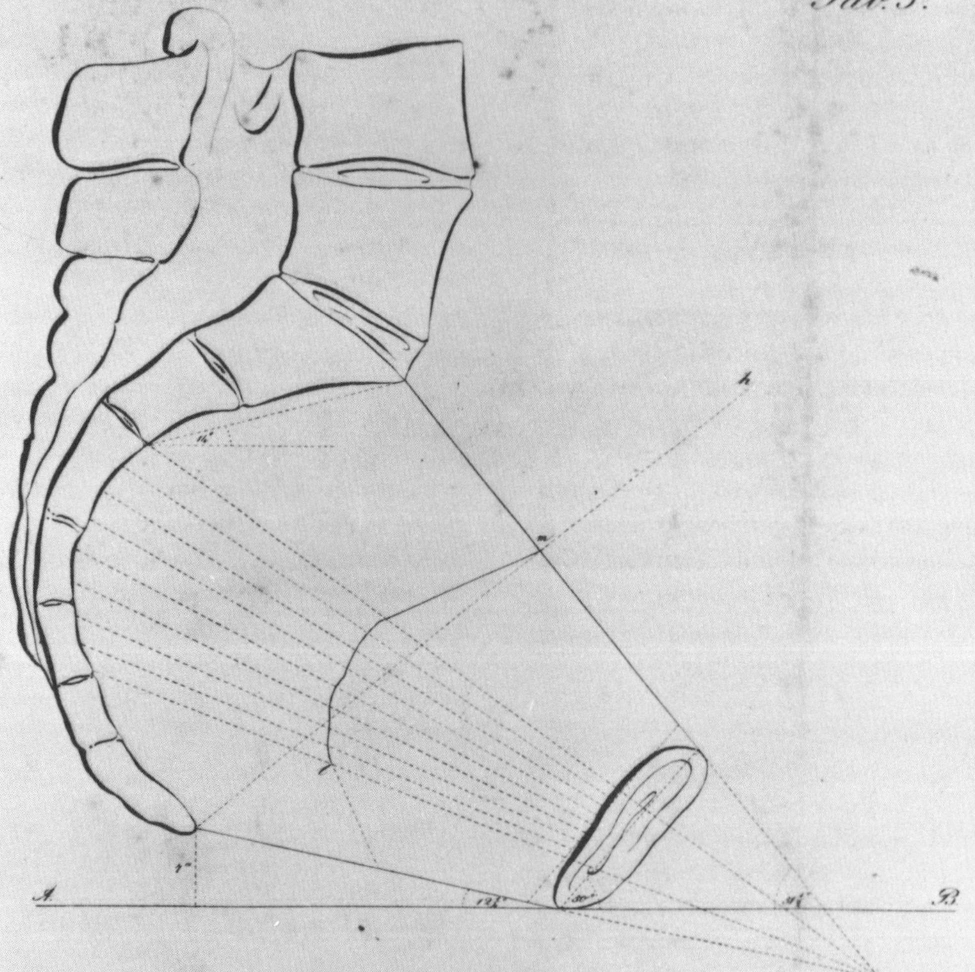

# Franz Carl Naegele

## THE FEMALE PELVIS

Franz Carl Naegele (1778-1851) was the second and ablest son of a prominent German army surgeon, Joseph Naegele, of Düsseldorf. His elder brother, Anton, also made his mark as a physician, and his younger brother, Joseph II, followed their father's calling and distinguished himself in care of the wounded after Waterloo.

Franz Carl was first appointed medical officer to the Institute for the Poor at Elberfeld-Barmen in the Rhineland, where he reformed the administration and medical service. He became professor of medicine at the ancient University of Heidelberg and in 1810 was named, in addition, director of the Lying-in Hospital there, a post he held for forty years.

Recognized as the best practicing obstetrician of his time, he improved the instruments of his specialty and made a number of significant contributions to the scientific literature. His papers on calculating the length of pregnancy and on the mechanism of birth provided a scientific basis for obstetric practice. He also wrote about various aspects of obstetric pathology.

His most important work concerned the anatomy of the pelvis and the problems presented by pelvic and spinal deformities in cases of difficult labor. This book, "The Female Pelvis Considered in Relation to Its Position and the Inclination of Its Curvature along with Contributions to the History of the Knowledge of the Pelvic Axis," based on his measurements of hundreds of patients and postmortem studies, gave a new precision to morphologic knowledge. The book comprises two parts. In the first, fourteen short anatomic chapters are devoted to his measurements and calculations undertaken to establish "detailed knowledge of the form and conditions of all the points which constitute a well-made pelvis." The second part contains a critical history of all that had been written on the subject of the pelvic axis since the pioneer study by Hendrik van Deventer, of Leyden, in 1701.

Naegele's work not only was useful in itself but also set the example for much research during the next hundred years, which culminated in the classification of pelvic variations and their effects on labor published by the American obstetricians Caldwell and Moloy in 1933. Naegele himself published a study of the obliquely contracted pelvis in 1839. In his later years, he was assisted by his son, Herman Franz Joseph, who advanced the use of auscultation in midwifery.

Franz Carl Naegele. *Das weibliche Becken betrachtet in Beziehung auf seine Stellung und die Richtung seiner Höhle nebst Beyträgen zur Geschichte der Lehre von den Beckenaxen.* Carlsruhe, 1825.

The first half of Naegele's book presents detailed information about the "well-made pelvis," but it is the obliquely contracted pelvis described by Naegele in 1839 that is named for him.

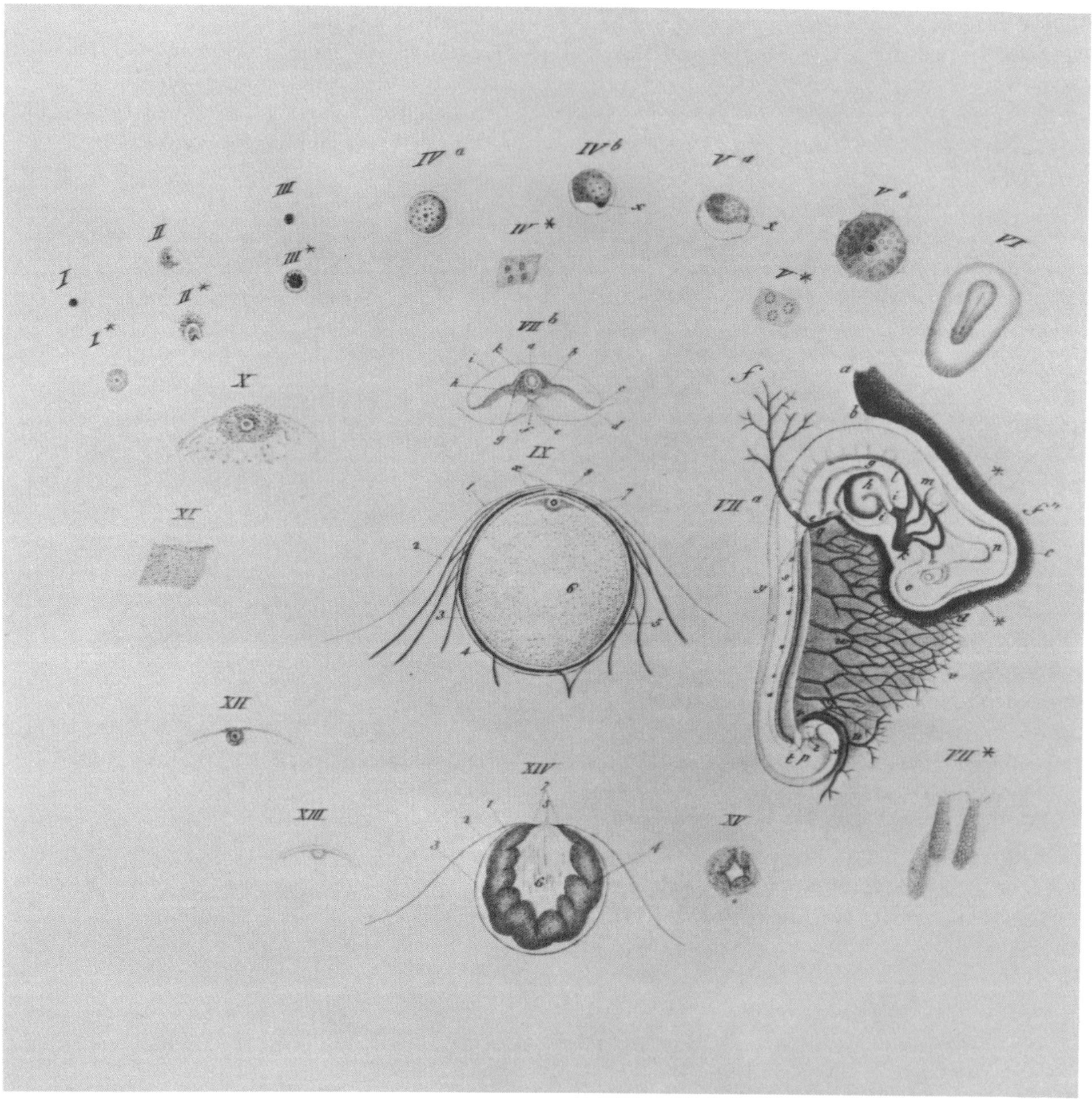
I
I*
II
II*
III
III*
IV a
IV b
IV*
V a
V b
V*
VI
VII a
VII b
VII*
IX
X
XI
XII
XIII
XIV
XV

# Carl Ernst von Baer

## ON THE GENESIS OF THE OVUM OF MAMMALS AND MAN

Born in Estonia of German parents, von Baer (1792-1876) spent the first half of his long life in Germany and the second half in Russia. His work was a link between the "nature philosophy" of the eighteenth century and the precise inductive science of the nineteenth. This many-sided biologist was trained in botany and zoology as well as medicine. From 1819 to 1834, he taught at Königsberg in East Prussia, where he made his original influential discoveries. He is best known for having found the mammalian ovum, which he detected in 1826 in the ovary of a dog and later in other mammals. He published this brief account of the formation of the egg of animals and man the next year.

The book describes the beginnings of the fetus in the dog, the genesis of the ovum, the Graafian vesicles, and the embryonic development of mammals. His announcement that "every animal which springs from coition of male and female is developed from an ovum, not from a simple generative fluid," cleared away many theoretical contrary opinions. The results of his infinite meticulousness in refining the then rudimentary techniques of microscopy laid the foundations for the new field of embryology and earned the profound admiration of his contemporaries.

Von Baer continued his observations and elaborated his "reflections" in the larger, unfinished two-volume work, *Über die Entwicklungsgeschichte der Thiere* (1828 and 1837). This title literally meant "the history of development of animals" but soon acquired the technical connotation of "embryology." He first distinguished the germ layers and discovered the notochord (chorda dorsalis), transient structures of great importance in understanding embryonic development and the common genesis of vertebrates. Von Baer recognized the neural folds as rudiments of the nervous system and described the primary brain vesicles. He showed that all vertebrate embryos are more alike than their adult forms, since development proceeds from the general to the special, and thus discredited the widely held theory that all characteristics of the organism were "preformed" in the ovum.

Von Baer's work provided a basis for systematic embryology. He was critical of Darwin's theory of evolution, but his ideas had considerable influence on the contributions of embryologists to evolutionary theory.

The last thirty years of his life were spent in Russia, where he devoted himself to studying the anthropology and physical geography of that country.

Carl Ernst von Baer. *De Ovi Mammalium et Hominis Genesi.* Leipzig, 1827.

Von Baer identified the mammalian ovum and the notochord in 1827. Later, using the rather primitive microscope then available, he traced the development of all principal organs from germ layers.

Pl. I.

Fig. 1.

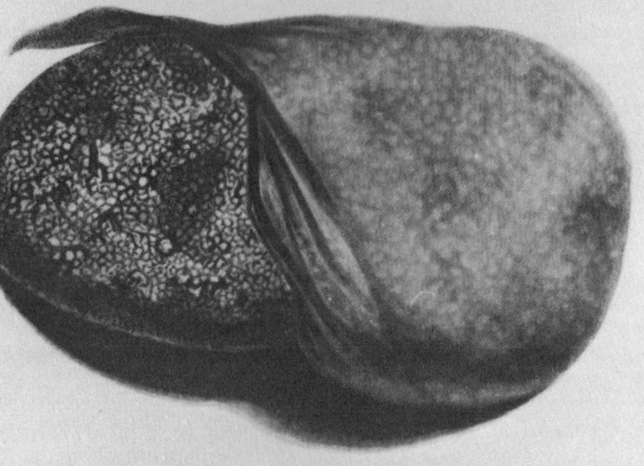

Fig. 2.

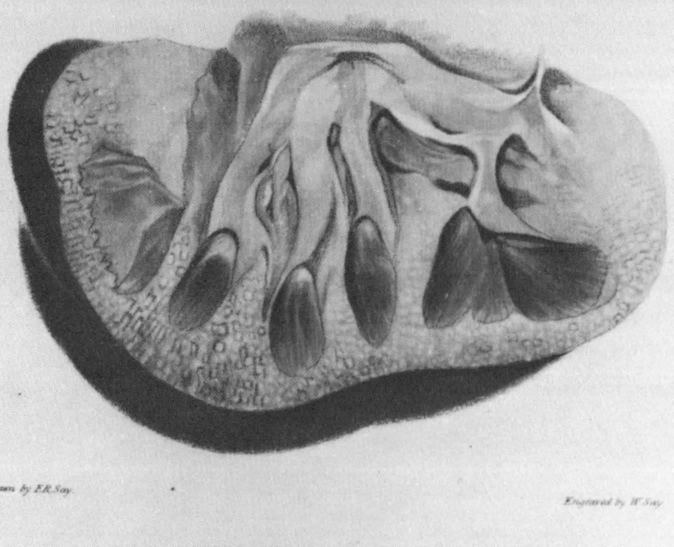

Drawn by F.R. Say. — Engraved by W. Say

London, Published Jan.y 1st 1827 by Longman Rees Orme & Brown.

# Richard Bright

## REPORTS OF MEDICAL CASES

Richard Bright (1789-1858), born in Bristol, was a brilliant and popular physician at Guy's Hospital, London, for twenty-three years. He also lectured on clinical medicine and therapeutics and enjoyed an illustrious reputation as artist, collector, Continental traveler, and writer as well as accomplished botanist and geologist.

His *Reports of Medical Cases,* published in two volumes, was a series of case histories that correlated clinical and pathologic findings. The first volume included twenty-three cases of kidney disease. In his preface, Bright noted that the book contained "statements and conjectures regarding the dependence of a peculiar class of dropsies on disease and irritation of the kidneys." Besides his historic differentiation of renal from cardiac dropsy, Bright established the symptomatology of chronic nonsuppurative nephritis, the "Bright's disease" that has immortalized his name. Although he had observed his first postmortem case of chronic nephritis in 1811, he published no reports on this disease until 1827, after being convinced by long and patient study of many cases that his findings were scientifically supportable.

The second volume was concerned mainly with diseases of the brain and spinal cord, including forty instances of cerebral hemorrhage. Bright presented cases of laryngeal tuberculosis, acne, and hydrocephalus, reported a relationship between chorea and rheumatism, and was the first to describe the administration of oxygen.

The *Reports* is a notable landmark in publishing, both for its important new knowledge and for its beautifully expressive colored engravings. Bright himself was an artist, but for these plates he supervised the drawings done for him by Frederick Richard Say and the aquatint engravings made from them by the artist's father, William Say.

"Utility is my object," Bright stated in his preface, "and the work which I now commence will not, in theory at least, be thoroughly completed until every disease which influences the natural structure, or originates in its derangements, has been connected with the corresponding organic lesion." He went a long way toward realizing this ambitious plan, with later reports in areas that comprised neurology, cardiac disease, metabolic disorders, and infectious diseases. As he neared retirement, he was instrumental in the establishment of a forty-two-bed renal disease unit at Guy's Hospital.

Richard Bright. *Reports of Medical Cases, Selected with a View of Illustrating the Symptoms and Cure of Diseases by a reference to Morbid Anatomy.* 2 vols. in three. London, 1827-1831.

These original engravings of the kidney appear in the book in vivid colors that have retained their vibrancy after one hundred and fifty years.

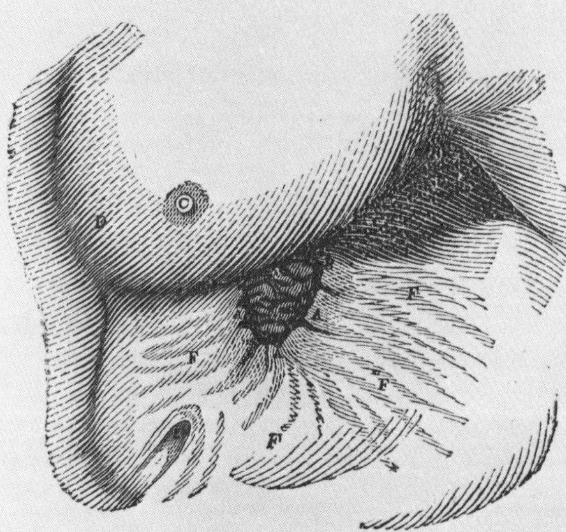

This engraving represents the ordinary appearance of the left breast and side, the aperture filled with the valve; the subject in an erect position.

A A A The circumference and edge of the aperture, within which is seen the valve.

B The attachment of the valvular portion of the stomach to the superior part of the aperture.

C The nipple.

D The anterior portion of the breast.

E The scar where the opening was made with the scalpel, and the cartilages taken out.

F F F F Cicatrice of the original wound, around the aperture.

# William Beaumont

## THE GASTRIC JUICE AND THE PHYSIOLOGY OF DIGESTION

Beaumont (1785-1853), a United States Army surgeon stationed at isolated Fort Mackinac in northern Michigan in 1822, was summoned to treat a French-Canadian *voyageur,* Alexis St. Martin, for a wound in the abdomen from an accidental musket shot at close range. A permanent gastric fistula formed in the wound, and Beaumont realized that St. Martin's case offered a unique opportunity to investigate the process of digestion. He was able to view the contents of the stomach during digestion through the opening and to watch the action of gastric secretions. He began his observations in the spring of 1825 and initially reported them in the *Medical Recorder* of Philadelphia.

During the next eight years, although St. Martin was often away hunting and fur trapping, sometimes deep in the Canadian wilds, and Beaumont was reassigned to remote posts in the Wisconsin wilderness, he was able from time to time to find St. Martin and continue his experiments. At one point, he persuaded his patient to travel to Plattsburgh, New York, where Beaumont was spending a leave, for a series of tests. Specimens of St. Martin's gastric juice were sent for analysis to chemists at the University of Virginia and at Yale University. Both found free hydrochloric acid.

The papers of 1825-1826 excited considerable interest, not the least in Europe, where Müller, Schwann, and Purkinje were influenced by the first report of Beaumont's discovery. His book describing his studies in detail was printed in Plattsburgh in 1833. It was reprinted in Boston and translated into German the next year and was published again in Edinburgh, Scotland, in 1838.

Beaumont realized the value of his observations for gastric function, digestion, and the pathology of gastritis and suggested that there was some special secretion in the stomach in addition to the hydrochloric acid. This was confirmed in 1836, when Schwann discovered pepsin. Beaumont eventually lost touch with St. Martin, who was said to have survived some forty-five more years and to have fathered twenty children.

This book, a remarkable example of brilliant clinical investigation performed under almost primitive conditions, represents a discovery that proved to be a major milestone in the field of physiology.

William Beaumont. *Experiments and Observations on the Gastric Juice, and the Physiology of Digestion.* Plattsburgh, 1833.

Beaumont followed the *voyageur* St. Martin across the wilds of North America to gather data on gastric secretions. A pioneer study in a pioneer country, the work preceded Pavlov's by sixty-five years.

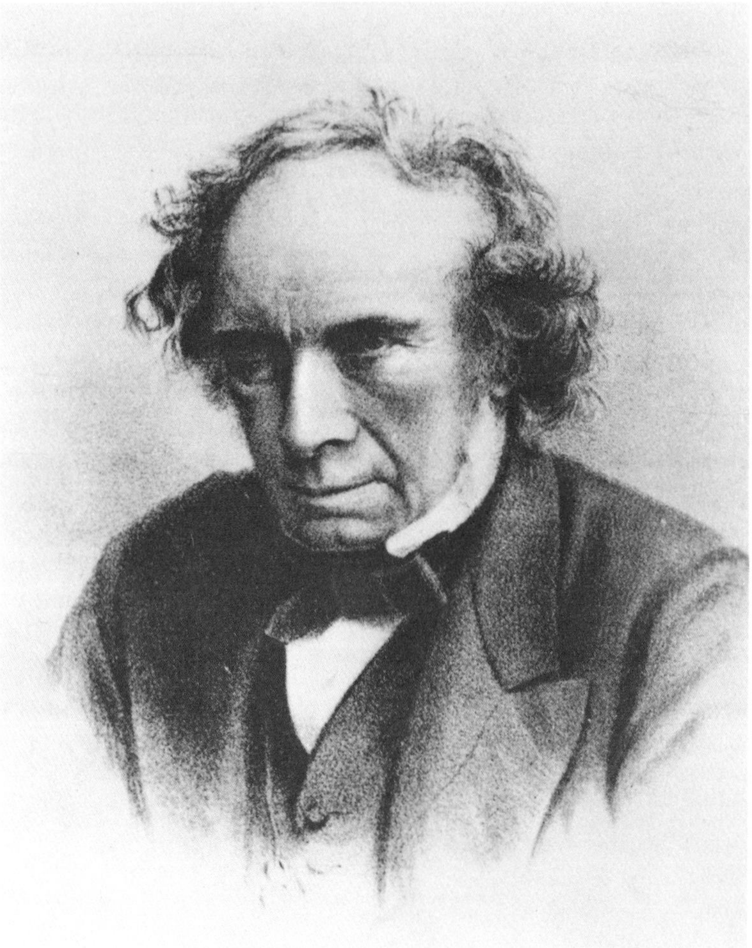

# William Stokes

## DISEASES OF THE CHEST

Stokes (1804-1878) was the son of a prominent Irish physician, intellectual, and political activist. During his career, he succeeded his father first as physician to the Meath Hospital in Dublin and later as regius professor of medicine at the University of Dublin.

As a boy, the younger Stokes often accompanied his father on archaeologic and scientific excursions into the Irish countryside and undoubtedly learned much about meticulous observation on these trips. At the age of twenty-one, while still a student in Edinburgh, he wrote *An Introduction to the Use of the Stethoscope,* the first systematic English treatise to follow Laënnec's book of 1819. It is credited with giving significant impetus to acceptance of the stethoscope as a diagnostic tool.

The masterly *Diseases of the Chest*, published when Stokes was thirty-three, was the fruit of twelve years' experience and established his reputation. Intending it to meet the needs of the practicing physician, he simplified the descriptions and explained the principles, rather than the details, of treatment. He extended the studies of Laënnec and Corvisart on the physical signs and symptoms of pulmonary illnesses.

After discussion of the diagnosis of thoracic disease, Stokes dealt in turn with disorders of the mucous membrane (including bronchitis in particular), the larynx, and the trachea; pneumonia; gangrene of the lung; and disease of the pleura. Among other new observations, he described paralysis of the intercostal muscles and diaphragm after pleurisy and the use of the stethoscope to detect foreign bodies in the air passages. His monograph was certainly one of the most famous contributions of the Irish school of medicine.

Although Stokes never wrote the projected second part of his treatise on the lungs, he made a notable addition in later years to medical literature and to the study of heart disease with publication of *The Diseases of the Heart and Aorta* (1854). His name has been perpetuated in the eponyms "Stokes-Adams syndrome" (heart block and syncope), "Cheyne-Stokes respiration," and Stokes' expectorant.

William Stokes. *A Treatise on the Diagnosis and Treatment of Diseases of the Chest. Part I. Diseases of the Lung and Windpipe.* Dublin, 1837.

Lithograph portrait of Stokes. Besides medicine, his interests included music, drama, and archaeology, especially that of Ireland, and he was a cofounder of the Dublin Zoo.

Plate IV.

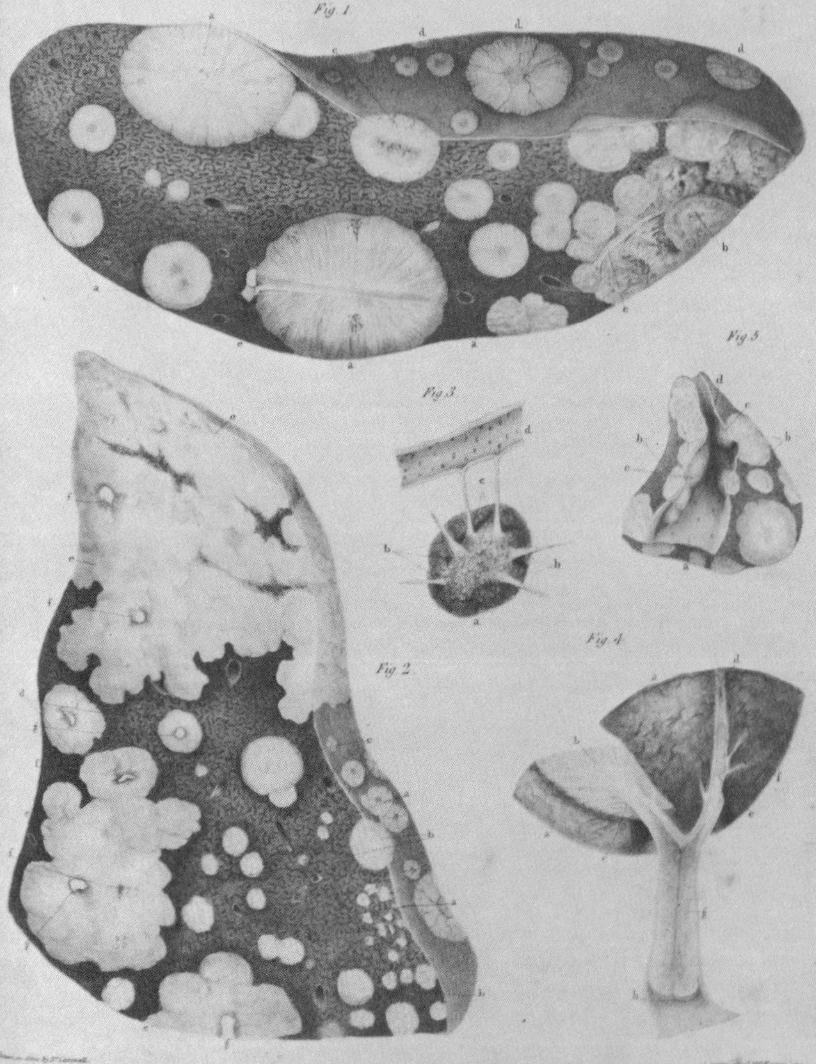

# Sir Robert Carswell

## ILLUSTRATIONS OF THE ELEMENTARY FORMS OF DISEASE

Robert Carswell (1793-1857) studied medicine at Glasgow, was granted his medical degree by Aberdeen, and became professor of pathologic anatomy at University College, London. He had spent five years in Paris, where he made watercolor drawings of diseased tissues. In his illustrations, Carswell pursued a different purpose from that of a Parisian contemporary, Jean Cruveilhier, whose pathologic plates appeared in forty fascicles between 1828 and 1842. Cruveilhier's work was an encyclopedia of case histories, fully described; Carswell's book was a selection of representative renderings of diseased structures from some 2,000 drawings that he himself had made and copied onto lithographic stones for reproduction. (The Lilly Library possesses two of his original drawings.)

Carswell was chiefly interested in etiology and the pathologic process in tissues. Some diseases he illustrated, such as disseminated sclerosis, had not yet been described clinically. He dealt with gross naked-eye pathology at a time when the microscopic researches of Schwann, Purkinje, Bowman, and others were just beginning to lay the foundation for Virchow's belief that pathology must be studied at the cellular level. Although it has been suggested that, without the microscope, Carswell did not properly understand complicated tissue, the accuracy and color of his illustrations have never been surpassed. This atlas is notable for the merit of its artwork.

The plate of osteomyelitis has been much admired, and among other markedly successful representations are those of bone sarcoma, cancer of the gall bladder, distention of the urethra, renal cysts, gastromalacia, bronchiectasis, and the scar tissue of burns. Each section of the atlas has a lengthy introduction on the etiology, character, and progress of the general condition which the drawings illustrate. Carswell made frequent references to contemporary English and French work and discussed the opinions of earlier authorities. In the dedication to James Jeffray, he recalled that he "first attempted to represent by coloured delineation the healthy and diseased appearances of the human body" while attending Jeffray's classes in Glasgow.

Carswell proposed to publish a second edition with his illustrations of calculi, entozoa, and monstrosities, but this was not achieved. At the time he was holding his professorship, he also practiced as a physician in London. He was knighted by Queen Victoria and in 1840 moved to Brussels as physician to King Leopold of Belgium, an uncle of the queen.

Robert Carswell. *Pathological Anatomy. Illustrations of the Elementary Forms of Disease.* London, 1838.

The various figures illustrate the gross appearance of carcinoma of the liver, the manner in which the disease develops, and its presence in the blood.

PL. 36

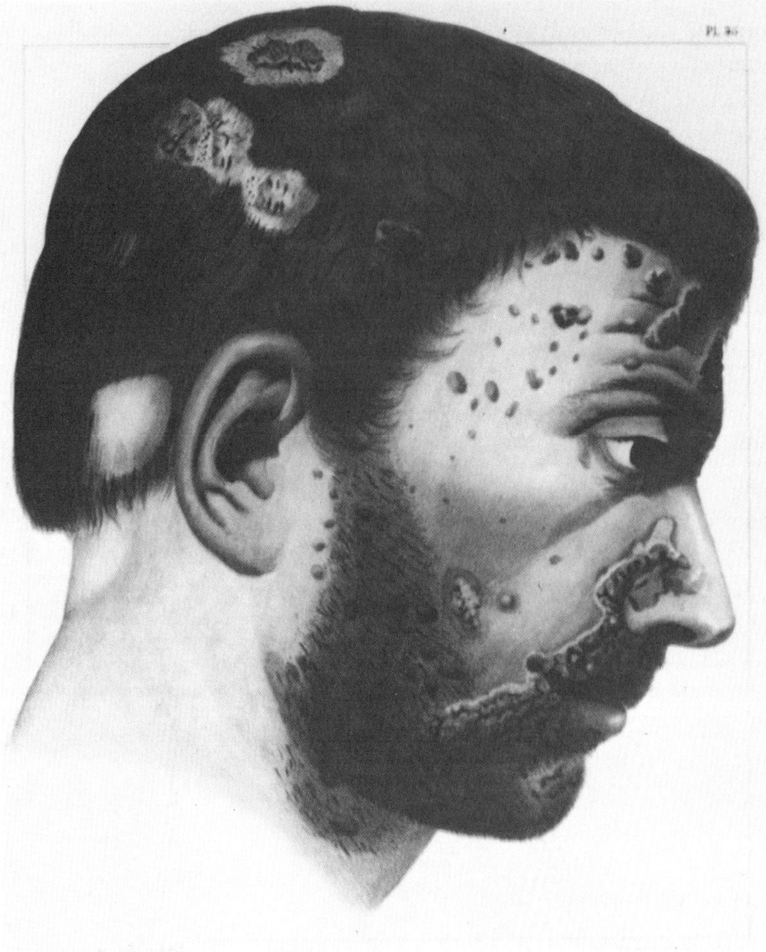

# Philippe Ricord

## VENEREAL DISEASES

In his authoritative *Treatise on the Venereal Disease* (1786), John Hunter declared that syphilis and gonorrhea were manifestations of a single disease. The error arose when he inoculated himself with syphilis without knowing that he had also infected himself with gonorrhea. Differentiation of the two diseases was established fifty years later by Philippe Ricord (1800-1889), whose experiments are recorded in his thorough "Practical Treatise on Venereal Diseases."

Ricord was born of French parents in Baltimore, Maryland, but went to France for his surgical training under Dupuytren, Lisfranc, and other great teachers of the Paris school. He was graduated with an M.D. degree in 1826 and spent his long, active career wholly in France as a specialist in venereal diseases. He was surgeon to the Hôpital du Midi in Paris, held a professorial chair, and conducted a large private practice. Possessed of a compassionate interest in alleviating suffering, he was renowned also as a wit and writer of light verse.

Ricord had already written books on gonorrhea and on chancre when he published this outstanding treatise. Beginning with a "critical and general" discussion, the book recorded his conclusions that there is a unique syphilitic "virus," that gonorrhea is a different disease, that syphilis can be divided into primary, secondary, and tertiary stages, and that prophylactic treatment against the later stages is available. He gave credit for first correcting Hunter's error to J. F. Hernandez, who had published an essay on the "Nonidentity of Syphilis and Gonorrhea" in French in 1812, but it was Ricord's own detailed presentation of his experimental results in this treatise that established the truth.

The central section of the book, giving his experiments in detail, demonstrated that the pus of a chancre produces syphilis but inoculation with a gonorrheal secretion does not. He went on to describe his method of treatment and appended a brief formulary of the mineral medications employed in his clinic. It was shown that mercury was not a universal specific and that some so-called secondary infections were due to mercury poisoning.

This lengthy work was completed in the first decade of Ricord's medical practice. His book achieved immediate success. It was revised many times and widely translated; thirteen American editions were published between 1843 and 1858. Ricord raised the treatment of venereal disease to a level not to be surpassed for seventy years.

Philippe Ricord. *Traité pratique des maladies vénériennes.* Paris, 1838.

This hand-colored lithograph, one of a series of fifty portraits of Ricord's syphilitic patients, appeared in his *Clinique iconographie*, which was published in 1851.

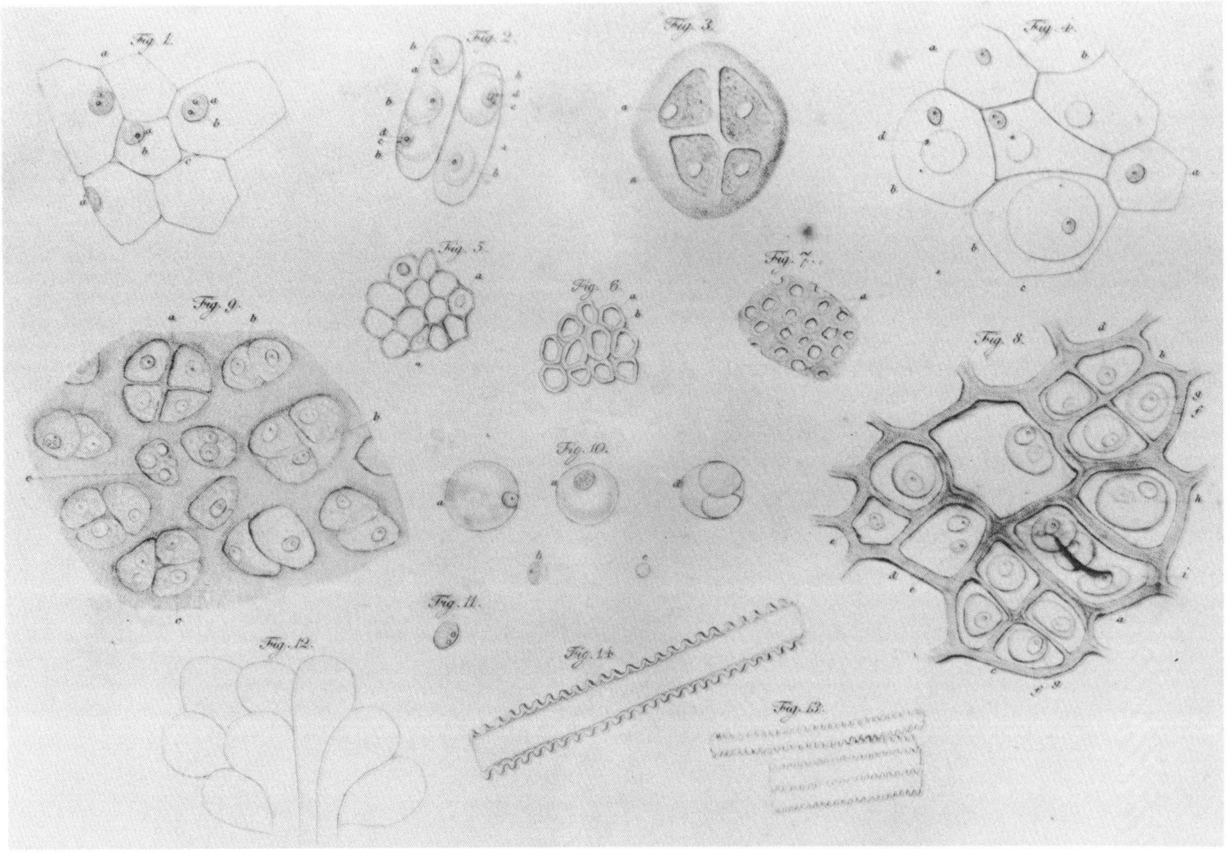
Fig. 1.
Fig. 2.
Fig. 3.
Fig. 4.
Fig. 5.
Fig. 6.
Fig. 7.
Fig. 8.
Fig. 9.
Fig. 10.
Fig. 11.
Fig. 12.
Fig. 13.
Fig. 14.

# Theodor Schwann

## THE STRUCTURE AND GROWTH OF ANIMALS AND PLANTS

Theodor Schwann (1810-1882), born into a devout Catholic family near Düsseldorf, Germany, studied under the great physiologist Johannes Müller at Bonn and at the University of Berlin. For the first five years after receiving his medical degree at Berlin, Schwann served as assistant in anatomy to Müller, and it was during this period that he made his great scientific contributions.

Schwann was one of a number of young researchers investigating animal tissue cells during the 1830's, when M. F. Schleiden, his botanist friend, demonstrated to him the importance of the nucleus in the development of plant cells. "I immediately recollected," Schwann wrote, "having seen a similar organ in the cells of the dorsal cord, and at the same moment grasped the extreme importance my discovery would have if I could show that this nucleus plays the same part as is played by the nucleus in vegetable cells." He pursued his microscopic research and was able to announce in his remarkable book in 1839 that "a similar cellular origin is common to everything living." He had already made some significant biologic observations, but they were overshadowed by the far-reaching influence of "Microscopic Research into the Conformity in the Structure and Growth of Animals and Plants," a carefully argued thesis on the universality of the cellular structure of all living tissues.

The book is in two parts. The first is a thorough, detailed description of the structure and growth of the spinal cord, with an elaboration of Schwann's thesis that the cells are the basis of all tissues in the animal body. The second part contains sections on the ovum, the cellular structure of other tissues, a summary, and a defense of the cell theory against criticisms made of it. Certain particulars were later corrected, but Schwann's general concept made possible the great advances in physiology and pathology of the later nineteenth century.

Although he is remembered primarily for his original discourse on the cell theory, his physiologic-histologic studies also led him to the discovery of pepsin, the recognition that bile is essential for digestion, and original observations on muscle contractility (the neurolemma is also called the "sheath of Schwann").

This publication of 1839 brought Schwann renown at the age of twenty-nine, and in the same year he was appointed professor of anatomy at the University of Louvain in Belgium. Nine years later, he assumed the chair of anatomy and physiology at Liège, where he taught until his death at the age of seventy-two.

Theodor Schwann. *Mikroskopische Untersuchungen über die Uebereinstimmung in der Struktur und dem Wachsthum der Thiere und Pflanzen.* Berlin, 1839.

With these delicate drawings,
Schwann demonstrated that the cell nucleus
is found in plants (Figures 1 through 3) and in cells of the
roach, the frog, and the swine fetus.

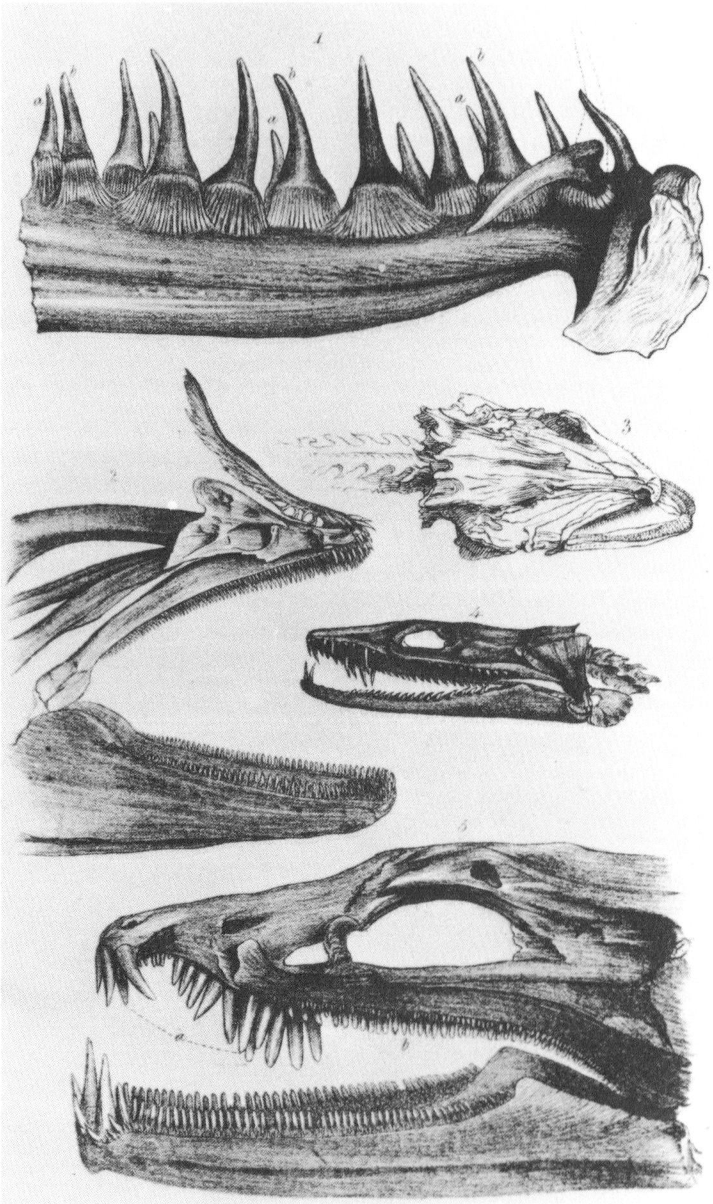
1
2
3
4
5

# Sir Richard Owen

## ODONTOGRAPHY

This vast storehouse of detail on the structure of teeth was the first large-scale original work by Sir Richard Owen (1804-1892). A native of Lancaster, England, and a pupil of physiologist John Abernethy in London, he had prepared the five-volume *Physiological Catalogue* of John Hunter's museum and had edited Hunter's posthumous papers on comparative anatomy and zoology. He was an associate and son-in-law of Hunter's secretary, William Clift.

The scope of Owen's writing, based on his own dissections and usually illustrated with his own drawings, has hardly been surpassed. He was forty-one when he completed this study, which was published in two volumes five years apart.

The work covered the whole range of the toothed vertebrates, fossil and extant, and discussed in detail the microscopic structure of the teeth and the physiology of dentition. After a long introduction, Owen described the dental system of fishes, reptiles, and mammals. The dentition of extinct large reptiles and mammals as well as that of the marsupials and cetacea was included in his survey. Human dentition was treated in the section on mammals. The illustrations by several artists (including the author) are particularly impressive. They comprise 168 full-page plates, mostly lithographs; a few are colored engravings of microstructure.

In a sense, dental anatomy and paleontology met here and were brought into the scientific limelight. Owen later wrote many long monographs and large-scale treatises on paleontology and comparative anatomy. One of these was *On the Archetype and Homologies of the Vertebrate Skeleton* (1848), written when he still held the belief that the identity of class, order, genus, and species could be traced back to the beginning of the universe. In his later years, he became involved in hot controversy with Huxley over Darwinism but eventually was won over to the theory of the evolutionary development of species.

He was Hunterian professor for twenty years at the Royal College of Surgeons and from 1856 to 1883 was superintendent of the natural history department of the British Museum. He died at the age of eighty-eight.

Richard Owen. *Odontography; or, a Treatise on the Comparative Anatomy of the Teeth; Their Physiological Relations, Mode of Development, and Microscopic Structure, in the Vertebrate Animals.* 2 vols. London, 1840-1845.

One of many lithograph plates in the book, this illustration reflects Owen's detailed observation of the teeth of fishes. The angler, broad-nosed eel, and moray eel are shown here.

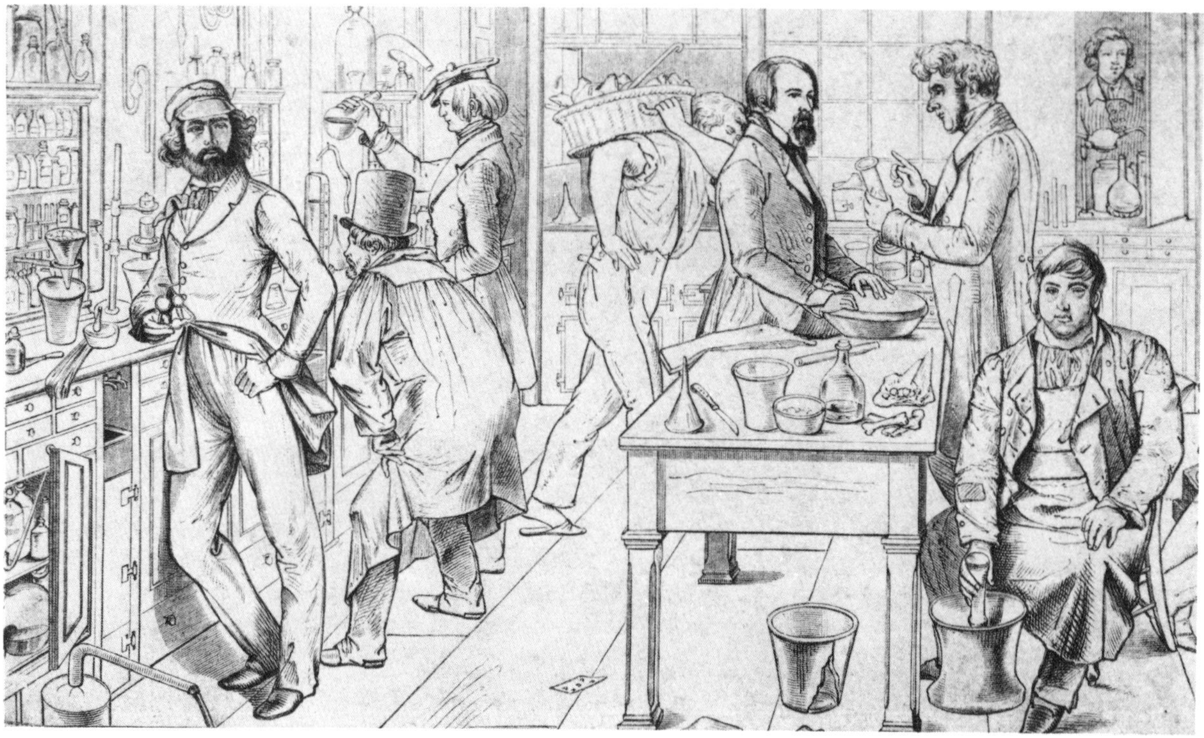

# Justus von Liebig

## ORGANIC CHEMISTRY

Von Liebig (1803-1873) became professor of chemistry at Giessen in 1825 when he was only twenty-two. He had studied first at the University of Bonn, then earned his Ph.D. at Erlangen, and continued his studies under Gay-Lussac in Paris. A pioneer in laboratory teaching and agricultural chemistry, he made his reputation as a pure chemist.

In 1825, Germany lagged behind other European countries in the field of chemistry. Von Liebig, by creating the first teaching laboratory, inaugurated Germany's era of brilliant chemical research. He became interested in the application of chemistry to agriculture and tried to introduce scientifically compounded fertilizers to replace local empirical methods of improving the soil. He was the first to suggest that overuse of the soil depleted its nutrients and that they should be replaced by nonorganic chemicals.

His interest later extended to medical needs, and he became the first modern chemist to apply the specialized techniques of organic chemistry to physiology, pathology, and pharmacy. He studied many reactions, including the metabolism of carbohydrates and fats and the degradation of proteins and purines to urea, uric acid, and hippuric acid. Paradoxically, despite von Liebig's inventive nature, he also was a conservative who could not accept Schwann's demonstration of living cells in yeast and the biotic cause of putrefaction.

Von Liebig wrote "Organic Chemistry in Its Application to Physiology and Pathology" at the age of thirty-nine. The treatise was dedicated to the doyen of contemporary chemists, the Swedish scientist John Jacob Berzelius, although Berzelius had criticized him severely. It contains three main sections: the chemical process of respiration and nutrition; the metamorphosis of forms, which carries as a running title on each page "The Chemical Process of the Change of Forms"; and the phenomena of movement in animal organisms, followed by discourses on the theories of disease and of respiration. The medical value of the book, beyond its somewhat theoretical formulation, consists in the clear explanation of the chemical process in respiration (including the importance of oxygen), the introduction of the concept of metabolism, and a classification of the organic foodstuffs. With these three sections, von Liebig laid the foundation of subsequent biochemical knowledge.

Von Liebig's resistance to the new living-cell theory and his conviction that all biologic processes could be explained as chemical reactions led him into some erroneous deductions, but his factual observations had lasting validity.

Justus von Liebig. *Die organische Chemie in ihrer Anwendung auf Physiologie und Pathologie*. Braunschweig, 1842.

An artist's concept of von Liebig's laboratory at Giessen. Here, in the first teaching laboratory associated with a university, von Liebig and his students carried out their basic research on metabolism.

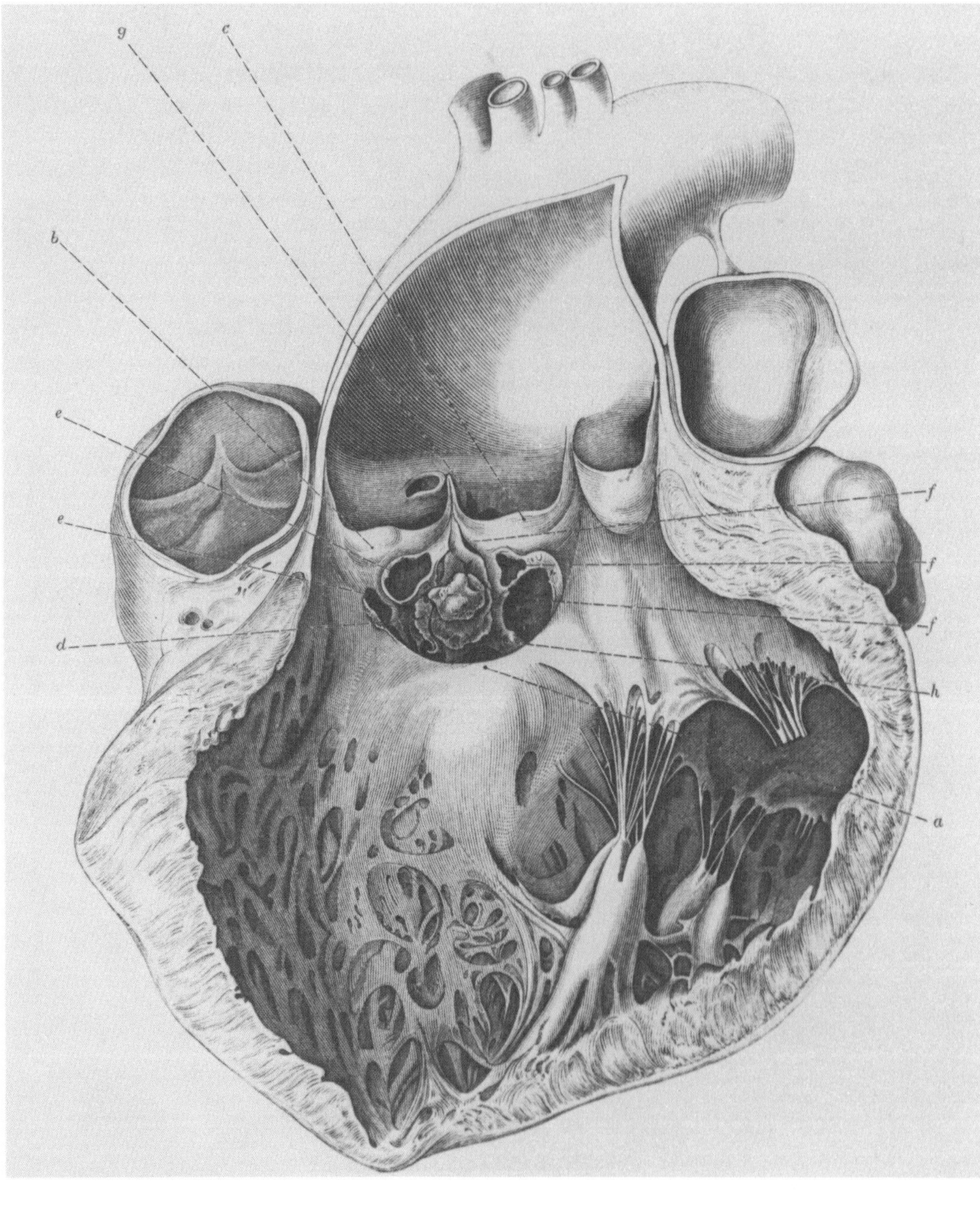

g
c
b
e
e
f
f
f
d
h
a

# Carl Rokitansky

## HANDBOOK OF PATHOLOGIC ANATOMY

Carl Rokitansky (1804-1878), born in Bohemia, was one of an illustrious group who were credited with reestablishing Vienna as an important center of medical research. He studied in Prague and Vienna, where he graduated in medicine, and then spent his entire career in the pathology laboratory. He and Josef Skoda, the clinician, were the leading founders of the revolutionary movement that became known as the New Vienna School.

Having access to the great hospitals of Vienna, where he was professor of pathology in the university, Rokitansky became the most thoroughly equipped pathologist of his time. By decree of Emperor Joseph II, all patients who died in hospitals were to be autopsied. This allowed Rokitansky to perform some thirty thousand postmortems himself during his lifetime and to have available the findings of more than thirty thousand others.

His "Handbook of Pathologic Anatomy" provided the nineteenth century with a fund of pathologic observation comparable in scope to Morgagni's in the previous century. The work is in three volumes, but they were published in reverse order. Volume III appeared first, in 1842, and dealt with abnormalities of the respiratory, digestive, urinary, and reproductive systems. Volume II, issued in 1844, contained sections on abnormalities of cellular, serous, and mucous tissues, the skin, fibers, bone, muscle, and the vascular and nervous systems. In these volumes were the first accounts of acute yellow atrophy of the liver and an improved concept of pneumonia. Congenital malformations were meticulously described. Volume I, containing the general survey, finally came out in 1846. Both volumes II and III were reissued without alteration, presumably because the publisher had underestimated their chances for success.

Rokitansky's observations and descriptions were original and impeccable. Some of his theories, however, especially his chemical hypothesis of tissue change, were misconceived and outdated. They were so sharply criticized by Virchow in the *Medizinische Zeitung* in 1846 that Rokitansky omitted them from later editions of his work. He has also been accused of divorcing pathologic from clinical observation and, with Josef Skoda, has been charged with encouraging therapeutic nihilism. Later in life, he published beautifully illustrated and detailed monographs on the pathology of the arteries and malformations of the heart.

Carl Rokitansky. *Handbuch der pathologischen Anatomie.* 3 vols. Vienna, 1842, 1844, and 1846.

Rokitansky's "Defects of the Valves of the Heart" (1875) was illustrated with fine engravings such as this one. The book represented fourteen years of research.

Let those now laugh, who never laugh'd before,
And those who always laugh, now laugh the more.

# A GRAND EXHIBITION

OF THE EFFECTS PRODUCED BY INHALING

NITROUS OXIDE, EXHILERATING, OR

# LAUGHING GAS!

WILL BE GIVEN AT *The Masonic Hall*

*Saturday* EVENING, *15th* 1845.

*30* **GALLONS OF GAS will be prepared and administered to all in the audience who desire to inhale it.**

**MEN will be invited from the audience, to protect those under the influence of the Gas from injuring themselves or others. This course is adopted that no apprehension of danger may be entertained. Probably no one will attempt to fight.**

THE EFFECT OF THE GAS is to make those who inhale it, either

**LAUGH, SING, DANCE, SPEAK OR FIGHT, &c. &c.**

according to the leading trait of their character. They seem to retain consciousness enough not to say or do that which they would have occasion to regret.

**N. B. The Gas will be administered only to gentlemen of the first respectability. The object is to make the entertainment in every respect, a genteel affair.**

Those who inhale the Gas once, are always anxious to inhale it the second time. There is not an exception to this rule.

No language can describe the delightful sensation produced. Robert Southey, (poet) once said that "the atmosphere of the highest of all possible heavens must be composed of this Gas."

For a full account of the effect produced upon some of the most distinguished men of Europe, see Hooper's Medical Dictionary, under the head of Nitrogen.

**The History and properties of the Gas will be explained at the commencement of the entertainment.**

The entertainment will be accompanied by experiments in

# ELECTRICITY.

**ENTERTAINMENT TO COMMENCE AT 7 O'CLOCK.**

**TICKETS *12½* CENTS,**

For sale at the principal Bookstores, and at the Door.

# Sir James Young Simpson

## ACCOUNT OF A NEW ANAESTHETIC AGENT

Sir James Young Simpson (1811-1870), who was elected professor of midwifery at the University of Edinburgh when he was only twenty-nine, is credited with introducing inhalation anesthesia into obstetrics. As a brilliant practitioner and pioneer advocate of the use of anesthesia in childbirth and surgical operations, he was one of the founders of modern obstetrics and gynecology.

At the age of thirty-five, he was appointed physician to Queen Victoria in Scotland, but the event was overshadowed by another of greater importance to him. "Flattery from the Queen is perhaps not common flattery," he wrote a few days later, "but I am far less interested in it than having delivered a woman this week without any pain while inhaling sulphuric ether. I can think of nought else."

However, he was not satisfied that ether, with its unpleasant side-effects, was the best anesthetic possible and continued to experiment with other chemicals. On November 4, 1847, he and two assistants tested a new one, chloroform, on themselves, and he was elated with the results. Almost immediately, he had the opportunity to deliver a colleague's wife of a baby girl under the new anesthetic. Within two weeks, the twenty-three-page pamphlet, *Account of a New Anaesthetic Agent,* was published. (The Lilly Library copy is bound with three other pamphlets by Simpson on the subjects of anesthesia and childbirth.)

Since midwifery, as then practiced, was based on the belief that labor pains were a "desirable, salutary, and conservative manifestation of life-force," Simpson became a focus of controversy. Although opposed by many of his colleagues on "moral" and "religious" grounds, he was the idol of his patients, who flocked to Edinburgh from throughout the British Isles. The debate with his peers began to die down only when, in 1853, Queen Victoria chose to take chloroform at the birth of Prince Leopold.

Several instruments and gynecologic procedures were also introduced by Simpson, who held strong and farsighted theories that infections were being transmitted from patient to patient within the hospitals. During his busy lifetime, he published some two hundred articles on medical subjects and found time to write about twenty more on another interest of his, archaeology.

After twice rejecting offers of royal recognition in the form of a title, Simpson finally accepted a baronetcy. Upon his death from heart disease at the age of fifty-nine, his family refused the offer of a tomb in Westminster Abbey, because he had wished to be buried among some of his children.

James Young Simpson. *Account of a New Anaesthetic Agent, as a Substitute for Sulphuric Ether in Surgery and Midwifery.* Edinburgh, 1847.

While Simpson was advocating the use of inhalation anesthesia to ease the pains of childbirth, his contemporaries were being entertained by the effects of nitrous oxide on "gentlemen of the first respectability."

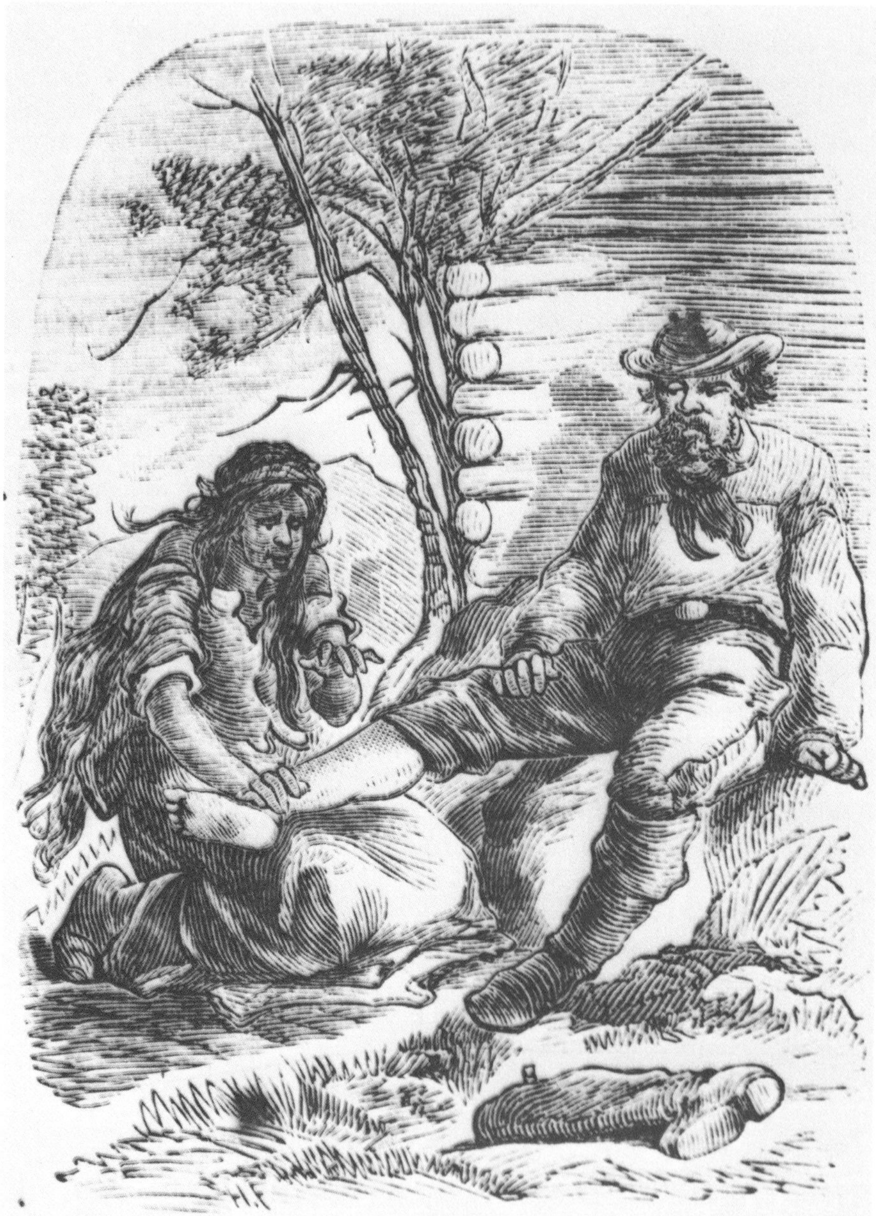

# Daniel Drake

## THE PRINCIPAL DISEASES . . . OF NORTH AMERICA

Drake's heroic subject was the North American continent—its topography, meteorology, and ethnology as they related to the health of its people. In the preface of his monumental work, he stated that he had begun forty years previously to make "personal observations from Florida to Canada of the causes, symptoms, pathology and treatment" of the diseases prevailing in the midlands of the continent, into which men of European origin and their African slaves were rapidly spreading. This is an epic record of the physical state of the nation during the decades of the westward movement and offers a physician's view of health and sickness among the peoples of a vast and diversified region.

Drake (1785-1852) died after only half his papers had been published; the second book was edited and issued posthumously in 1854. The first volume surveyed the "topographical and hydrographical etiology" of disease in twelve areas that extended north and east from the Delta of the Mississippi through the Ohio and St. Lawrence basins and from the Great Lakes to the Arctic. He discussed the climate (including the prevalent winds and storms) and its effects on health, dealing particularly with the central areas around St. Louis and Cincinnati. He also described "physiological and social etiology," population, and the modes of living of the inhabitants, such as their occupations and recreations. This book included the first part of Drake's strictly medical reports, with chapters on "autumnal fever." The twenty-seven chapters of the posthumous volume contained the remainder of these medical reports, classified under five different types of fever.

Drake was a picturesque character. Restless, critical, and combative by nature, he was a crusader for improved medical education in the frontier lands. He filled successively seven teaching positions in the Midwest and founded two medical faculties—the Medical College of Ohio (1821) and the medical department of Cincinnati College (1835). He established a western medical journal, and in it appeared his celebrated series of essays on medical education, eminently readable even today. In these, he strongly criticized the way physicians were being prepared for their profession.

Tall, commanding, and dignified in appearance, he lectured with fiery eloquence but was also endowed with a gentle sense of humor, as can be seen by his entertaining writings on pioneer life.

Daniel Drake. *A Systematic Treatise, Historical, Etiological, and Practical, on the Principal Diseases of the Interior Valley of North America, as They Appear in the Caucasian, African, Indian, and Esquimaux Varieties of Its Population.* Cincinnati, 1850.

——. *A Systematic Treatise . . . Second Series,* edited by Drs. S. Hanbury Smith and Francis G. Smith. Philadelphia, 1854.

An injured frontiersman receives treatment from an Indian woman in this drawing by an unknown artist. The scarcity of trained physicians prompted Drake's efforts to improve frontier health care.

Fig. 2.

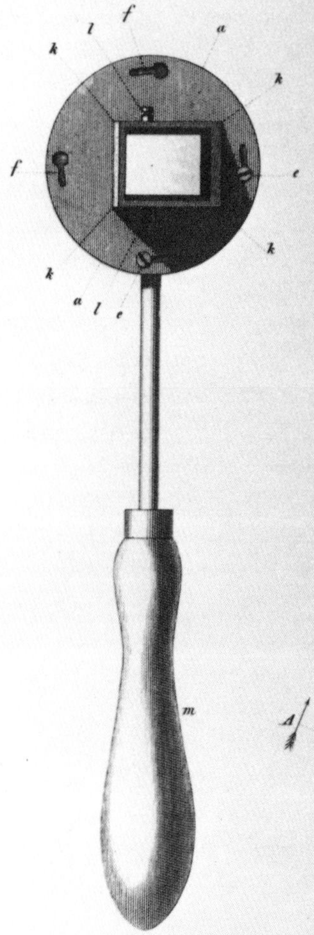


Fig. 3.

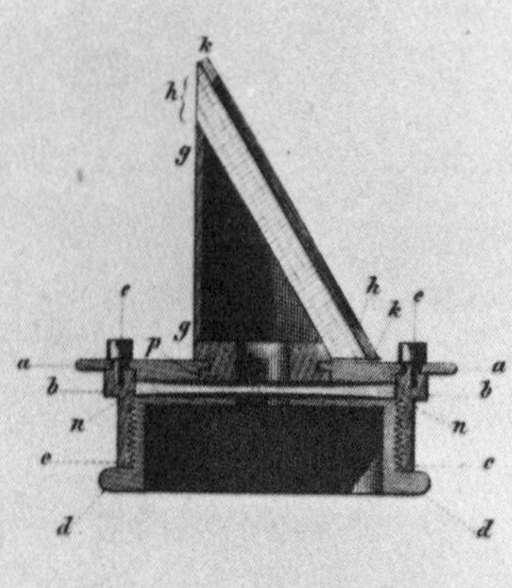


Fig. 1.

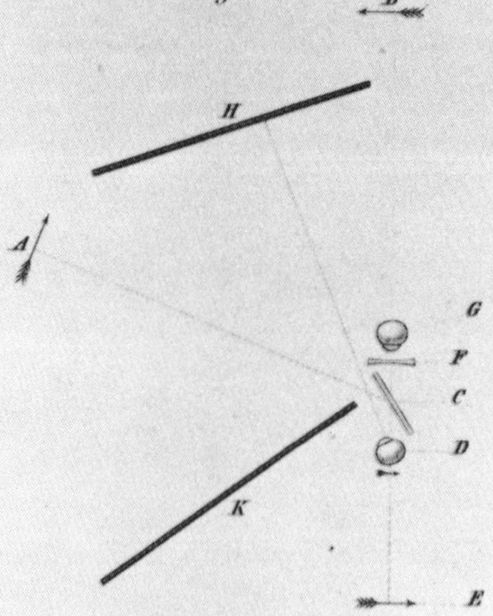

# Hermann von Helmholtz

## DESCRIPTION OF AN OPHTHALMOSCOPE

Ophthalmology, physics, acoustics, physiology, clinical medicine, thermodynamics, and nerve energy—von Helmholtz (1821-1894) was at home in all of these fields and contributed significantly to each. In 1851, he invented his "eye-mirror," or ophthalmoscope, a tool of immense importance for the diagnosis of pathologic conditions in the eye, and introduced the device in this forty-nine-page booklet.

In his monograph, von Helmholtz comments, "We need a source of light to observe sufficiently the part of the retina at which we look through the pupil, and we can see the background of the eye only through a refractive medium." The mechanism of the instrument is described and clarified by means of a diagram.

Von Helmholtz was thirty when he invented the ophthalmoscope. Four years earlier, he had presented his theoretical conclusions on the conservation of energy to the Physical Society of Berlin, and publication of his essay established the first law of thermodynamics. In 1852, using a pendulum-myograph he had invented, he measured the velocity of the nervous impulse; the mean of his observations was about thirty meters per second, a value accepted today.

Von Helmholtz had been educated in Berlin as a surgeon for the Prussian army. He was of German, French, and English extraction; his mother was a direct descendant of William Penn. It was in the barracks laboratory at Potsdam, the city of his birth, that he conducted his research on the conservation of energy. At the age of twenty-nine, he was appointed professor of physiology and pathology at the University of Königsberg. Later, he occupied the chairs of anatomy and physiology at Bonn and then the chair of physiology at Heidelberg. Finally, when he was fifty, he became professor of physics at Berlin, where he remained until his death. In his laboratory, Heinrich Hertz discovered the electrophysical principles that led to the development of wireless telegraphy, and Henry Augustus Rowland did the basic work on colloid chemistry.

Von Helmholtz never practiced ophthalmology or otolaryngology, but his "Handbook of Physiologic Optics" (published in three parts between 1856 and 1867) has remained a permanent classic, and his study of the tympanum and ossicles of the middle ear contributed greatly to understanding of the phenomenon of audition. His *Tonempfindungen* ("Sensations of Tone") (1863) dealt exhaustively with acoustics.

Although most of von Helmholtz's later life was devoted to physics (and he is regarded as a giant in this field), he always remembered that he was a physician. "Medicine was once the intellectual home in which I grew up," he said, "and even the emigrant best understands and is best understood by his native land."

Hermann von Helmholtz. *Beschreibung eines Augen-Spiegels zur Untersuchung der Netzhaut im lebenden Auge.* Berlin, 1851.

The precision and economy of von Helmholtz's drawing of the first ophthalmoscope reflect his aptitude for mathematics and physics, which he further expressed in major contributions to thermodynamics, electrodynamics, and hydrodynamics.

VIII

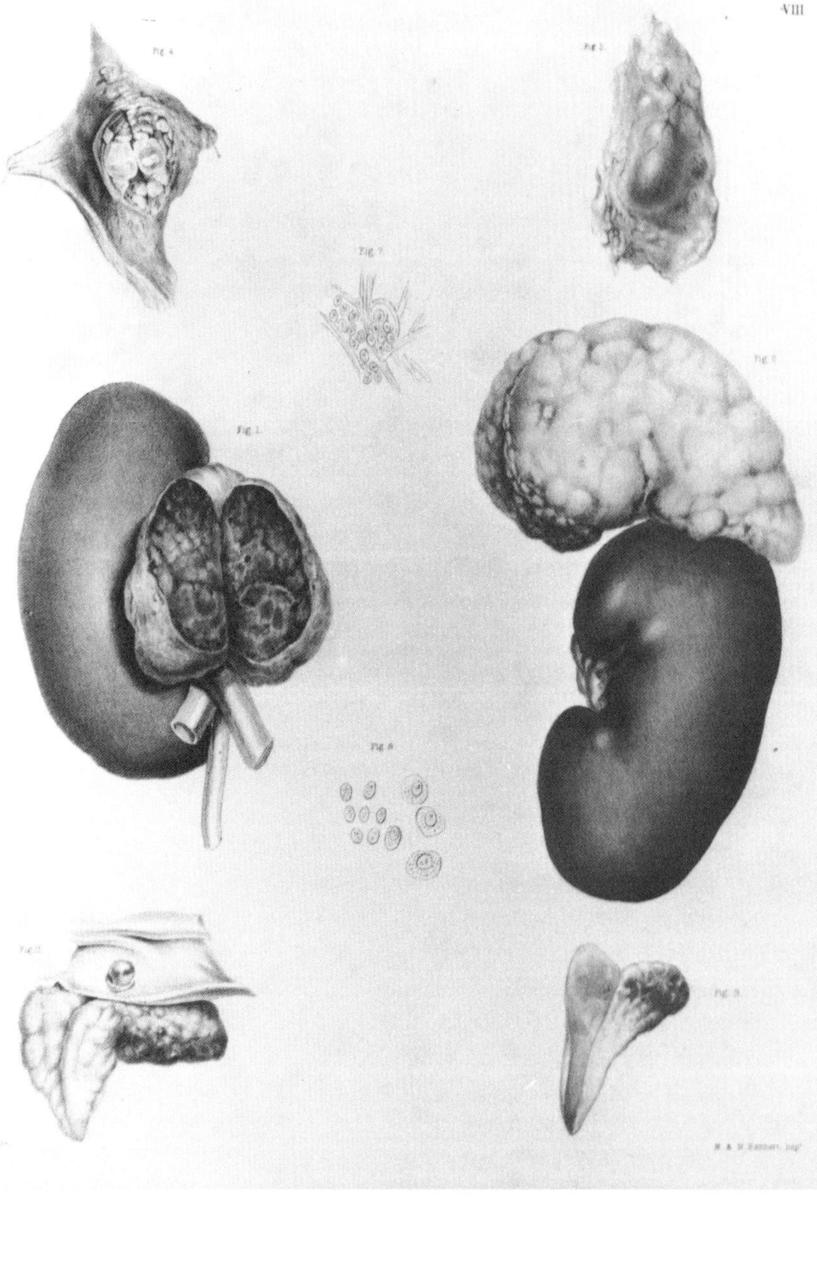

# Thomas Addison

## DISEASE OF THE SUPRA-RENAL CAPSULES

After receiving a medical degree from the University of Edinburgh in 1815, Addison (1793-1860) joined the staff of Guy's Hospital in London, where he was Richard Bright's colleague as physician and lecturer on medicine. He was a man of masterful but cold and haughty personality, more interested in the diagnosis of disease than in the treatment of his patients. It was even said that "he sometimes forgot to prescribe"! Understandably, his practice never became large, and he was able to spend most of his time in teaching and in pathologic research. He had many medical interests. For example, he was the coauthor of the first English book on poisons, he first described xanthoma, and he was a pioneer in the use of static electricity in the treatment of neuromuscular disorders. Addison and Bright collaborated in writing an elementary textbook on medical practice but did not complete it.

Addison is best known for his brilliant clinical accounts of pernicious anemia and Addison's disease. He first defined the syndrome of pernicious anemia to the South London Medical Society in 1849, although no formal report was printed. Later in the same year, he contributed a paper to the *London Medical Gazette* in which he described cases of pernicious anemia (until recently called "Addisonian pernicious anemia"). In the same paper, he presented three cases of weakness and pigmentation in which postmortem examination revealed destruction of the adrenal glands. He revised and expanded this paper and published the new version as a slim monograph, *Disease of the Supra-Renal Capsules,* six years later when he was sixty years old. At that time, Addison's account of the condition he called "melasma suprarenale" was regarded as a scientific curiosity, but its importance to medical practice was soon realized, and his discussion of the "suprarenal syndrome" became a foundation stone of modern endocrinology. Trousseau, his famous contemporary and a generous interpreter of other men's ideas, gave the syndrome the name "Addison's disease."

This notable book is based on a series of detailed histories of eleven cases and is illustrated with accurate but rather coarsely drawn full-page colored plates.

Thomas Addison. *On the Constitutional and Local Effects of Disease of the Supra-Renal Capsules*. London, 1855.

The adrenal disorders illustrated in Addison's monograph include fungoid and cancerous growths. This black-and-white reproduction is far less striking than the original colored drawings.

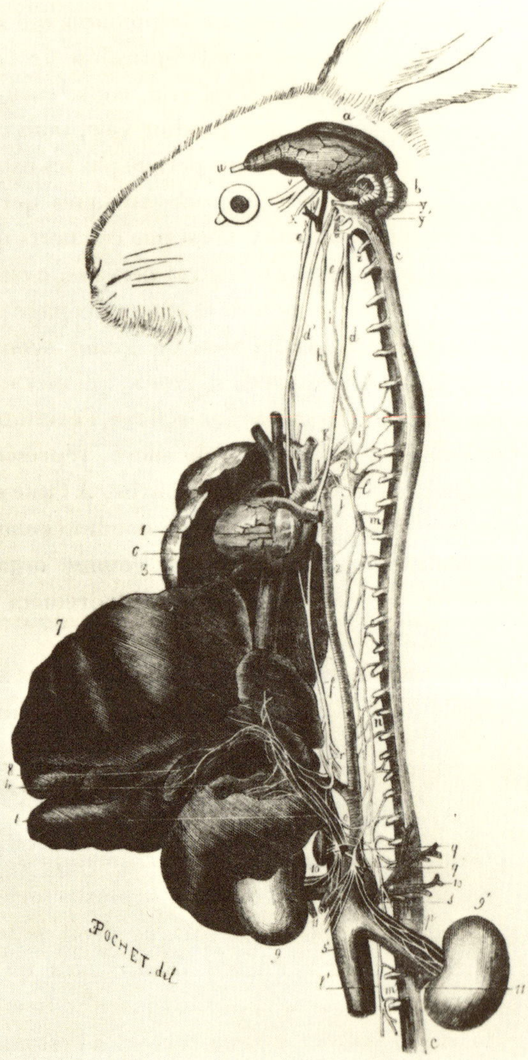

**Fig. 18.** ***Appareil nerveux cérébro-spinal et splanchnique du Lapin, pour montrer les rapports nerveux qui existent entre le foie, le poumon et le rein, et pour comprendre le mécanisme du diabète artificiel.***

# Claude Bernard

## EXPERIMENTAL PHYSIOLOGY

Claude Bernard (1813-1878) was the pupil of and assistant to François Magendie, whom he succeeded as professor at the Collège de France in 1855. There he continued Magendie's physiologic research with even greater intellectual power. He had started as a pharmacist's assistant in Lyons and, before qualifying as a physician, had had some success as a poet and playwright. The greatest of French physiologists, Bernard was the first scientist in his country to be honored with a public funeral at the cathedral of Notre-Dame de Paris.

Bernard combined Magendie's objectivity with enormous curiosity about the facts uncovered. That attitude is well summed up in his own words: "Put off your imagination, as you take off your overcoat, when you enter the laboratory; but put it on again, as you do your overcoat, when you leave the laboratory. Before the experiment and between whiles, let your imagination wrap you round; put it right away from you during the experiment itself lest it hinder your observing power." A contemporary of Charcot, Pasteur, Virchow, Addison, and Darwin, he lived during a period of intense scientific ferment.

His classic book on experimental physiology laid the foundation for today's understanding of physiology, metabolism, and endocrinology. It was based on his lectures, which were given in two courses in 1854 and 1855. In the first, after a preliminary exposition of the indivisibility of physiologic and pathologic research, Bernard described his investigation of glucose production, with special reference to diabetes. He had studied the chemistry of the liver and the blood and announced his discovery of the glycogenic function of the liver. The second course discussed the mechanical and chemical aspects of digestion, with emphasis on the chemistry and the digestive role of saliva and the properties and function of the pancreas.

Bernard introduced the concept of "internal secretions" and showed that all the relevant organs of the body cooperate in the general functions. He later elaborated his concept of the *"milieu intérieur."* His subsequent lecture courses presented his discoveries on the effect of poisons, the pathology and physiology of the nervous system (particularly of the vasomotor nerves), body fluids, and anesthesia. Much of our understanding of diabetes, gastrointestinal physiology, and, especially, the experimental method in science stems from Claude Bernard.

Claude Bernard. *Leçons de physiologie expérimentale appliquée à la médecine.* 2 vols. Paris, 1855-1856.

Here Bernard pictures the rabbit to illustrate a facet of diabetes; the drawing shows the cerebrospinal and splanchnic nerves and demonstrates the relationship of the liver, lung, and kidney.

265.—Nerves of the Left Upper Extremity. Front View.

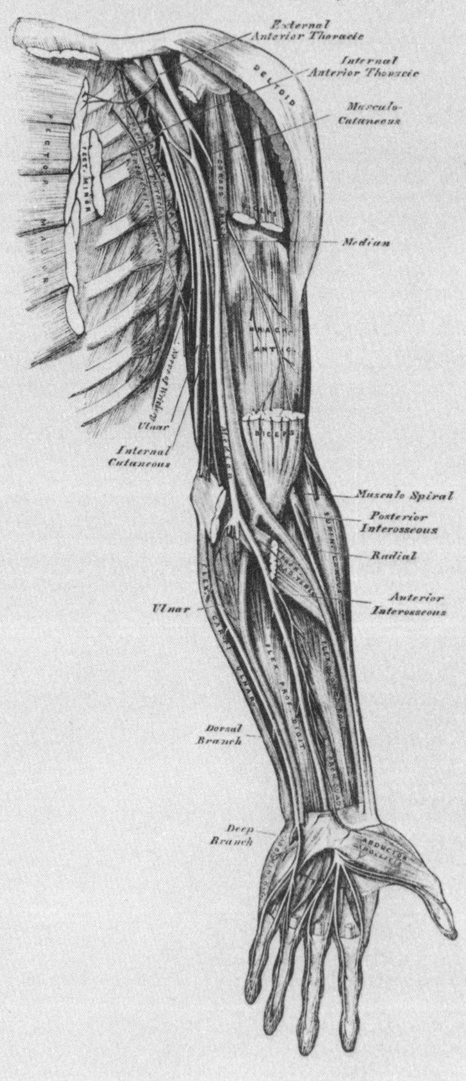

# Henry Gray

## ANATOMY, DESCRIPTIVE AND SURGICAL

Gray (1825-1861) was thirty-three when he wrote his *Anatomy,* which since then has been extensively revised and remains the standard handbook on this subject for English-speaking students. The work was superior to other treatises on anatomy in three areas—the lucid and logical arrangement of a mass of detailed description; clear new drawings based on dissections by the surgeon-author and the artist, a physician; and sections on the surgical anatomy of defined areas, such as the axilla, the elbow, the popliteal space, the perineum, and the laryngotracheal region. Even today, the book is considered a standard reference on anatomy; the thirtieth edition appeared in 1949.

Gray was a surgeon who was engaged chiefly in anatomic research and teaching at St. George's Hospital in London. He had published original studies on the ocular and auditory nerves, on the development of the retina and the labyrinth, and on the adrenals, the thyroid, the thymus, and the spleen. By discussing the embryologic development of these glands and classifying them as ductless, he laid a foundation for the specialty of endocrinology. He was awarded the triennial prizes of the Royal College of Surgeons for his research on the optic nerve and the spleen. Later, he became interested in pathology but unfortunately died of smallpox at the age of thirty-five.

The physician-artist who assisted Gray in his dissections was Henry Vandyke Carter. Among the superb drawings he prepared for "Gray's *Anatomy"* are those of the muscles of the hand, the superficial lymphatics of the head, the upper surface of the tongue, the nerves of the nasal septum, and the mucous membrane of the stomach. Most of these illustrations were reproduced in later editions. Carter outlived Gray by thirty-six years and died in 1897. He enjoyed a distinguished career as a physician and research worker in India.

Henry Gray. *Anatomy, Descriptive and Surgical.* London, 1858.

This drawing by H. Vandyke Carter
has served medical students for more than a century.
It appeared in the original edition of Gray's *Anatomy* and is
retained, virtually unchanged, in the 1966 edition.

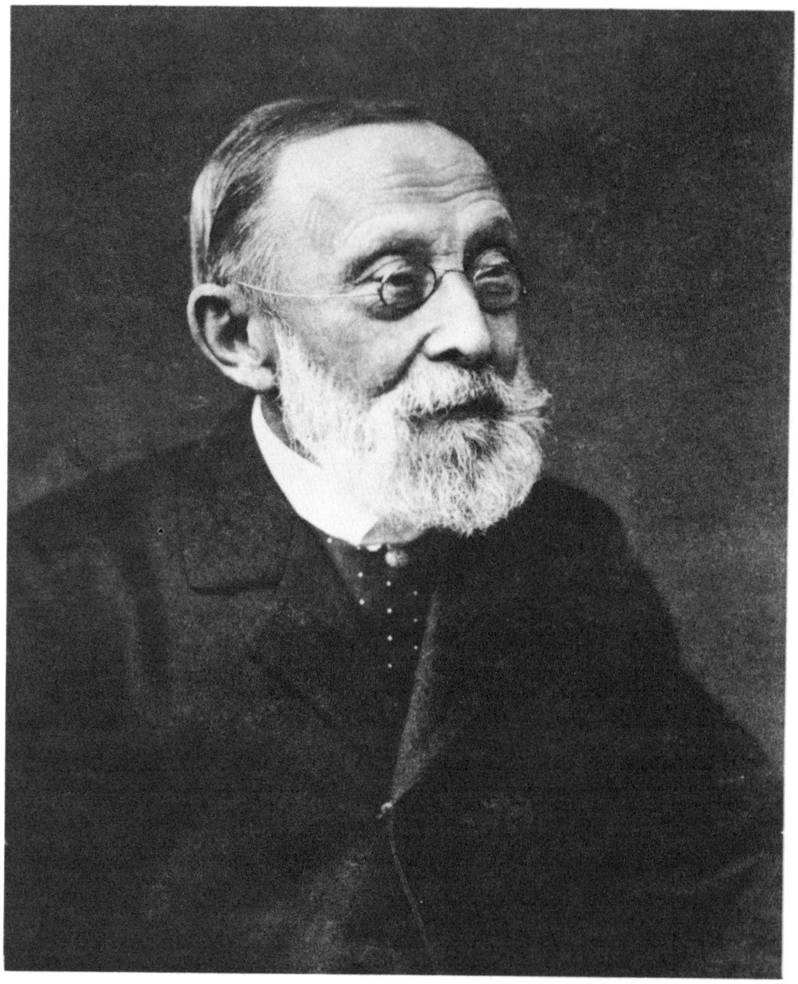

# Rudolf Virchow

## CELLULAR PATHOLOGY

Virchow (1821-1902) was one of the greatest medical men of the nineteenth century, excelling as teacher, physiologist, pathologist, and practical hygienic expert, with an added interest in anthropology. He was an active politician whose liberal sympathies led him into trouble with the authorities in 1848, the year of abortive revolution. Because of this, he had to resign his position at the University of Berlin and leave the city. He was forgiven later, asked to return, made professor of pathology at the university, and given the directorship of the Pathologic Institute, a position created for him. He served as a member of the Reichstag from 1880 to 1893.

Virchow's impressive list of achievements includes his observations and definitions of leukocytosis and leukemia and his descriptions of the many types of thrombosis and embolism, which he saw as a sequel to phlebitis.

This book was the foundation of all subsequent work in pathology. Virchow accepted the theory of the cellular structure of living tissue that had been advanced by Schwann but disagreed with his concepts of protoplasm, the cytoblast, and the origin of cells. He enunciated the dictum that "every cell arises from a cell" and regarded the body as "a cell-state in which every cell is a citizen," disease being "merely a conflict of citizens in this state, brought about by the action of external forces."

The book was based on twenty lectures delivered in April, 1858, at the Pathologic Institute. Beginning with a survey of the development of the cell theory from Bichat to Schwann, Virchow discussed the physiology and pathology of tissues in general and went on to describe the cellular conditions of disease processes in nutrition, circulation, the blood and lymph, and the nervous system. In addition, he dealt with the cellular basis of disturbances of function, irritability of tissues, fatty degeneration and metamorphosis, inflammation, normal and pathologic regeneration, and the character of regenerated tissue. The book was revised several times, without marked alteration, and was translated into English by Frank Chance in 1860.

Late in his life, many honors were bestowed on Virchow. He dedicated the Pathologic Museum in 1899 and gave it his personal collection of more than twenty-three thousand specimens, each of which he had personally prepared and labeled. On his eightieth birthday he received a gold medal from Kaiser Wilhelm II and, shortly before he died in 1902, witnessed the completion of the new Berlin municipal hospital, which is named for him.

Rudolf Virchow. *Die Cellularpathologie in ihrer Begründung auf physiologische und pathologische Gewebelehre.* Berlin, 1858.

"A Life Filled with Toil and Work Is Not a Burden, but a Blessing," the title of Virchow's graduation thesis, was a prophetic statement of his philosophy and dedication.

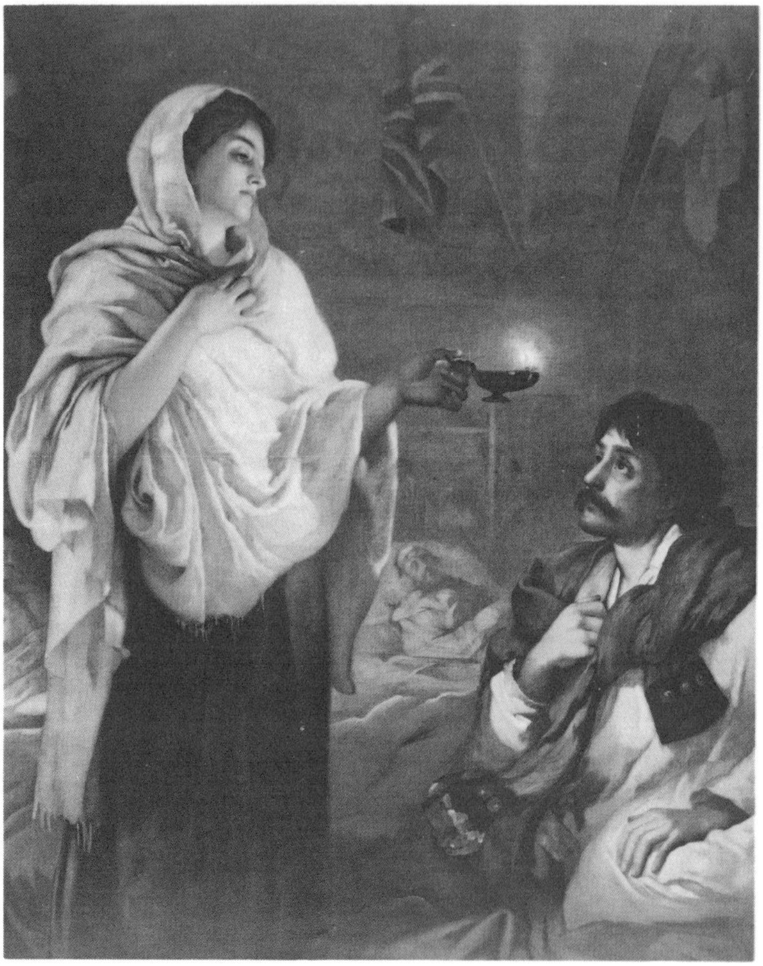

# Florence Nightingale

## NOTES ON NURSING

Florence Nightingale's seventy-nine-page monograph, *Notes on Nursing,* reflects the intelligence, efficiency, and administrative talent of the woman who inaugurated the professional training of nurses in England and, indirectly, in the United States. As a young woman, she had sought the best training for a nursing career then available. She chose the Institute of Protestant Deaconesses at Kaiserswerth, Germany, where she learned both nursing and hospital and training-school administration.

The need for radical reform in the care of the sick was made evident to Miss Nightingale (1820-1910) not only through her work in a London hospital but also through service in the barracks hospital in Scutari during the Crimean War.

So effectively did she cut through ancient regulations in establishing a clean and efficiently run army hospital that, on her return to England, she was asked to establish a training school for nurses. The school opened at St. Thomas's Hospital in 1860 with fifteen probationers, who lived at the hospital and were instructed by staff and visiting physicians. Graduates of the school were much sought after; many of them subsequently started nursing schools in England and the United States.

*Notes on Nursing* was written with simplicity and direct common sense, enlivened by occasional sharp wit. After an introductory chapter in which she stated that "nursing ought to assist the reparative process of disease," she discussed the conditions necessary for good nursing: ventilation and warmth; the "health of the house," or domestic hygiene; management ("being in charge means that the work you do is not undone when your back is turned"); freedom from noise; selection of food; bed and bedding; personal cleanliness and the cleanliness of rooms and walls; and observation of the sick. In conclusion, she pointed out that her rules for nursing the sick applied even more to the care of children and puerperant women. In an appendix, she added statistics on the number of nurses employed at that time in England.

A disciple of the pioneer Belgian statistician, Adolphe Quetelet, Florence Nightingale supported all her writings with statistical evidence; she was the first to display this material in colored diagrams with proportioned areas. *Notes on Nursing* is one of the seminal books of the modern world. It was published a few weeks after another significant work, Darwin's *Origin of Species.*

Florence Nightingale. *Notes on Nursing: what it is, and what it is not.* London, 1859.

Henrietta Rae's romantic painting shows Florence Nightingale caring for a wounded soldier of the Crimean War at an army hospital. As a hospital administrator, she introduced sweeping improvements in military nursing services.

the tube, and held there by the left hand of the surgeon, one end of the explorer is to be placed in his mouth, and the other in the catheter, and held there also by the left hand. With his right hand thus left at liberty, the surgeon is now to take the *otoscope* and introduce one end of it into the ear of the patient, who may hold it there, the other end being held by the surgeon in his own ear; or the tube may be made so light as to

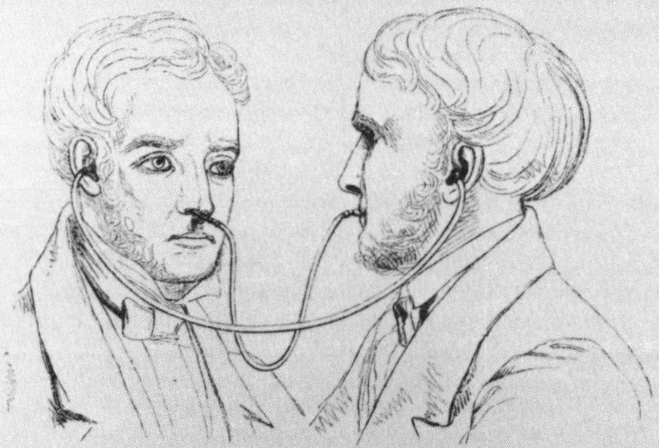

THE SURGEON USING THE EUSTACHIAN CATHETER AND THE EXPLORER.

remain there without being held, leaving the operator's right hand still free.

The medical man next proceeds to blow air gently through the explorer, at the same time that he listens through the otoscope to ascertain whether the air enters the ear, and if it does, what is the peculiar sound it produces. When the tympanum is unobstructed by mucus, the air is heard to pass in a stream against the inner surface of the membrana tympani, but when mucus is present, a peculiar gurgling is heard; and if the mucous membrane itself is thickened, a peculiar squeak or bubbling is also perceptible. It is not advisable to blow with force into the ear, but rather to make a few gentle successive puffs, attentively listening during each, to detect the kind of sound that may be heard in the tympanum. Sometimes no air enters, the mucous membrane being too thick to allow it to pass; and, under such circumstances, it is unwise to attempt to force

# Joseph Toynbee

## THE DISEASES OF THE EAR

Joseph Toynbee (1815-1866) had been a pupil of Benjamin Brodie, surgeon and physiologist; his own first paper, written at the age of twenty-one, was on the physiology of the ears. He wrote this practical treatise after he had spent eight years as aural surgeon at St. Mary's Hospital, London. During the previous two decades, he had published a series of reports on his clinical and pathologic observations, including those made during some two thousand dissections. A list of these papers appeared in his book.

From careful autopsies of the deaf, Toynbee was able to establish the association of several hearing problems (including various types of deafness) with specific lesions in parts of the external, middle, and inner ear. He was the first to describe immobilization of the foot-plate of the stapes and the accompanying clinical symptoms of what is now called "otosclerosis"; this laid the foundation for its cure by fenestration. He also made a great contribution to therapy of deafness with his invention of an artificial drum with which he was able to replace a chronically immobilized or perforated membrana tympani. This remained in wide use until comparatively recently, when it was superseded by the modern tympanoplasty operation.

This book's nineteen chapters detail the structure and function of each part of the ear, with accounts of its diseases and indications for treatment, illustrated by case histories. The surgical procedures are particularly well presented, and Toynbee reported on a new operation for removal of the temporal bone. The treatise was intended to be useful rather than encyclopedic and was the first one of merit since Jean-Marc-Gaspard Itard published his French treatise on diseases of the ear in 1821. Earlier studies of the ear had been done largely by Italians, but there was a wider awakening of interest in the 1860's. Ménière in France and von Tröltsch, Helmholtz, and Politzer in Germany and Austria all contributed new knowledge immediately after Toynbee's significant book appeared.

Toynbee was a man of deeply felt sociologic interests, active in improving the health and housing of the poor. He died tragically in 1866, at the age of fifty-one, during an experiment he performed on himself with the then-new chloroform anesthesia.

Joseph Toynbee. *The Diseases of the Ear: Their Nature, Diagnosis, and Treatment.* London, 1860.

In this drawing from Toynbee's book, the patient on the left and the physician on the right demonstrate a method of diagnosing an obstruction of the eustachian tube.

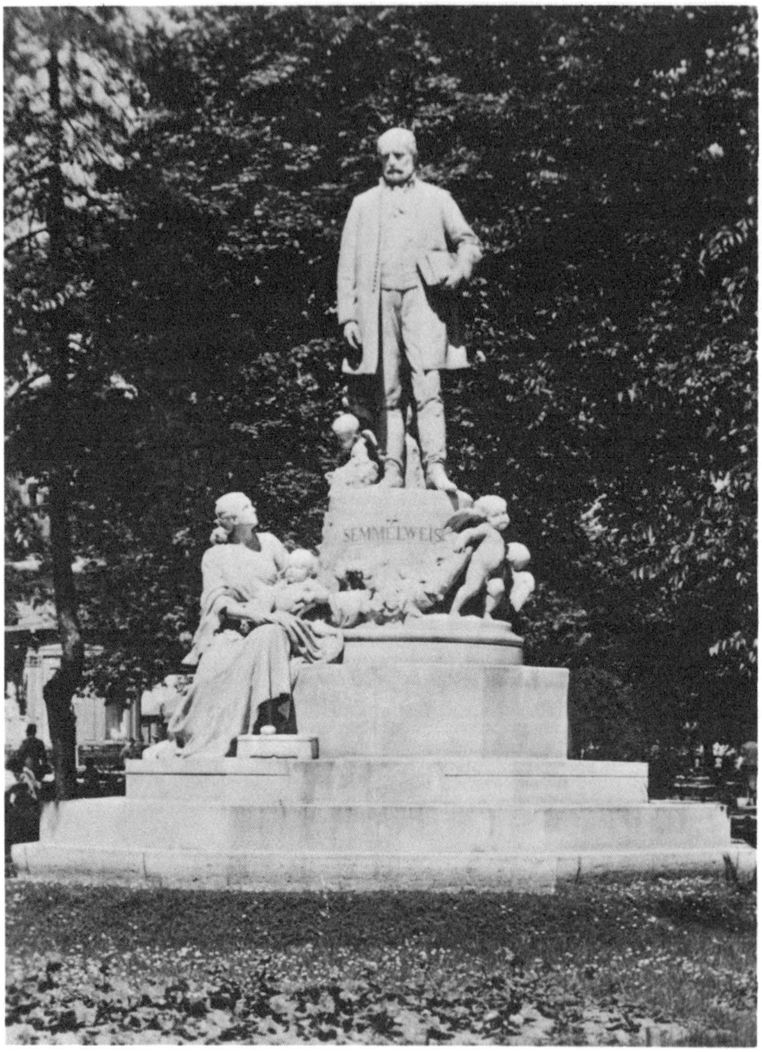
SEMMELWEIS

# Ignaz Philipp Semmelweis

## THE ETIOLOGY OF CHILDBED FEVER

In the 1840's, Semmelweis (1818-1865), a young Hungarian assistant in the obstetric clinic at the General Hospital in Vienna, noted a startling difference between the mortalities of the hospital's two maternity wards. In 1847, the mortality of the first ward, which was staffed by medical students who moved freely from the morgue to the maternity wards, was 11.4 percent; in the second ward, staffed by midwives, who were not permitted to work in the morgue, the mortality was 2.7 percent. Semmelweis reasoned that puerperal fever was brought into the first ward by the medical students, who had been conducting postmortem examinations on cadavers in the morgue.

A twelve-month trial was initiated to test his thesis. During that time, the medical students were required to wash their hands in a chlorinated lime solution before touching or examining a pregnant woman. At the end of the test period, the mortality in the first ward had declined strikingly and was slightly lower than that in the second ward.

Semmelweis was not only a pioneer of asepsis in obstetrics; he recognized that puerperal fever is a form of septicemia. He was not the first to point out that puerperal fever is contagious; Oliver Wendell Holmes, in America, had read a paper on the contagiousness of puerperal fever to the Boston Society for Medical Improvement in 1843. Holmes and Semmelweis apparently did not know of each other's work.

Semmelweis's theory was violently resisted by many orthodox obstetricians of the day, just as that of Holmes had been opposed in America. So strong was the opposition to Semmelweis that he returned to Hungary, where he became professor of obstetrics at the University of Pest and director of St. Rochus Hospital. In 1861, almost fifteen years after he had begun to document his observations, he published his treatise on "The Cause, Treatment, and Prophylaxis of Puerperal Fever."

Unfortunately, nearly half of the long book consists of a controversial survey of other men's opinions of his work. He pursued the controversy in his scathing "Open Letters to Sundry Professors of Obstetrics," which appeared in three pamphlets in 1861. (Two of these exceedingly rare items are also in the Lilly Library.)

The rejection, opposition, and controversy were more than Semmelweis could bear. In 1865, when he was forty-seven, friends committed him to a mental hospital in Vienna. There he died within two weeks from a dissection wound. Ironically, his death has been attributed to septicemia, a variant of the disease he had tried to eradicate during his professional life.

Ignaz Philipp Semmelweis. *Die Aetiologie, der Begriff und die Prophylaxis des Kindbettfiebers*. Pest, Vienna, and Leipzig, 1861.

A monument in Budapest commemorates Semmelweis's contribution to the life and health of childbearing women. Many had died of puerperal fever before Semmelweis's theories of asepsis were finally accepted.

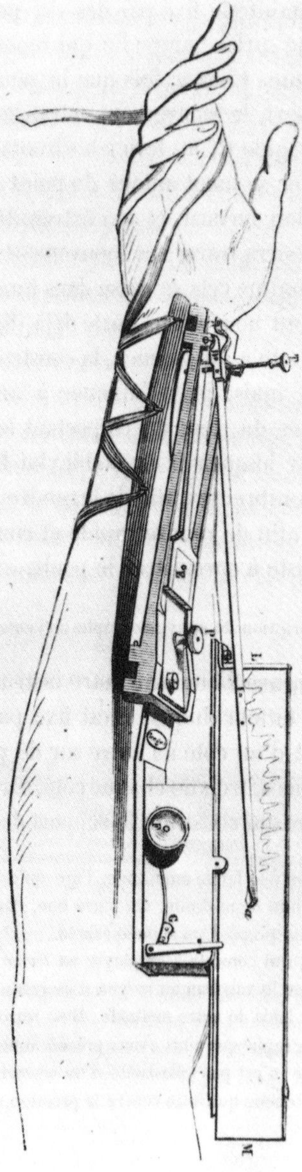

Fig. 23.

# Etienne-Jules Marey

## THE PHYSIOLOGY OF CIRCULATION

Marey's work on blood circulation in relation to the diagnosis of vascular disease followed that of the Weber brothers in Germany and J.-L.-M. Poiseuille in France, who had begun to study the hydrodynamics of blood flow and pressure. Their instruments had been improved by Carl Ludwig, inventor of the kymograph, and Karl Vierordt, who applied graphic methods to study of the pulse.

Marey (1830-1904), in Paris, built on these foundations and, in 1860, described an improved sphygmograph. The instrument was portable and, by use of a stylus of the lightest possible weight, minimized errors from inertia in the recording system. Separate prints of his article are now excessively rare, but the description of his apparatus was included in "Medical Physiology of the Circulation of the Blood" *(Physiologie médicale de la circulation du sang)*, published in 1863 when he was thirty-three.

Marey is remembered also for discovering the cardiovascular reflex that has been named for him. In explaining the reflex, he stated that the heart rate is inversely proportional to the blood pressure in the arch of the aorta and in the carotid sinus.

This book was, he wrote, "an attempt to determine the influence of respiration on blood pressure and flow, reconciling the opinions of Ludwig and Vierordt, since opposite effects can be produced by respiration according to the state of the lungs." He described "apparatus and experiments for recording the heart movements," including his cardiograph and his sphygmograph, which was an improvement on Vierordt's instrument. He also supplied much new information about the distribution of heat by the circulating blood, with an explanation of the equilibrium of body temperature. He reported on changes of color and temperature in the superficial organs, showed that the pulse varies according to the arterial tension, and discussed changes of frequency in the heartbeat, claiming that improved methods of diagnosing vascular disease were provided by his research, in which he made experimental heart lesions in animals and artificial working models.

The book includes the first graphic records of the pulse, and for it Marey was awarded a medical prize in 1864 by the Academy of Sciences. He published another large book on circulation (*La Circulation du sang à l'état physiologique et dans les maladies*) in 1881 but meanwhile became more interested in animal movement, on which he wrote three important monographs in 1867, 1873, and 1894.

Etienne-Jules Marey. *Physiologie médicale de la circulation du sang.* Paris, 1863.

Marey's device for recording pulse waves used smoked paper for the tracing.

Fig. 25.

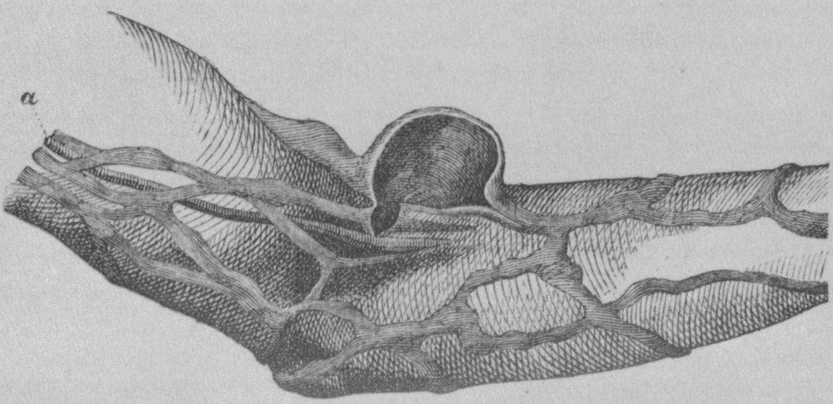


Varix aneurysmaticus. a. Art. brachialis; nach Bell. Froriep, Chirurg. Kupfert. Bd. III. Taf. 263.

Fig. 26.

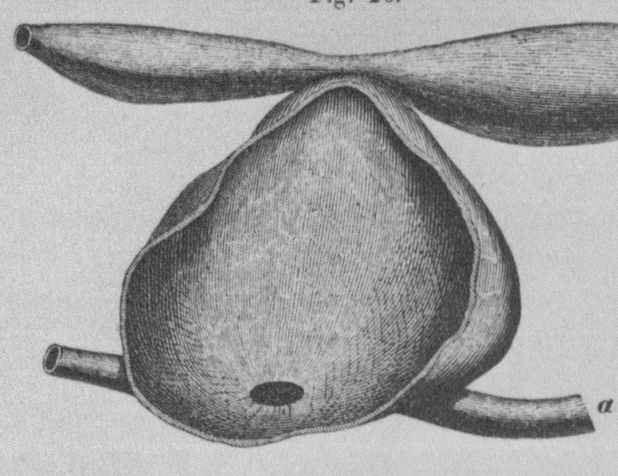


Aneurysma varicosum. a. Art. brachialis. b. Ven. mediana. Der aneurysmatische Sack ist aufgeschnitten; nach Dorsey. Froriep, Chir. Kupfert. Bd. III. Taf. 263.

# Theodor Billroth

## GENERAL SURGICAL PATHOLOGY AND THERAPEUTICS

Billroth (1829-1894) graduated from the University of Göttingen in 1852 and showed interest in many branches of medicine before he settled into a career of surgery and pathologic anatomy. He was also an accomplished artist and musician. Three years after he had been appointed professor of surgery at Zürich in 1860, he published his course of lectures on surgical pathology and treatment in this "handbook for students and doctors," a work that was translated into many languages.

Billroth was particularly concerned with wound infections and discussed the surgical care of various classes of injuries and the diseases of the tissues arising from them. The book is arranged in twenty chapters that encompass the subject matter of fifty lectures. It describes the pathology and cure of all sorts of lesions and is exceptionally complete.

In 1867, Billroth moved to Vienna, where he was professor of surgery for more than twenty years. There he raised the medical school to a new peak of fame and taught many students who became leading surgeons of the next generation. He was a pioneer in surgery of the gastro-intestinal tract and devised gastric operations for resection of the intestine in ulcers and in carcinomas of the stomach, surgical techniques that now bear his name. He was also the first surgeon to resect the esophagus and the first to perform a total laryngectomy.

Curiously, this methodical man did not readily accept Lister's findings and only belatedly appreciated the significance of the new science of bacteriology in relation to surgical sepsis.

In addition to medicine, Billroth made contributions to the arts both as a poet and a composer. His charming *Briefe* was written as a memorial to his lifelong friend, the composer Johannes Brahms, with whom he had played chamber music.

Billroth's book is regarded as important because, more than any other, it linked the practice of surgery to the study of pathologic anatomy. No one else had so carefully studied the tissues removed surgically, and his operations truly earned their description as "autopsies *in vivo,*" a phrase that was coined in compliment.

Theodor Billroth. *Die allgemeine chirurgische Pathologie und Therapie*. . . . Berlin, 1863.

Billroth is usually identified with gastrointestinal surgery. However, he is also recognized for significant contributions linking surgery with pathologic anatomy, as he does in this drawing of an aneurysm.

person down to the lower edge of it, *c c*, whether for a digital or speculum examination. Afterwards the patient moves again up on the centre or seat of the chair, the uprights, *a*, *a*, are drawn back, and the chair almost voluntarily assumes its proper form.

For a speculum examination the patient is to lie on the left side. The thighs are to be flexed at about right angles with the pelvis, the right being drawn up a little more than the left. The left arm is thrown behind across the back, and the chest rotated forwards, bringing the sternum very nearly in contact with the table, while the spine is fully extended, with the head resting on the left parietal bone. The head must not be flexed on the sternum nor the right shoulder elevated. Indeed, the position must simulate that on the knees as much as

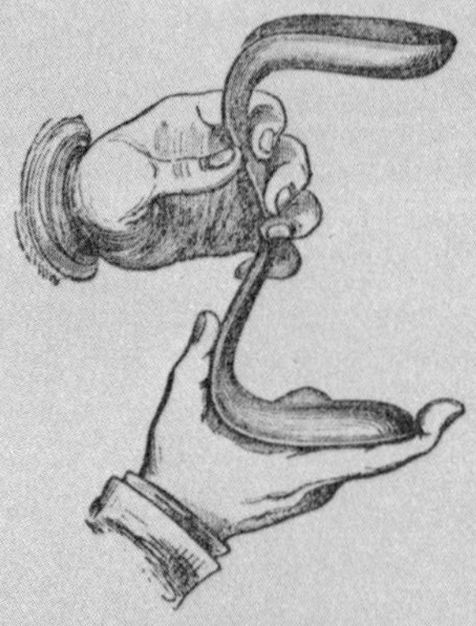

FIG. 8.

possible, and for this reason the patient is rolled over on the front, making it a left lateral semiprone position. The nurse or assistant standing at her back pulls up the

# James Marion Sims

## UTERINE SURGERY

Sims (1813-1883), a graduate of Jefferson Medical College in Philadelphia, became the founder of modern gynecologic surgery in the United States. His operative techniques were perfected when, as a young man practicing in Alabama, he undertook to treat slave girls suffering from vesicovaginal fistula. He applied his new methods in curing these young women who, without his attention, would have been allowed to die. The operation for closure of vesicovaginal fistula, in which he used silver wire sutures, has been named for him.

He moved to New York in 1853 and there distinguished himself as the leading gynecologic surgeon. In 1861, he introduced his operation for amputation of the uterine cervix and later invented the duckbill vaginal speculum, which was also named for him. In addition, he discovered that the left lateral position—Sims's position—is more convenient for gynecologic procedures than the knee-chest position. The speculum, this position, and a good light, he wrote, "are all that are necessary for obtaining an accurate view of the parts. If the vagina and outlet are ordinarily capacious, a good strong northern light, of a clear day, from a large solitary window, is all-sufficient. But if this canal has been narrowed by cicatrices after extensive sloughs, or from other causes, then sunlight is absolutely necessary for every stage of the operation from first to last."

During the War between the States, Sims, a Southern sympathizer, was in Europe. "In 1862," he wrote, "I voluntarily left my own country, on account of its political troubles." He introduced his successful methods in London and Paris, where he was entertained by Napoleon III and had the Empress Eugénie for his patient. "After three years in a most favourable position in the highest circles of practice in Europe," as he wrote in his dedication, he published this masterly account of his work, first in London and then in New York. It was soon translated into German and proved to be a major contribution to gynecology.

The book is written in clear and simple language. After detailing his new method of uterine examination, Sims deals in eight sections with the physiology, anatomy, and surgery of the female pelvic organs, including an account of their pathology and abnormalities and the mechanism of conception. He also records a method of artificial fertilization that he had employed. The book is well illustrated and thoroughly indexed.

James Marion Sims. *Clinical Notes on Uterine Surgery with Special Reference to the Management of the Sterile Condition.* New York, 1866.

Sims fashioned his first duckbill speculum from a bent silver spoon. His contributions to gynecologic surgery were memorialized by a statue placed near the New York Academy of Medicine.

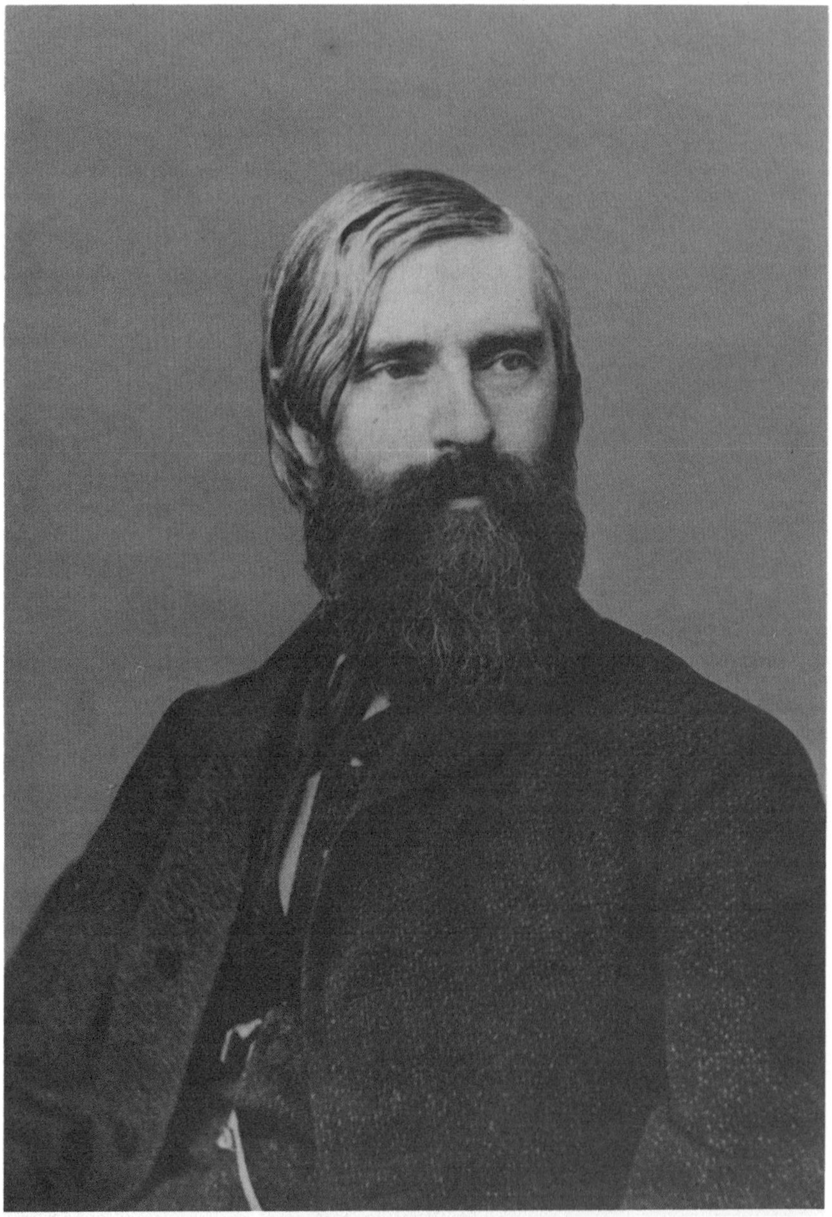

# Albrecht von Graefe

## PARALYSES OF THE EYE MUSCLES

This comparatively short, unillustrated book provided the first thorough account of paralysis of the eye muscles and the basis for their surgical treatment. Albrecht von Graefe (1828-1870), the son of a wealthy surgeon, was educated in Berlin, Prague, Paris, Vienna, and London. He was professor of ophthalmology at the University of Berlin from 1857 until his death from tuberculosis at the early age of forty-two.

Prepared by study in the great medical centers of Europe, he was the leading eye surgeon of his time and introduced many invaluable technical improvements. Owing to his reputation, the ophthalmology clinic at the University of Berlin was frequented by ophthalmologists who came from all over the world to learn about the eye. Nearly all of the notable ophthalmologists of the nineteenth century were included in this group. Most of von Graefe's work was published in the important journal that he founded in 1854, the *Archiv für Ophthalmologie*. The first volume alone contains von Graefe's papers on glaucoma, diphtheritic conjunctivitis, mydriasis, keratoconus, disorders of the oblique eye muscles, and double vision following the operative correction of squint.

"Von Graefe's sign" is the eponymous name given to the tardy and jerky downward movement of the upper eyelids that occurs when exophthalmic goiter patients lower their eyes. A special knife used by ophthalmic surgeons is also named for him. His most significant contributions were iridectomy for glaucoma, a report on conical cornea, and work on the pathogenesis of embolism of the central retinal artery.

The first seventy pages of his book "Paralyses of the Eye Muscles" describe conditions that can result from injuries to the eye muscles and the methods to be used in their diagnosis and in determining the extent of the injury. Special consideration is given to paralytic diplopia. The second part, some hundred pages, outlines the physiologic laws governing eye movements and then details the effects of impaired function in each of the ocular muscles.

Albrecht von Graefe. *Symptomenlehre der Augenmuskellähmungen*. Berlin, 1867.

Portrait of von Graefe. In the forty-two years of his life, he became the greatest of eye surgeons and numbered among his students most of the famous ophthalmologists of the nineteenth century.

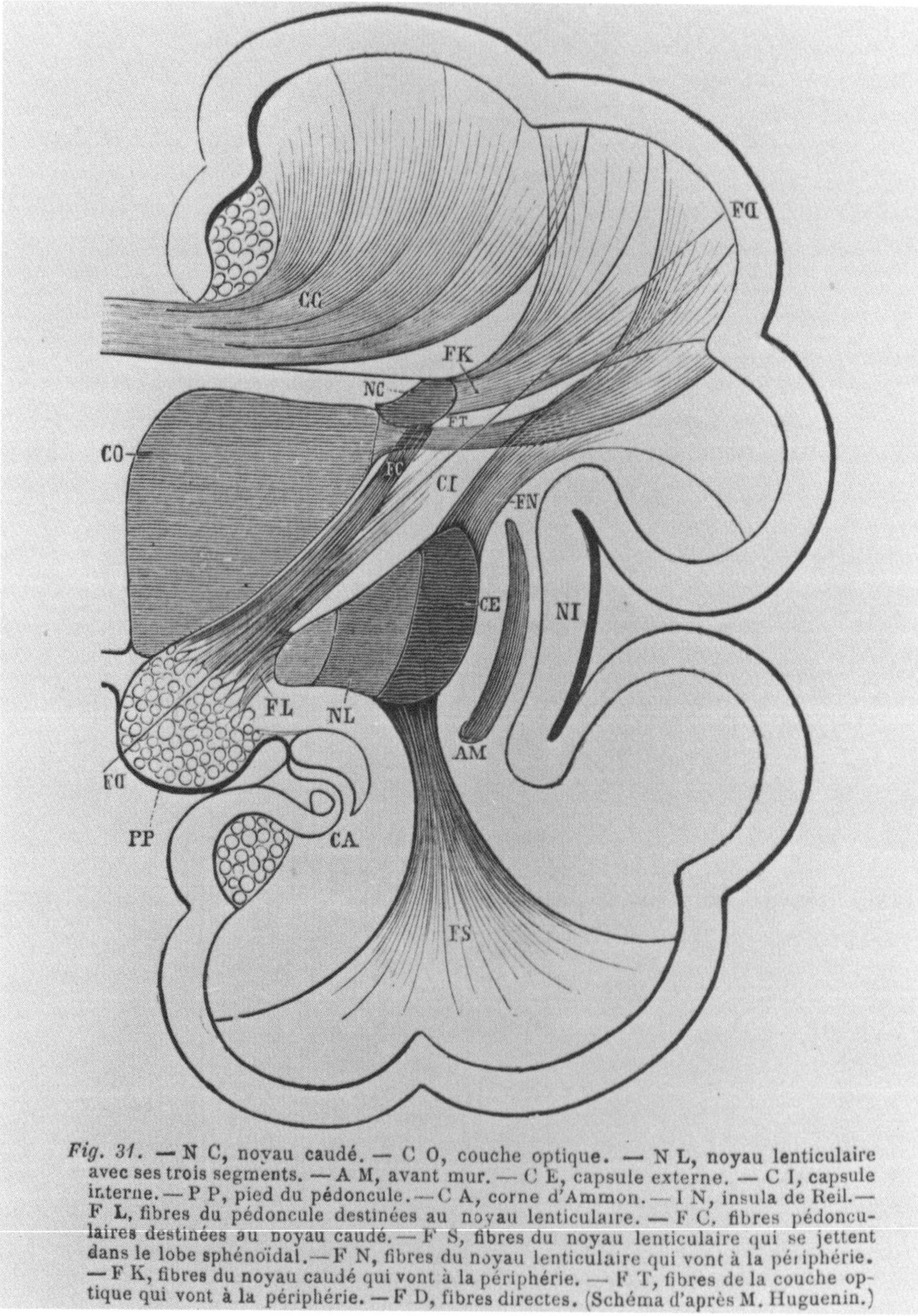


*Fig. 31.* — N C, noyau caudé. — C O, couche optique. — N L, noyau lenticulaire avec ses trois segments. — A M, avant mur. — C E, capsule externe. — C I, capsule interne. — P P, pied du pédoncule. — C A, corne d'Ammon. — I N, insula de Reil. — F L, fibres du pédoncule destinées au noyau lenticulaire. — F C, fibres pédonculaires destinées au noyau caudé. — F S, fibres du noyau lenticulaire qui se jettent dans le lobe sphénoïdal. — F N, fibres du noyau lenticulaire qui vont à la périphérie. — F K, fibres du noyau caudé qui vont à la périphérie. — F T, fibres de la couche optique qui vont à la périphérie. — F D, fibres directes. (Schéma d'après M. Huguenin.)

# Jean-Martin Charcot

## LOCALIZATION OF FUNCTIONS IN CEREBRAL DISEASE

Charcot (1825-1893) was thirty-seven when he was appointed senior physician to the hospital of La Salpêtrière in 1862; in ten years' time, his contributions helped usher in the age of modern neurology. Before his death at the age of sixty-eight, he had transformed La Salpêtrière from a women's prison—an asylum for the aged, infirm, and insane—into the greatest neurologic clinic of modern times.

Although he is remembered primarily for his contributions to neurology, Charcot's first areas of interest were rheumatism, gout, and the diseases of the elderly. At the age of twenty-eight, he completed his doctoral thesis on the differential symptoms and lesions of gout and arthritis. His first professional post at La Salpêtrière was in pathologic anatomy; in 1882, when the department of neurology was created, he became its first professor and chairman and remained in that position until his death eleven years later.

In 1876, Charcot published his work on the localization of functions in cerebral and spinal disease. The book is clinically oriented and deals with such topics as hemiplegia and spinal lesions. Cerebral disorders are discussed in the first part and spinal disorders in the second. Small black-and-white illustrations clarify the text.

Charcot's far-reaching interests and contributions are commemorated in the wide range of clinical entities that bear his name. Among these are the Charcot triad (intention tremor, nystagmus, and staccato speech) that occurs in multiple sclerosis; Charcot's joint, a neuropathic arthropathy seen in diabetic polyneuritis, syringomyelia, and tabes dorsalis, in which articular cartilage and subjacent bone degenerate and result in joint instability; and Charcot-Marie-Tooth disease, or peroneal muscular atrophy.

Charcot brought order into the classification of nervous diseases and was a pioneer in psychotherapy. Freud worked with him for a few months in 1885 and later translated Charcot's lectures into German. Charcot defined hysteria as "a condition induced by purely mental processes"; it depended, he said, on the subject's susceptibility to suggestion and did not arise from organic lesions in the central nervous system.

Not only was Charcot a superb teacher who could mimic tics, spasms, rigidity, and other symptoms for his students, but his skill as a clinician was recognized internationally. He described multiple sclerosis, amyotrophic lateral sclerosis, tabetic arthropathies, and spastic paralysis. Other areas of interest included exophthalmic goiter and intermittent claudication.

Jean-Martin Charcot. *Leçons sur les localisations dans les maladies du cerveau.* Paris, 1876.

This diagram from Charcot's book is one of the early attempts at clarifying the complexities of cerebral neuroanatomy. Charcot's inspired teachings came at a time of rapid ferment in neuropsychiatry.

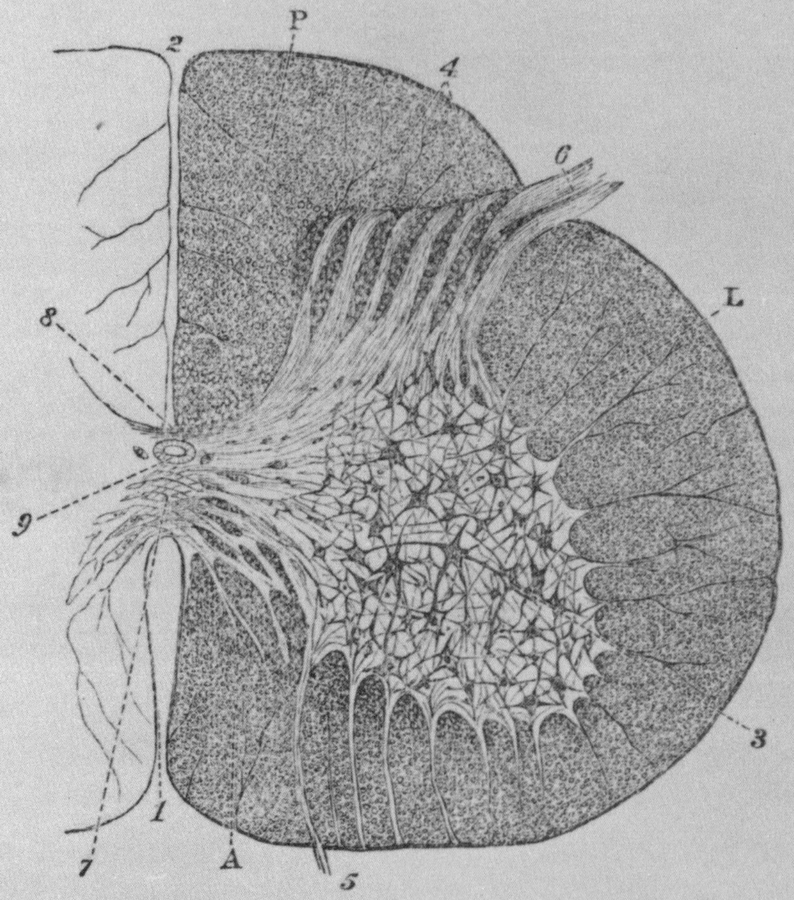


FIG. 2.—Section of Spinal Cord in the Lumbar Region, magnified.—A. The anterior column. L. The lateral column. P. The posterior column. 1. The anterior fissure. 2. The posterior fissure. 3. The anterior cornu with multipolar cells. 4. The posterior cornu, the letters placed on the *substantia gelatinosa*. 5. The anterior roots of the spinal nerve. 6. The posterior roots. 7. The anterior commissure. 8. The posterior commissure. 9. The central canal of the spinal cord lined with epithelium.

# Sir David Ferrier

## THE FUNCTIONS OF THE BRAIN

At the beginning of the nineteenth century, the theory that nervous control of function is localized in special areas of the brain was elaborated, without genuine anatomic evidence, in the pseudoscience of phrenology. Research by Flourens in the 1820's had suggested that such localization was general, not specific. During the 1860's, the problem was explored in England, France, and Germany. The discoveries made there were extensively corroborated by David Ferrier in the 1870's, before he made his own contribution to our knowledge of the central-nervous-system functions.

Born in Scotland, Ferrier (1843-1928) became professor of forensic medicine at King's College, London. In 1873, while working at the West Riding Lunatic Asylum at Wakefield in Yorkshire, he combined clinical observation of nervous diseases with experimental research on many species of animals, utilizing electrical stimulation of the brain cortex. He summarized his work in the Croonian lectures before the Royal Society in 1874. These lectures were ultimately published in his book, which he characterized as "a systematic exposition of the bearing of my own experiments."

The volume consists of thirteen chapters. Ferrier sketched the structure of the brain and then described the functions he had located in its various parts. He discussed the phenomena of electrical irritation, the physiologic and psychologic aspects of the brain hemispheres (including the problem of mind, with aphasia and inhibition), and then the functions of the basal ganglia. He concluded with a diagrammatic survey of cerebral and cranial topography and, from his clinical and pathologic discoveries, noted the homologies between his observations in man and his experimental findings in animals.

His Gulstonian lectures on *The Localization of Cerebral Disease* (1878) provided the clinical and pathologic complement to Ferrier's mainly experimental work, and in 1889 he was appointed to a professorship of neuropathology at King's College. Ultimately, he received a knighthood for his contributions to neurology, which have come to be regarded as the foundation upon which all of our present knowledge concerning the localization of cerebral functions has been built.

David Ferrier. *The Functions of the Brain*. London, 1876.

This magnified section of the spinal cord in the lumbar region shows the anterior and posterior nerve roots. The drawing is from Ferrier's book and accompanies one of the earliest detailed descriptions of the spinal cord.

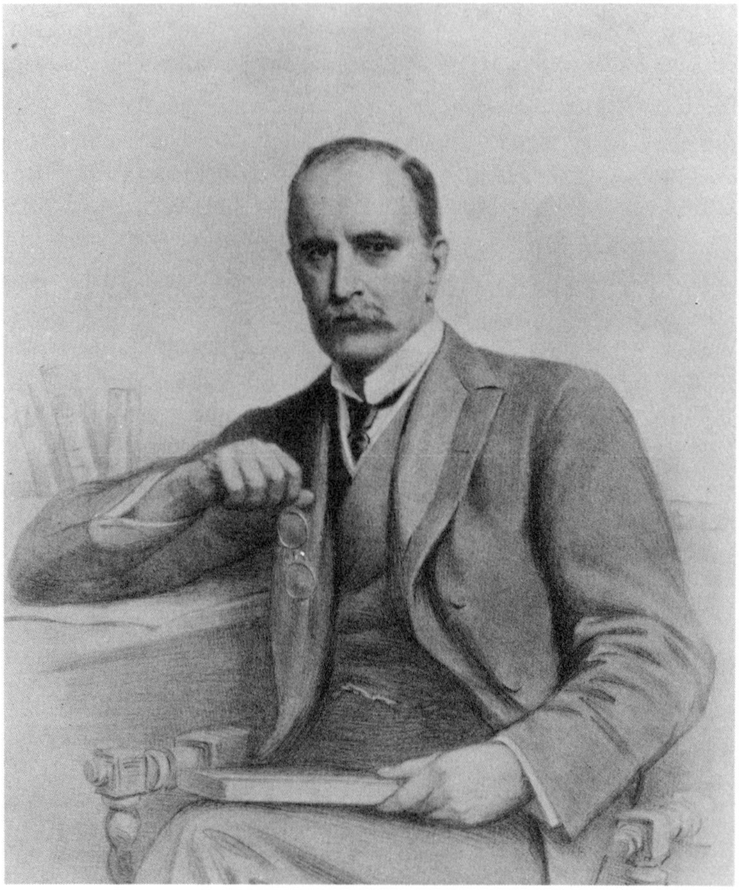

# Sir William Osler

## THE PRINCIPLES AND PRACTICE OF MEDICINE

Osler (1849-1919) was the outstanding physician of the English-speaking world at the end of the nineteenth and the beginning of the twentieth century. Canadian by birth, he trained in medicine at Toronto and McGill universities, taught for twenty years at the University of Pennsylvania and at Johns Hopkins University, and then, during his last fifteen years, was regius professor of medicine at Oxford.

He is remembered as clinician, pathologist, and historian of medicine; the personal magnetism that he exerted on colleagues and pupils was widely spread by his *Principles and Practice of Medicine*. He wrote the book in fourteen months when he was forty-two, and it appeared in February, 1892. Meeting a widely felt need, it provided a rigidly systematized text on internal medicine as well as relevant information from the great advances in the laboratory sciences, particularly bacteriology, that had done so much to revolutionize medicine in the previous decades. Three thousand copies were sold in a month; through triennial revisions, the book became a standard text for students and practitioners over a period of thirty years, not only in English, but also in German, Spanish, French, and Chinese translations. Osler completed the eighth edition in 1912, and further editions were published for many years after his death in 1919. The chapters describe specific diseases by systems, a pattern since followed by most standard textbooks.

Osler is also remembered for his research in infectious and cardiovascular diseases (e.g., Osler's nodes, Osler's disease), as a founding editor of the *Quarterly Journal of Medicine*, and as the author of *Aequanimitas* (1904) and *An Alabama Student* (1908). Both books address themselves to the philosophic, social, and ethical aspects of medical life. While at Oxford, Osler became curator of the Bodleian Library. He was one of the greatest medical book collectors and the first to concentrate attention on the outstandingly influential books of successive centuries. He bequeathed his library to McGill University, Montreal, where he had graduated and held his first professorship.

Osler's warm and charming personality, his great skill as a physician, his innovative restructuring of the medical school curriculum, and his many significant writings have made him the most important figure of his time in both English and North American medicine.

William Osler. *The Principles and Practice of Medicine....* New York, 1892.

This pencil drawing of Osler captures the dignity and stature of the man who has been an unparalleled example and inspiration to the medical students of this century.

FIG. 53.—FACIAL EXPRESSION IN CAVERNOUS SINUS THROMBOSIS.

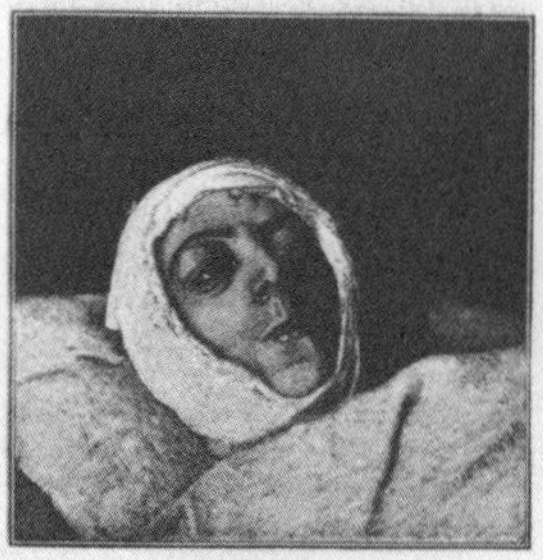

Exophthalmos, with internal strabismus œdema of right eyelids and corresponding side of nose in an early stage of thrombosis of cavernous sinus (Case LII.).

FIG. 54.—FACIAL EXPRESSION IN CAVERNOUS SINUS THROMBOSIS.

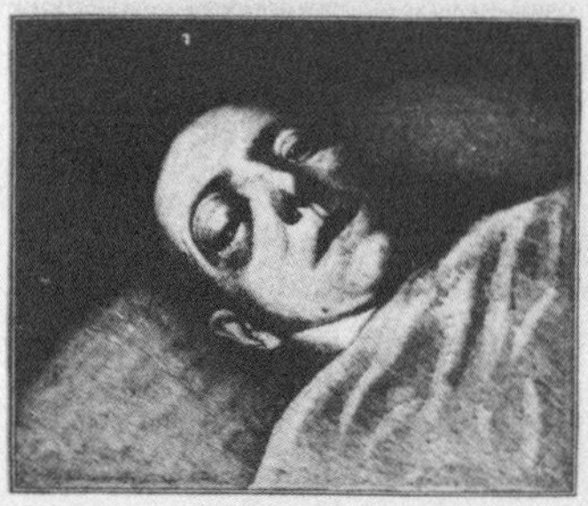

The same as above, a few days later. The œdema of the right eyelids, side of nose, brow, and face has greatly increased. The left eyelids are still free (Case LII.).



the exophthalmos may arise within a few days—occasionally twenty-four hours—and subsides to a marked extent when the collateral circulation is established. It is especially marked when there is ophthalmic phlebitis and retro-orbital abscess (see Case LII.). Œdema of the eyelids and chemosis frequently accompany the exophthalmos originating in thrombosis of the cavernous sinus, and they are due to the same causes as the exophthalmos.[1] "Choked disc" does sometimes arise from

FIG. 55.—FACIAL EXPRESSION IN CAVERNOUS SINUS THROMBOSIS.

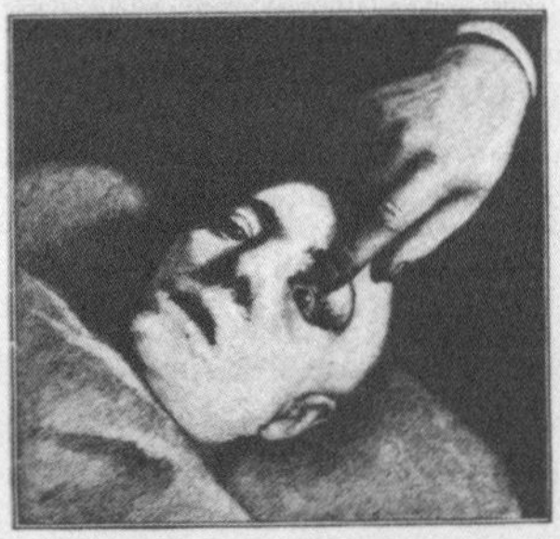

The same patient, later stage. The right eyelids comparatively free from œdema, while the left have become affected to a very marked extent, the œdema extending over brow, face, and neck. Proptosis was also marked (Case LII.).

thrombosis of the cavernous sinus, though it is of course due immediately to obstruction of the retinal and ophthalmic vessels.

Besides these, swelling of an œdematous kind is occasionally found in the pharynx and tonsil on the same side, when the thrombosis in the cavernous sinus has extended into the pterygoid plexus, and possibly into the pharyngeal vessels. Œdema of the corresponding side of the face, due to obstruction of the facial vein, may be seen occasionally, arising from extension of the thrombosis, but may be also due to extraneous causes. In obstruction of the cavernous sinus, which has pursued

[1] In the four cases seen by the author the œdema of the eyelids was distinct along with the exophthalmos, and in all the others there was chemosis, but in variable degrees.

# Sir William Macewen

## PYOGENIC INFECTIVE DISEASES OF THE BRAIN

Sir William Macewen (1848-1924) was professor of surgery at the University of Glasgow and the first surgeon to apply in practice the recent discoveries of Sir David Ferrier and John Hughlings Jackson concerning cerebral localization. In 1876, he made a diagnosis (subsequently proved correct at postmortem examination) of an abscess in the left frontal lobe of a boy. In 1879, he successfully evacuated and excised a hematoma of the brain, and, in a third case, he removed a tumor from the dura mater and another from under it. This was almost certainly a meningioma. By the time of Sir Rickman John Godlee's widely noted excision of a brain tumor in London in November, 1884, Macewen had successfully treated a series of no fewer than seven neurologic cases by surgery.

Before this book was published, he was already well known for his improved treatment of aneurysm, his radical method of curing oblique inguinal hernia, and his use of osteotomy for genu valgum, and he had made successful transplantations of bone. In 1895, he also became a pioneer in the field of thoracic surgery by removing a tuberculous lung.

Macewen begins with a clear account of the surgical anatomy and pathology of the brain, the spinal cord, and their coverings. He goes on to present a description of his new surgical methods and the results obtained in treating pyogenic infections of the meningeal coverings of the brain, sixty-five cases of brain abscess, and infective sinus thrombosis. He comments, "Since the majority of pyogenic infections of the brain arise from neglected otitis media, they ought to be regarded as preventable diseases, and their prophylaxis scrupulously attended to."

The book is a record of triumphant achievement resulting from the most imaginative application of the newest surgical techniques to a region previously considered unreachable. This innovative work was the beginning of the modern specialty of neurosurgery.

William Macewen. *Pyogenic Infective Diseases of the Brain and Spinal Cord: Meningitis, Abscess of Brain, Infective Sinus Thrombosis.* Glasgow, 1893.

This series of photographs shows the development of eye edema in a case of cavernous sinus thrombosis. Macewen's other publications included works on lung surgery and inguinal hernia.

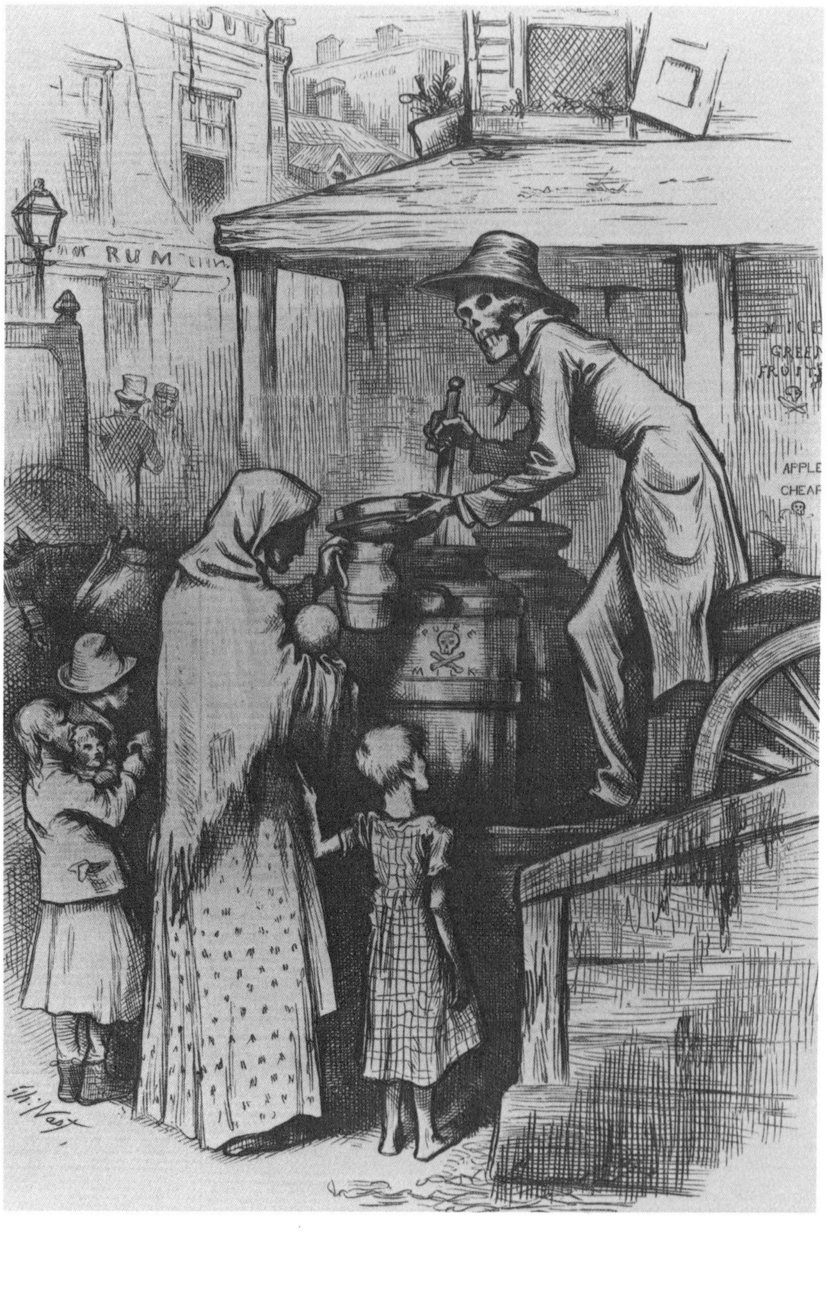
RUM
GREEN
FRUIT
APPLE
CHEAP
PURE MILK

# Luther Emmett Holt

## THE CARE AND FEEDING OF CHILDREN

Holt (1855-1924) exerted an outstanding influence on child health throughout America by his work at the Babies Hospital in New York, where he was physician from 1889 to 1923. At the suggestion of Mrs. Robert Chapin, a patroness of the hospital, he started a training school for nursemaids, providing a course of four to six months that led to a diploma. The basic teaching was described in his small book written for these students as well as for mothers and untrained children's nurses. In it he discusses the differing nutritional needs of the newborn and older infants; the methods whereby cow's milk should be pasteurized and modified to simulate human milk in its concentrations of carbohydrate, protein, and fat; and ways in which cereals and other foods should be introduced with and later given as substitutes for milk. The book achieved an unrivaled popular success and revolutionized child care in the United States. The field of pediatrics was never the same.

Holt was concerned with helping not merely the well-to-do. He campaigned successfully for a pure milk supply in New York City and spent nearly six years between 1890 and 1896 writing a masterly textbook on pediatrics, *The Diseases of Infants and Children,* which remained the best of its kind through many editions and instructed several generations of pediatricians. As professor of the diseases of children at the College of Physicians and Surgeons of New York, Holt exerted a stern but inspiring influence on his students. He brought to the United States in 1908 the new European understanding and surgical treatment of pyloric stenosis, which saved the lives of innumerable infants. In 1918, together with W. H. Howell, he isolated and named heparin from a crude anticoagulant preparation first discovered by Howell's pupil, Jay McLean.

Holt revised *The Care and Feeding of Children* twelve times, expanding it to three times its original length, and the book was translated into many foreign languages.

Luther Emmett Holt. *The Care and Feeding of Children; A Catechism for the Use of Mothers and Children's Nurses.* New York, 1894.

In this woodcut from *Harper's Weekly* (1878), Death distributes contaminated milk to the poor. Holt helped to abolish such dangers in New York City by actively campaigning for a pure milk supply.

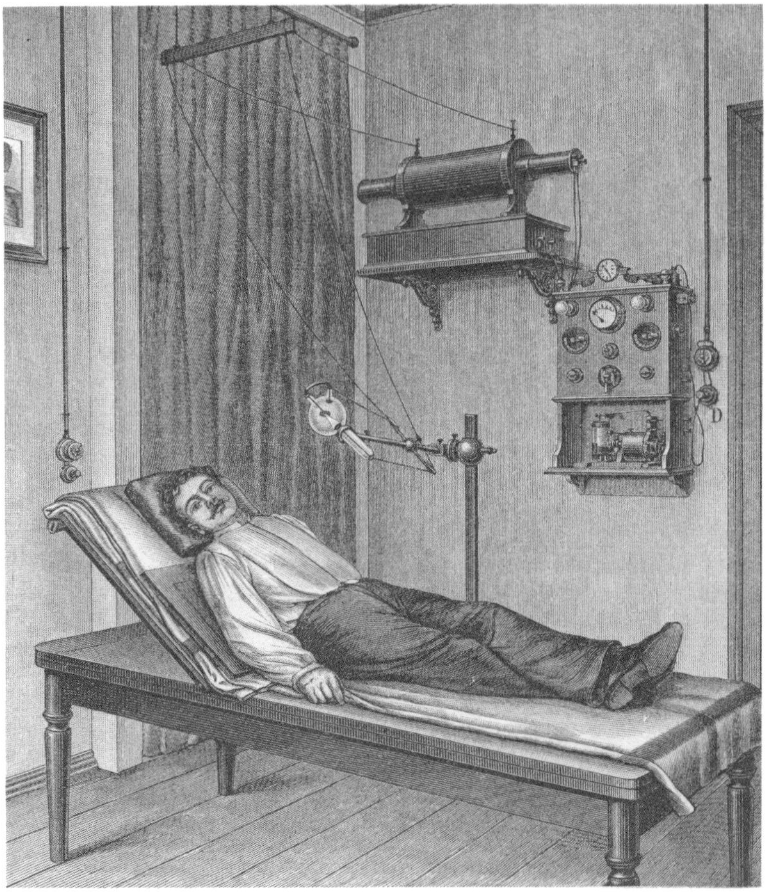
D

# Wilhelm Conrad Röntgen

## A NEW KIND OF RAY

Röntgen (1845-1922) was a professor of physics, not a physician, but his discovery of x-rays was of such immediate value to medicine, directly for diagnosis and indirectly through the development of radium treatment, that this small pamphlet must be counted as one of the classics of medicine.

His discovery was made accidentally, but the accident befell a receptive mind. While experimenting with a lightproof Crookes tube as a source of cathode rays, Röntgen was surprised to find that he could produce shadows of solid objects and a fluorescent light upon a screen several feet away. He correctly ascribed this phenomenon to the effect of a previously undiscovered type of radiation. On further investigation, he found that these rays passed through the soft parts of his hand more readily than through the bones and that the shadows of bones and tissue could be captured on a photographic plate.

He announced the results to the Würzburg physical and medical society in December, 1895, and the report to the meeting was promptly issued as a separate pamphlet. This account of "a new kind of ray" is organized into seventeen numbered sections. Its first section contains the statement that "the fluorescence is noticeable even two meters away from the apparatus." Farther on, the report points out that "one soon finds that all bodies are translucent for these rays, but in very different degree."

The "shadow-picture" is described toward the end. Since this report was quickly translated into many languages, knowledge and application of x-rays spread rapidly around the world. Although Röntgen used the name "x-ray" for the "new kind of ray" he had detected, it was soon rechristened "Roentgen ray" by the great histologist, Rudolph Albert von Kölliker, and the term "roentgenology" was widely employed for several decades.

Röntgen received the Nobel Prize in Physics for 1901. In spite of this award and his international reputation, the discovery of x-rays was attributed by some to his assistant. Always modest and never a seeker of publicity, Röntgen was greatly saddened by this rumor, became increasingly withdrawn, and died at the age of seventy-seven, lonely and neglected.

Wilhelm Conrad Röntgen. *Ueber eine neue Art von Strahlen*. Würzburg, 1895.

The practical uses of x-rays in surgery and medicine were well established within twenty years of Röntgen's discovery, in spite of the crude instruments of the time. Further applications of radiotherapy continue to be explored today.

Fig. 2.

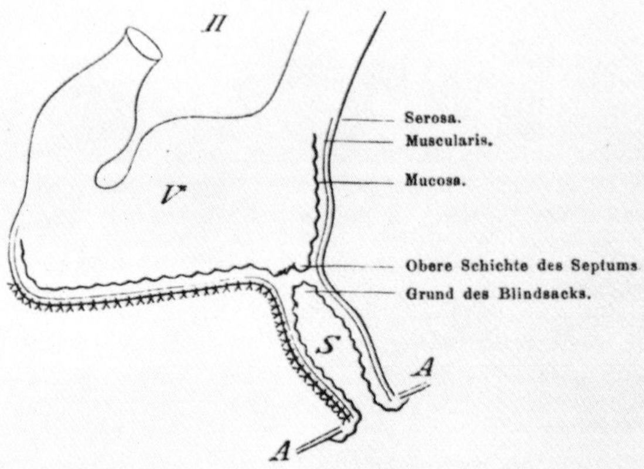


*V* — Magenhöhle. — *S* — Blindsack. — *A* — *A* — Bauchwand.

Oesophagotomie schon deshalb bedeutende Vorteile vor dem Verfahren Frémonts, weil sie operativ unvergleichlich einfacher ist und bei geeigneten Operationsbedingungen keine nutzlosen Opfer erfordert; überdies erfreuen sich unsere Hunde jahrelang einer blühenden Gesundheit. Ist dieses wohl mit den Hunden des Dr. Frémont der Fall?

Das übliche Verfahren, den Saft aus dem kleinen Magen aufzufangen, ist folgendes: In den Blindsack wird ein Röhrchen von Glas oder Gummi eingeführt, das an seinem inneren Ende vielfach durchlöchert ist. Das Röhrchen hält entweder von selbst oder wird durch eine elastische Schnur fixiert, die um den Leib des Tieres geführt wird. Der Saft wird entweder in liegender oder in stehender Stellung des Tieres aufgefangen.

Soviel ich augenblicklich beurteilen kann, muss diese Methode, einen isolierten kleinen Magen zu bilden, als einzig mögliche und im Prinzip richtige anerkannt werden; es bleiben zwar noch kleine Übelstände bestehen, die jedoch zum Detail der Sache gehören, so z. B. die Maceration der Wundränder und die Verluste an Magensaft; doch lassen sich diese Übelstände leicht ausgleichen

# Ivan Petrovich Pavlov

## THE WORK OF THE DIGESTIVE GLANDS

Pavlov's lectures detailing his famous experiments on digestion were first published in Russian in 1897. The following year, a German translation appeared—*Die Arbeit der Verdauungsdrüsen*. It is the German translation that is in the Lilly collection. Pavlov (1849-1936) was director of the Institute for Experimental Medicine in St. Petersburg when his book was published. By virtue of his ambidexterity and skill in handling laboratory dogs, particularly his operative formation of fistulas with intact nerve supply, Pavlov was able to acquire entirely new knowledge about the stimulation of gastric and pancreatic secretions. Discovering that the vagus controls these secretions, Pavlov and his assistants next studied nervous reflexes and showed that they depend on reactions integrated in the cerebral cortex. He was awarded the Nobel Prize in Medicine for 1904.

Pavlov's book of lectures was soon translated into French and English as well as German. After a general survey of the subject and his methods, he described the output of the digestive glands in response to feeding, the vagal efferent nerve supply of the gastric glands and pancreas, and a general scheme of the reflex pathways involved, including their relation to the salivary glands and appetite. His most original observations are reported on the period of occurrence and the importance of the "psychic," or appetitive, juice in gastric secretion in contrast to the relative inefficiency of merely mechanical stimulation by food.

After studying higher nervous functions, in 1912 he enunciated his concept of "conditioned reflexes," the effect of repeated sensory or psychic stimuli on reflex action. Pavlov used the term "telephone exchange" in depicting the central-nervous-system connections between a dog's senses and the organs of digestion. By conditioning the animal, he was able to elicit salivation from the parotid gland in response to pain and the ringing of a bell. Furthermore, he found that the salivary reflex could be conditioned not only to discriminate between the frequencies of beats of a metronome above and below 100 per minute but also to distinguish one-eighth variations in the tone of sound vibrations within and above the range of human hearing.

Pavlov's work continued after establishment of the Soviet regime, but he later resigned from several scientific organizations in protest against their political involvement. He died at the age of eighty-seven.

Ivan Petrovich Pavlov. *Die Arbeit der Verdauungsdrüsen.* Wiesbaden, 1898.

Pavlov shows the construction of a small stomach, or "blind sac" (S), from which intestinal juices can be obtained. One end of a glass or rubber tube is inserted into the opening (A-A); the other end extends to the outside of the animal.

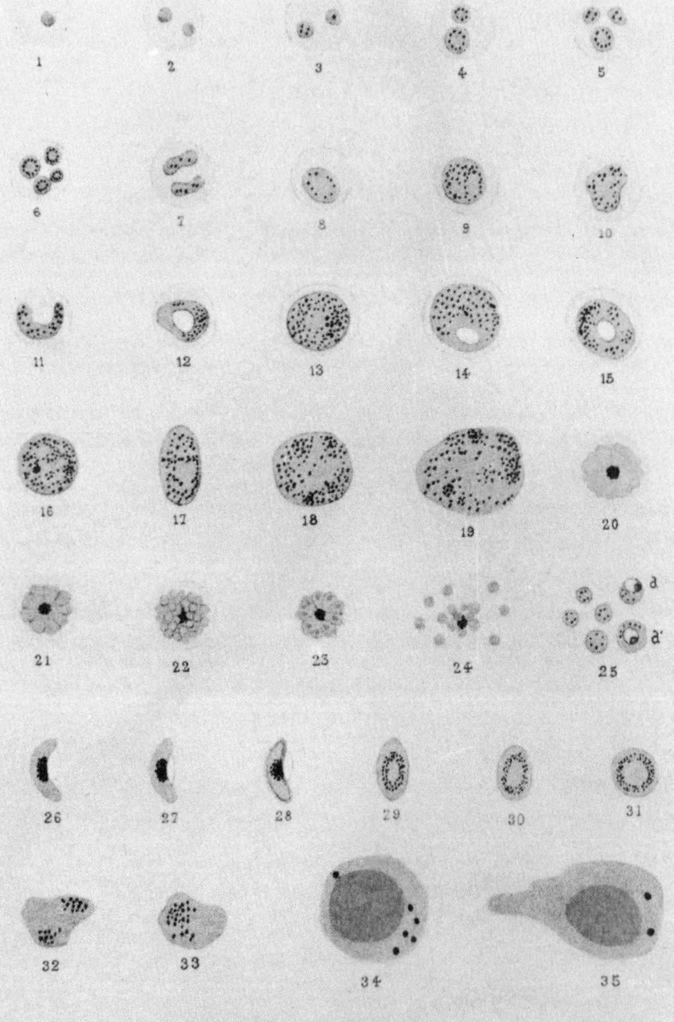

Dr Laveran del. V. Roussel, lith.

Hématozoaire du Paludisme

Sang coloré par l'éosine et le bleu de méthylène

# Alphonse Laveran

## MALARIA

Laveran (1845-1922), who detected the parasite that causes malarial fever, was born in Paris and graduated in medicine at Strasbourg. After postgraduate studies in bacteriology, he enlisted in the French army as a medical officer. While on a tour of military duty in Algeria in 1880, he took blood samples from acutely febrile patients suffering from malaria. In this way, by luck, he happened to be examining the blood of his patients at the time when the protozoan source of the disease was most in evidence. His first announcement of the discovery of the cause of "paludism," or marsh fever, was made to the Société Médicale des Hôpitaux de Paris. Thereafter, he continued his research on malaria for another twenty years and published four separate treatises on the disease in 1884, 1891, 1892, and 1898 as his knowledge increased. Laveran is also remembered for important contributions to military medicine and hygiene and for *Trypanosomes et trypanosomiases* (1904).

Patrick Manson, who had already found that mosquitoes carry the *Filaria sanguinis,* suggested that Laveran's malarial parasite must be carried in the same way. In 1897, the vector of Laveran's *Plasmodium* was eventually identified as the *Anopheles* mosquito by another British pathologist and parasitologist, Sir Ronald Ross, in India.

Laveran's final monograph, *Traité du paludisme* ("Treatise on Malaria"), published in the year following Ross's discovery, surveys the long history of the study of malaria. He describes his own discovery of the "hematozoon," gives an extensive account of this plasmodium, and then discusses the mosquito carrier of the disease, acknowledging the work of Manson and Ross. The remaining two-thirds of his book cover the clinical, pathologic, and therapeutic aspects of malaria with a lengthy chapter on prophylaxis that includes recommendations for the drainage and clearing of marshes and other bodies of stagnant water. The concluding chapters deal with related parasitic diseases and problems that were still to be explored. For these contributions, the Nobel Prize was awarded to Ross in 1902 and to Laveran in 1907.

Alphonse Laveran. *Traité du paludisme.* Paris, 1898.

The parasites of marsh fever, stained with eosin and methylene blue. Laveran's initial discovery of these malarial parasites in 1880 may have been fortuitous, but the stages of development shown here represent eighteen years of research.

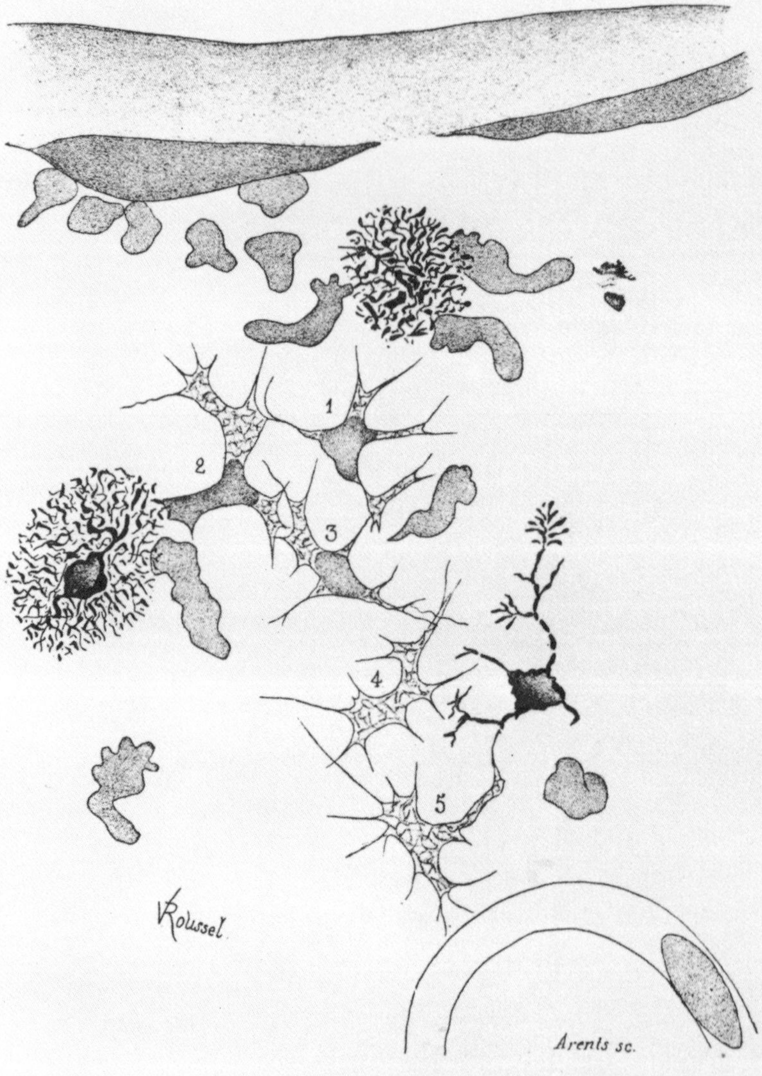


Fig. 50. — Le même point, cinq heures après la cautérisation.

1-5. Les mêmes cellules fixes que dans les fig. 47, 48.

# Elie Metchnikoff

## THE PATHOLOGY OF INFLAMMATION

Metchnikoff (1845-1916), born in Russia and trained as a zoologist, will always be identified with the fields of inflammation and immunity.

"One day when the whole family had gone to a circus to see some extraordinary performing apes," he wrote, "I remained alone with my microscope, observing the life in the mobile cells of a transparent star-fish larva....It struck me that similar cells might serve in the defense of the organism against intruders....if my supposition was true, a splinter introduced into the body of the star-fish larva, devoid of blood-vessels or of a nervous system, should soon be surrounded by mobile cells as is to be observed in a man who runs a splinter into his finger....I fetched...a few rose thorns and introduced them at once under the skin of some beautiful star-fish larvae as transparent as water....Very early the next morning I ascertained that it fully succeeded."

From this beginning, he went on to show that dilatation of the circulatory bed in an inflamed part of the body is a secondary rather than a primary event and that the basic cause of inflammation is the conflict between invading organisms and the mobile or fixed phagocytic cells of the mesoderm which are concerned with defense. Immunity, he suggested, fails whenever local or general conditions within the body impair or prevent this phagocytic response.

In 1891, after ten years of research, Elie Metchnikoff expounded his theory of phagocytosis in a series of lectures. They were published as a book in French and in Russian the next year and translated into English by the eminent physiologist E. H. Starling in 1893. The work begins with the statement, "Infection is a conflict of organisms for whose understanding a study of comparative pathology is essential." Metchnikoff traced intracellular digestion through the animal kingdom from unicellular forms to vertebrates, showing the phagocytic role of the leukocytes and the evolution of inflammation. He discussed chronic inflammation (with tuberculosis as its type), serous inflammation, and the antitoxic property of serum.

Although the concept of immunity had been intuitively grasped by earlier workers from Jenner to Pasteur, the new science of immunology was launched with Metchnikoff's "Immunity in Infective Diseases," published in 1901. For his contributions, he was awarded many honors from around the world, including the Nobel Prize in Medicine for 1908, which he shared with Paul Ehrlich, the German bacteriologist.

Elie Metchnikoff. *Leçons sur la pathologie comparée de l'inflammation faites à l'Institut Pasteur en Avril et Mai 1891*. Paris, 1892.

Inflammatory reaction of tissue to cauterization five hours after injury, as shown in Metchnikoff's book. In simple sketches such as this, he demonstrated the dynamic processes of the immunologic response.

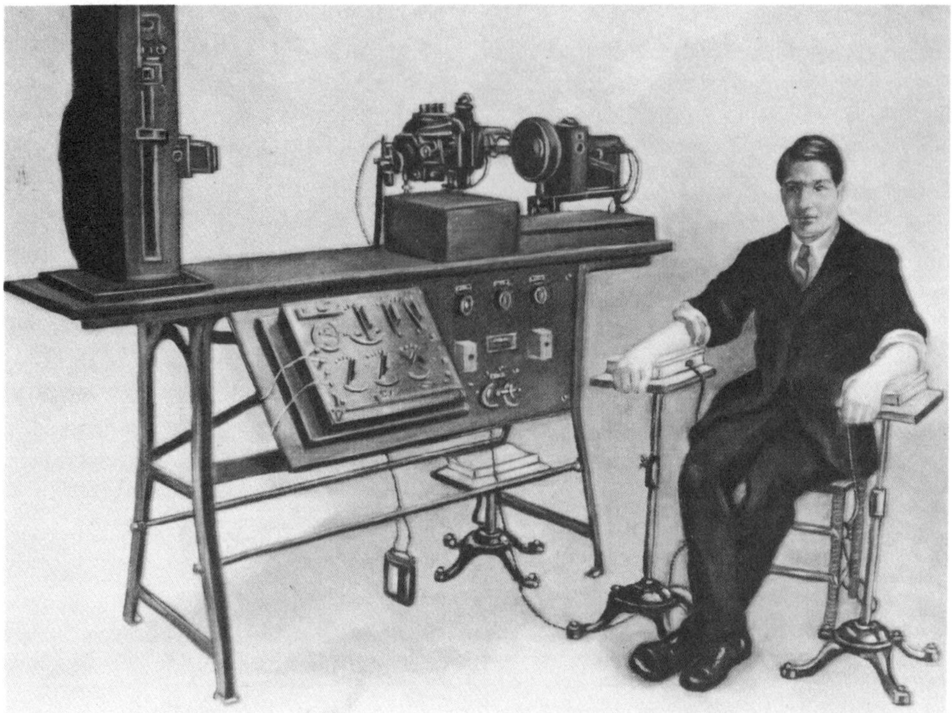

# Karel Frederik Wenckebach

## ARRHYTHMIA OF THE HEART

A native of The Hague, Wenckebach (1864-1940) studied medicine at Utrecht, where his interests focused on embryology and hematology. The discovery that he was color-blind caused him to change his plans. Turning to physiology, he spent long hours in the laboratory studying the fundamental properties of the frog heart.

When economic circumstances compelled him to leave the university, he entered practice in a small Dutch village. One day, while auscultating a patient, Wenckebach found a strange arrhythmia that reminded him of the irregularity he had frequently observed in his earlier frog experiments. After analyzing sphygmograms recorded from this patient and others, he was able to describe extrasystoles in man for the first time. His discovery of periodic dropped beats, often called "Wenckebach's periods," soon followed. The deductive analysis of sphygmograms must be considered a remarkable achievement when one recalls the crude apparatus then in use.

"Arrhythmia as an Expression of Certain Functional Disturbances of the Heart," published in German in 1903, was the first comprehensive account of his research. Wenckebach detailed his observations of the physiologic basis of arrhythmias and then discussed their clinical manifestations, noting that various problems of physiology and pharmacology would need to be solved before his findings could be applied clinically.

Some of these problems were being resolved by the time he wrote his later monographs—an expanded one on arrhythmias in 1914 and the monumental "The Irregular Action of the Heart," coauthored with Heinrich Winterberg in 1927.

Wenckebach derived much of the inspiration for his research from pupils and patients, and he was candid in acknowledging this fact. His report on the beneficial effect of quinine in certain arrhythmias established the clinical basis for the use of quinidine in cardiac therapeutics. With characteristic honesty, he disclosed that he had first become aware of the effect of quinine on stimulus formation when it was suggested by one of his patients, a Dutch sea captain with auricular fibrillation. The captain had reported that his cardiac irregularity disappeared when he took quinine to prevent malaria. After a pupil aroused Wenckebach's interest in the circulatory disturbances encountered in beriberi, he traveled to the Dutch East Indies, and his findings there led to a classic contribution to the recognition of nontropical beriberi.

At the age of thirty-seven, Wenckebach had given up private practice to accept an appointment at the University of Groningen. He subsequently became associated with the University of Strassburg and then the First Medical University Clinic at Vienna, from which he chose to retire at the age of sixty-five. He continued his research, however, until his death eleven years later.

Karel Frederik Wenckebach. *Die Arhythmie als Ausdruck bestimmter Funktionsstörungen des Herzens: eine physiologisch-klinische Studie*. Leipzig, 1903.

Electrocardiography became practical when Wenckebach's contemporary, Einthoven, developed the string galvanometer (right). Electromotive forces generated by the heart caused the string to move, and these movements were photographed by the camera (left).

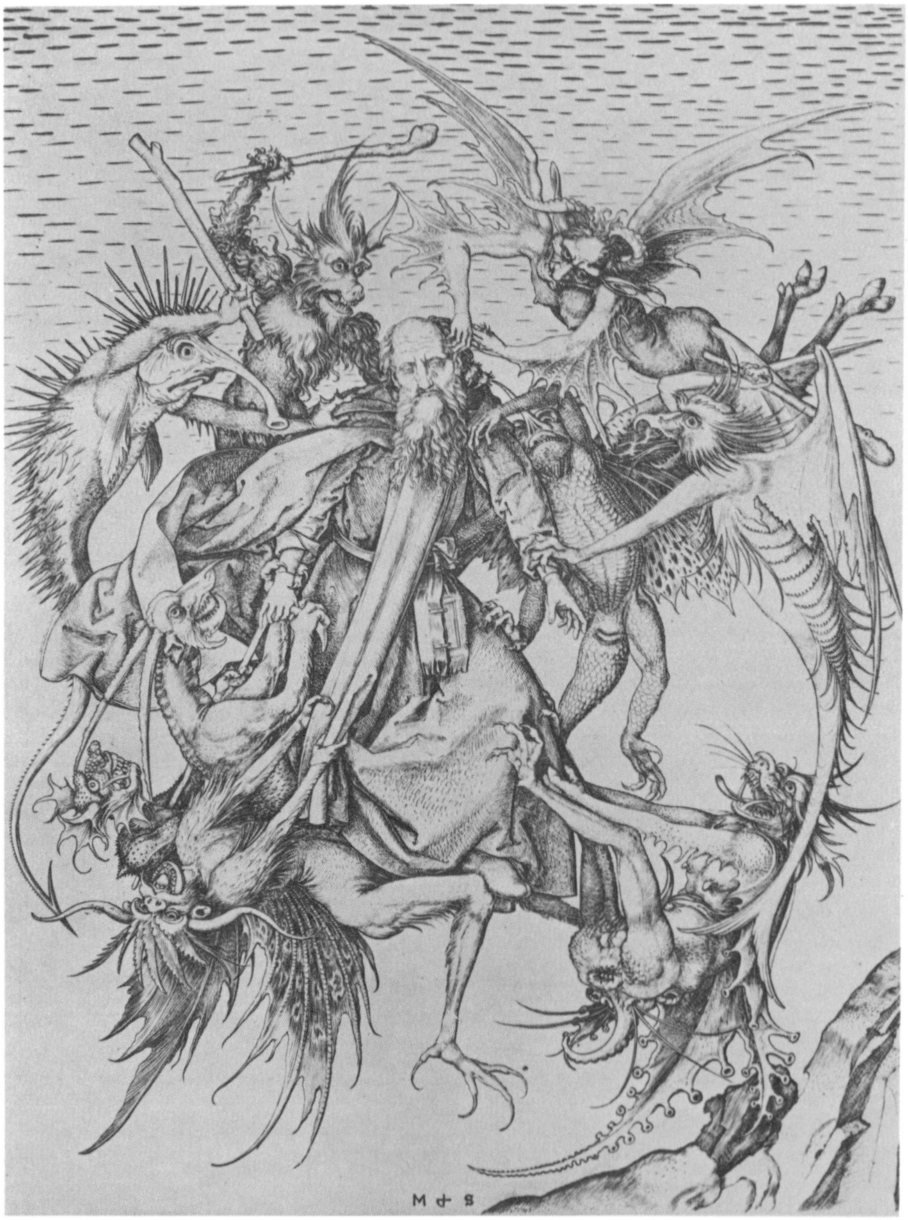

# Sigmund Freud

## THE PSYCHOPATHOLOGY OF EVERYDAY LIFE

Freud's name and work became known to a wide public through this book, in which he showed that many of the small mistakes in speech and memory of normal people differ in degree rather than in kind from the abnormal behavior of the mentally ill. After graduating in medicine and working for some years at the General Hospital in Vienna, Freud (1856-1939) obtained a traveling scholarship that enabled him to visit Paris and study at the clinic of Charcot (q.v.), the eminent French neurologist. On returning home in 1885, Freud became lecturer in neuropathology at the university and began his private practice in neurology, a specialty that then included psychiatry.

Freud had been impressed by Charcot's theory that hysteria was a thought disturbance rather than a disease of the nervous system and also was greatly influenced by his senior colleague, Josef Breuer, who had had some success in relieving the symptoms of hysteria with hypnosis. These experiences stimulated Freud's interest in the subconscious mind and led to his method of "psychoanalysis," in which, by "free association," his patients unburdened themselves of their repressed emotions and almost-forgotten thoughts. He made this discovery public in "Studies on Hysteria," written with Breuer in 1893, and explained his method in "Interpretation of Dreams" (1900).

Freud built a theory about neurotic behavior and its origin in repressed erotic urges. To him, these were not necessarily physical and included normal love for parents, spouse, children, friends, and self. This new book of 1904, incorporating his ideas in an analysis of mistakes of speech he had observed in himself and in his friends and patients, led to the "Theory of Sexuality" (1905), in which his chief conclusions were finally elaborated. Freud's doctrines effected a liberalization of general attitudes toward mental and sexual abnormality, but his rejection of criticism and his intolerant insistence that he alone was right lessened his influence on medical psychology.

The easy narrative style of "Psychopathology" made it acceptable to a wide public. After writing about the almost universal forgetfulness of proper names, Freud went on to discuss other forms of verbal error, such as substitution of words in speech, reading, and writing, and, through careful retracing of unconscious thought processes, related them to hidden memories or fears. He dealt similarly with mistaken impressions, neglected resolutions, and "unconscious" acts and ended with a general chapter on determinism and on actions apparently influenced by chance or superstition.

Sigmund Freud. *Zur Psychopathologie des Alltagslebens. (Über Vergessen, Vergreifen, Aberglaube und Irrtum.)* Berlin, 1904.

Ancient beliefs in superstition, demons, and the occult as influences on overt behavior, represented by this fifteenth-century Martin Schongauer engraving, were scientifically repudiated by Freud's theory of the role of the subconscious.

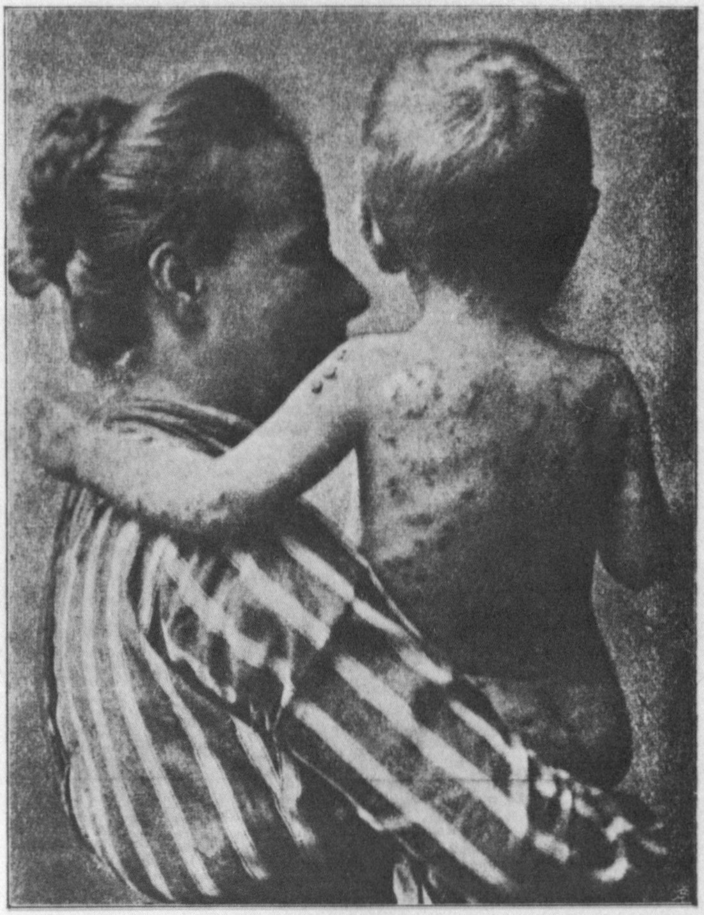

Abb. 18.

Kuhpockenexanthem auf Hals, Rücken, Unterarm. Die Umgebung der normal abgetrockneten Impfpusteln auf der linken Schulter ist frei von Exanthem. (Rehousek, 15. Tag.) Gleichzeitig mit der Photographie wurde die Moulage aufgenommen, die in Dreifarbendruck reproduziert ist. (Tafel Fig. 1.)

# Clemens Peter Pirquet

## VACCINATION AND ALLERGY FROM VACCINATION

The Austrian pediatrician Pirquet (1874-1929) introduced the term "allergy" and established immunology as a new specialty in medicine. In the Children's Clinic at the University of Vienna, he studied infectious diseases and was the first to postulate that the incubation period ends with the formation of antibodies. He devised the tuberculosis test named for him, in which a small area of skin is scarified through a drop of tuberculin, and, with Bela Schick, he established the concept of serum sickness. Later he developed the theory of autoimmunity.

His book on vaccination is the first work in immunology to involve the scientific analysis of a large series of clinical cases. It begins with a summary history of the hypotheses concerning reactions to vaccination and a statement of the objects and methods of immunization. The main text is divided into three parts: vaccination, revaccination, and theory. The first and second parts are based on the statistical evaluation of many case histories from the Children's Clinic.

The section on theory describes Pirquet's concept of allergy and undertakes to explain the differences between early and delayed reactions to vaccination. After discussing pock exanthema and the agglutination theory, he points out the diagnostic value of "allergy," which he defined as "an altered susceptibility to reaction in regard to the whole group of pock diseases, but not an immunity in the strict sense." He further described it as "the bridge between hypersensitivity and immunity."

Although most of Pirquet's career was spent in the medical centers of Austria and Poland, he came to the United States in 1908 and held the chair of pediatrics at Johns Hopkins University for two years. Upon his return to Europe, he filled similar positions at Breslau and Vienna.

Pirquet became interested in nutrition after 1910 and was a commissioner for food distribution during the famine in Vienna following World War I. In this capacity, he was credited with innovative programs to aid the starving infants, especially in providing them with an adequate milk supply. In his last years, he studied the allergies of old age and the role of aging in the incidence of cancer.

Pirquet's intellectual brilliance was marred by emotional instability. At the age of fifty-five, seemingly in good physical and mental health, he took his own life.

Clemens Peter Pirquet. *Klinische Studien über Vakzination und vakzinale Allergie*. Leipzig and Vienna, 1907.

This photograph from Pirquet's book shows a cowpox eruption on the child's neck, back, and armpits. The area around the dried vaccination pustules on the left shoulder is free of the eruption.

*B B* are the two tambours, and *F F* their levers. The writing pens are narrow-grooved wires, one end fixed to the bottom of a small cistern at the free extremity of the lever. The other end of the grooved wire is adjusted to barely touch the paper. The ink is put into the tiny cistern, and it flows along the groove to the pen point by capillary attraction. If the pens are kept clean, and the ink is free from dust, they serve their purpose most admirably, and are ever ready for use. As the radial pulse is the most serviceable of standards, a pecial method is employed to record it. A splint (*C* 1) is

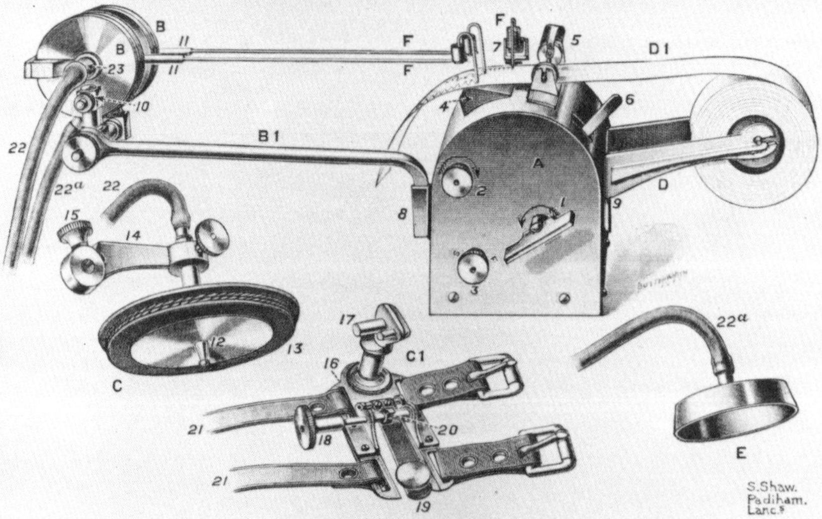


FIG. 18. The Ink Polygraph.

fastened to the wrist in such a manner that the pad of the steel spring falls on the radial artery, and is pressed down by an eccentric wheel (18) until a suitable movement is transmitted to the spring by the artery; then the broad tambour (*C*) is fitted on to the splint so that the knob (12) falls on the moving spring. This wrist tambour is connected to the tambour *B* by india-rubber tubing (22, 22), and the movements of the radial pulse are recorded by the lever *F*. The shallow cup (receiver) *E* is placed on the pulsation which it is desired to record, and the movement is conveyed to the lever *F* of the other tambour. In this way, simultaneous with the radial pulse, a record can be obtained of the apex beat, carotid, jugular, or other pulses.

# Sir James Mackenzie

## DISEASES OF THE HEART

Sir James Mackenzie (1853-1925), one of the giants of cardiology, was perhaps unique among the scientists represented in this collection, because he practiced general medicine and surgery for twenty-five years in a small English village and simultaneously carried out some highly significant clinical and experimental research. He had received his M.D. from the University of Edinburgh and spent a year as a house physician before going into practice. Mackenzie was essentially a self-taught investigator. Despite his isolation from the medical research community, he did original work in differentiating cardiac arrhythmias, pioneered in making devices for recording pulse waves, and reported his findings in the scientific literature. He first described his graphic recording instruments in 1892 and published a major treatise, *The Study of the Pulse,* in 1902. He moved to London at the age of fifty-four and the next year (1908) published *Diseases of the Heart.* Soon he became internationally famous as an outstanding clinician, teacher, and researcher.

This large volume, comprising thirty-five chapters and four appendices, summed up his work. Mackenzie pointed out that his approach had been essentially clinical and that the pathology needed more exhaustive study.

The book is logically arranged. After a general survey of the developmental, anatomic, and physiologic background (including that of the muscle cells), Mackenzie dealt with examination of the patient, giving details of special symptoms. He described his own instruments for simultaneously recording the arterial pulse at the wrist and the jugular pulse in the neck and for studying arterial pressure and the condition of the liver. Many of his historic tracings of abnormal pulse waves are reproduced.

Mackenzie explained the heart's action and the varieties of irregular function, particularly his concept of "nodal rhythm," which later was termed "auricular fibrillation." An appendix to this discussion recorded his observations on "contraction starting at a place other than the normal."

Chapters are also devoted to secondary alterations in heart function (for example, those in acute febrile disorders) and to other special aspects of heart disease. In addition, he described valvular defects, such as mitral stenosis. Recognition of this defect led to successful surgical treatment half a century later.

Toward the end of his life, Mackenzie resumed general practice in Scotland, where, to help young physicians, he established the Institute for Clinical Research at St. Andrews. In recognition of his achievements, he received a knighthood and many other honors. He greatly advanced the science of cardiology in the era preceding general use of the electrocardiogram.

James Mackenzie. *Diseases of the Heart.* London, 1908.

The writing pens (F) of Mackenzie's ink polygraph simultaneously recorded movements of the radial pulse and, by means of the cup receiver (E), of the apex beat, carotid, or jugular pulse.

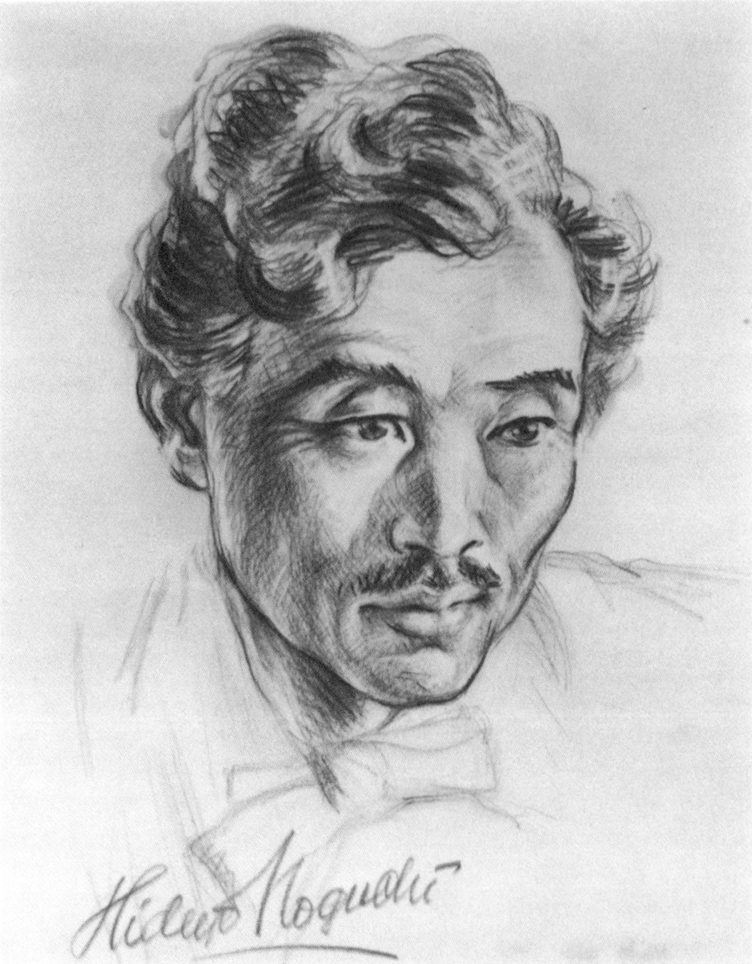
Hideyo Noguchi

# Hideyo Noguchi

## SERUM DIAGNOSIS OF SYPHILIS

Noguchi (1876-1928) came from Japan to the University of Pennsylvania as a research student in 1900. Young, poor, and alien, he was befriended by Simon Flexner, whom he followed to the new Rockefeller Institute in New York in 1904. His first work in this country was a study of all types of snake venom, their effects on the body, and the means by which snakebites should be treated. Noguchi elucidated the causes of many infectious diseases, studying in particular spirochetes and the vaccinia virus. In 1910, together with Flexner, he confirmed Schaudinn's discovery that syphilis was due to *Treponema pallidum*. Three years later, by finding these spirochetes in an impressively large series of autopsy specimens, he was able to establish that tabes dorsalis and general paralysis result from advanced syphilis of the spinal cord and brain.

His study of Oroya fever, establishing *Bartonella bacilliformis* as its agent and *Phlebotomus* as the vector, was a major contribution to tropical medicine. In his last ten years he worked on yellow fever; he succumbed to this disease soon after Adrian Stokes, who had discovered the causative virus just before his death.

Dedicated to Simon Flexner, the *Serum Diagnosis of Syphilis* contains in its preface the statement that "the author endeavored to make it suitable for use by practicing physicians and students and at the same time with sufficient comprehensiveness to render it useful to laboratory workers." Noguchi explained in the first chapters how in-vitro hemolysis can be utilized to demonstrate antibodies in serum and how complement, antigens, and antibodies affect the hemolytic process. Later chapters provide step-by-step instructions for conducting the Wassermann reaction for syphilis and an appraisal, based on clinical and autopsy findings, of the value of that test. In the last chapter, Noguchi digresses to describe the butyric acid test, a simple procedure carried out on cerebrospinal fluid, which he devised for the diagnosis of advanced syphilitic disease of the central nervous system.

Characteristically, Noguchi took pains to present every relevant detail on the subjects about which he wrote and included in his book a discussion on the quantitative relationships of all factors playing a part in the Wassermann reaction. As he put it, this was "an aspect of the subject that has not perhaps received the consideration that it deserves." The book sets an example of explicit thoroughness that few others have matched.

Hideyo Noguchi. *Serum Diagnosis of Syphilis and the Butyric Acid Test for Syphilis*. Philadelphia, 1910.

Portrait of Hideyo Noguchi drawn by C. L. Baldridge in Accra. The drawing was made in Africa ten days before Noguchi died of yellow fever while engaged in research on that disease.

taken are not restricted. In eighteen or twenty days ordinary food can be taken and enjoyed. I discourage

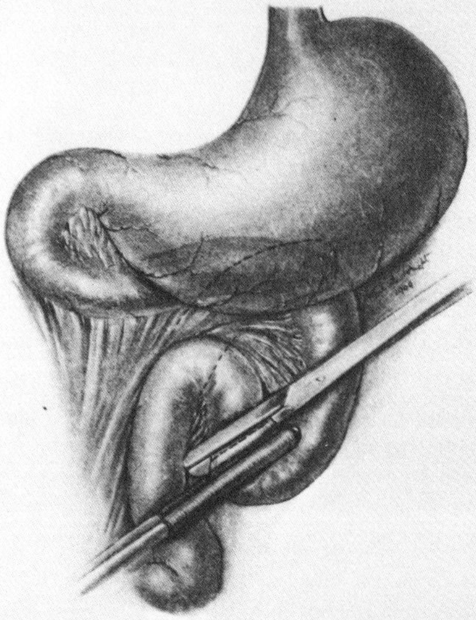

FIG. 47.—MODIFICATION OF ROUX'S OPERATION AS PERFORMED BY THE AUTHOR.

The jejunum is divided between a rubber-covered clamp and a Parker-Kerr clamp. It is cut across with the knife passed as close as possible to the latter. The division is carried on into the mesentery.

pastry, fresh fruits, and green vegetables in all cases for some time, for these things are without value as foods.

On the night of the operation the patient may be allowed $\frac{1}{6}$ gr. of morphine hypodermically. There is

# Sir Berkeley Moynihan

## DUODENAL ULCER

Moynihan's monograph on *Duodenal Ulcer,* though primarily a textbook of surgical treatment, gave a clear report of a disease syndrome that had previously been overlooked or misunderstood. "Through generations," he wrote in his preface, "the symptoms, first described in 1817, had been ascribed to a purely functional disturbance." Moynihan (1865-1936) showed that, according to "the accumulating experience of a few surgeons," the symptoms were due to structural changes in the duodenum. His work was called by the eminent English physician Arthur Hurst "as much a piece of original research as the discovery of a new element or a new star, and equally deserving of recognition."

The various chapters of the book pertain to ulceration of the duodenum, uremic ulcer, tuberculous ulcer, melena neonatorum, and duodenal ulcer. The symptoms, with their sequence of "pain, food, ease," were elucidated, as was the differential diagnosis of chronic duodenal ulcer. Another chapter deals in detail with treatment, "which should always be surgical." After describing various surgical methods, Moynihan concluded that "gastroenterostomy is by far the most satisfactory procedure." Chapters on perforation and pathology are followed by an appendix giving histories of 189 cases Moynihan saw between 1900 and the end of 1909. Although the mortality in the series was 1.6 percent, he wrote that "among the last 121 cases there was no death."

When this book appeared, he had already published many other influential surgical texts and articles, including a large volume on *Abdominal Operations.*

Moynihan was a man of abounding, masterful vitality. As professor of surgery at the University of Leeds in England, he had great technical skill, good judgment, and vision. If, while operating, surgeons would seek causes for all their patients' symptoms, he maintained, possibly they would discover more about disease than do pathologists by autopsy.

He wrote and spoke with clarity and was an able organizer and an enthusiastic encourager of cooperative effort and continuous education. He founded the *British Journal of Surgery* and played a major role in surgical training in England. Honors came to him in abundance for his many contributions to surgical diagnosis and to the operative treatment of abdominal disease and for his great abilities as a teacher and medical administrator. He became president of the Royal College of Surgeons, received a knighthood, and later, as Baron Moynihan of Leeds, became the first practicing physician since Lister to enter the House of Lords.

Berkeley Moynihan. *Duodenal Ulcer.* Philadelphia, 1910.

Moynihan devised, modified, and improved surgical methods for the treatment of duodenal ulcers. He was recognized as an authority on visceral surgery by virtue of his technical skill, broad experience, and sound judgment.

*a*

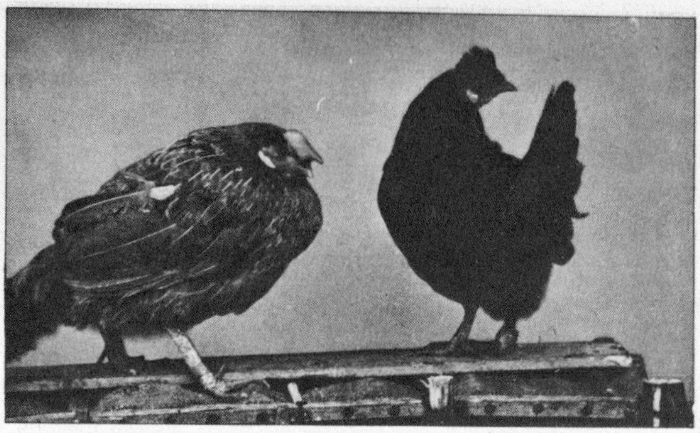

4 Tage nach Infektion.

Unbehandelt. Behandelt 2 Tage nach Infektion.

*b*

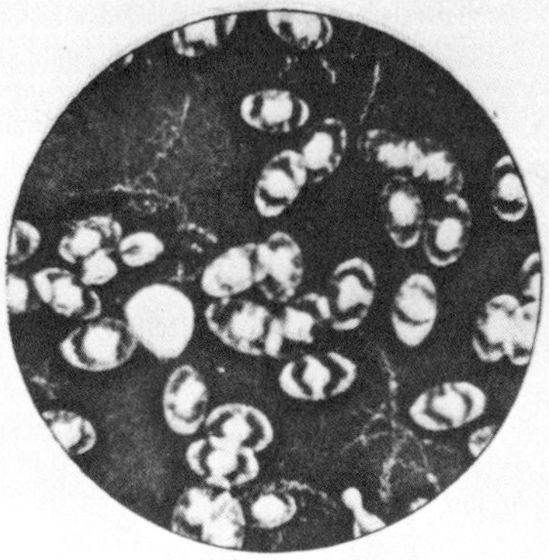

Kontrolle mit Spirillen.

*c*

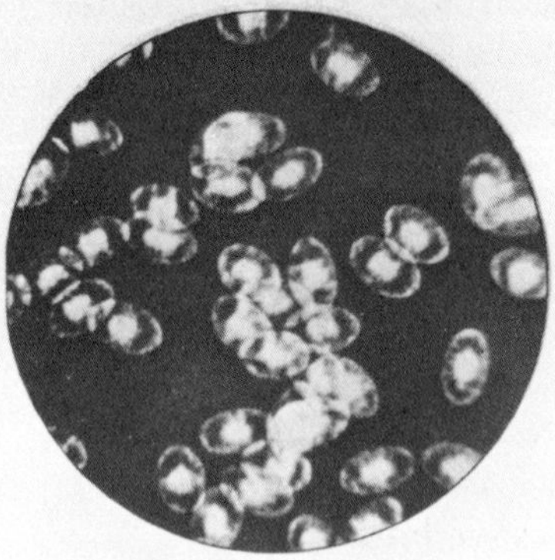

Behandeltes Huhn.
Spirillenfrei!

Verlag von Julius Springer in Berlin.

# Paul Ehrlich and Sahachiro Hata

## THE EXPERIMENTAL CHEMOTHERAPY OF SPIRILLOSES

Ehrlich (1854-1915), the great German pathologist and bacteriologist, combined medical and chemical interests in his histologic studies with aniline dyes. While examining sputum samples for the bacilli that cause tuberculosis, he accidentally discovered that the organisms would stain readily if the slides were exposed to heat during the staining procedure. Characteristically modest, he gave credit for the finding to the cleaning woman who, when tidying the laboratory, had inadvertently placed his slides on a hot stove. Ehrlich developed the differential white-blood-cell count as a tool for the diagnosis of leukemia and was the first to recognize aplastic anemia and to describe the red-blood-cell inclusion bodies seen in toxic hemolytic disorders. From hematology, he turned to antitoxins and the problems of immunity. Ehrlich's side-chain theory, in which he postulated the production of immunologically specific antibodies against invading microorganisms, ultimately won him universal recognition. For his contributions to the study of infectious disease and immunity, he was awarded the Nobel Prize in Medicine for 1908, which he shared with Elie Metchnikoff.

In 1899, he moved to the Institute of Experimental Therapy in Frankfurt and was later appointed its director. Here he worked on cancer, experimenting with tumor grafts, but gradually turned to the logical outcome of his earlier work—the search for synthetic chemical substances that would be toxic specifically to disease-producing microorganisms. His influential pioneer work in this field was of the first importance and paved the way for the discovery of the sulfonamides and nonsynthetic antibiotics.

After the cause and means of transmission of syphilis had been recognized (1903-1905), a specific against this disease became Ehrlich's main ambition. The effectiveness of arsphenamine ("Ehrlich's 606," or Salvarsan) was reported in this notable book. Written by his Japanese assistant, Sahachiro Hata, it contains a fifty-page essay by Ehrlich himself, in which he discusses the chemistry and practical use of his arsenical compound. In the first part of the book, Hata presents the experimental basis of chemotherapy and gives an account of studies on recurrent fever, chick spirillosis, and syphilis in rabbits.

Ehrlich's last four years were expended in meeting the worldwide demand for Salvarsan, in working with compulsive energy to find a safer alternative, and in facing bitter and unjust criticism. He was an inspired research worker and laboratory chief, a genius yet a simple soul, modest and not self-seeking but completely confident of the value of his work.

Paul Ehrlich and Sahachiro Hata. *Die experimentelle Chemotherapie der Spirillosen (Syphilis, Rückfallfieber, Hühnerspirillose, Frambösie)*. Berlin, 1910.

Ehrlich demonstrated conclusively that arsphenamine could eliminate the spirochetes of syphilis. The blood sample at the lower right, drawn from an infected chicken after two days of treatment, is free of spirochetes. The threadlike organisms are still present in the untreated chicken (left).

**Case 1.**—(J. H. H. Surgical No. 27140) Minnie G., an unmarried Russian Jewess, aged 23, referred by Dr. Stetten of New York, was admitted to the Johns Hopkins Hospital on *December 29, 1910.*

*Clinical history.*—One of a numerous and healthy family, though slight and undersized, she was well until sixteen years of age, having escaped the customary children's ailments.

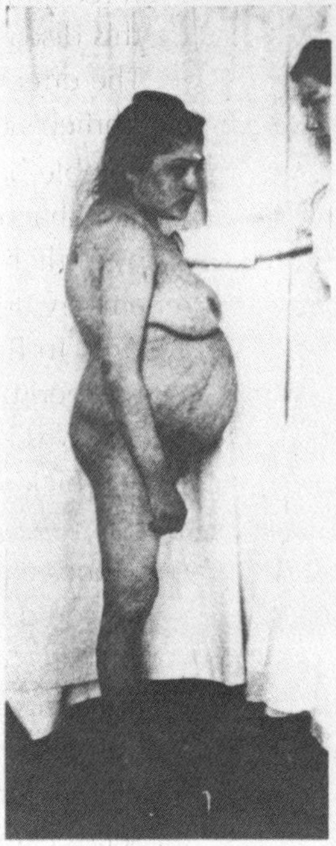

FIG. 34.—Case 1. The original example (1902) of basophil (unverified) obesity.

Her menses which started at the age of fourteen were regular for two years and then suddenly ceased. She began to grow stout and in the two years prior to admission her weight had increased from 112 to 137 pounds. She suffered greatly from headaches, nausea and vomiting sometimes accompanying the more severe attacks. She complained also of aching pains in the eyes which latterly had become prominent, and there had been occasional periods of seeing double.

Other noteworthy symptoms were insomnia, tinnitus, extreme dryness of the skin, frequent sore throats, shortness of breath, palpitation, purpuric outbreaks, recurring nose-bleeds, and marked constipation accompanied by bleeding piles. A definite growth of hair had appeared on the face with thinning of hair on the scalp. She had become increasingly round-shouldered having lost at least 4 inches in height. Muscular weakness had become extreme and there was constant complaint of backache and epigastric pains.

*Physical examination.* — This showed an undersized, kyphotic young woman 4 feet 9 inches in height (145 cm.), of most extraordinary appearance (Fig. 34). Her round face was dusky and cyanosed and there was an abnormal growth of hair, particularly noticeable on the sides of the forehead, upper lip and chin. The mucous membranes were of bright colour despite her history of frequent bleedings. Her abdominous body had the appearance of a full-term pregnancy. The breasts were hypertrophic and pendulous and there were pads of fat over the supra-clavicular and posterior cervical regions. The cyanotic appearance of the skin was particularly apparent over the body and lower extremities (Fig. 35) which were "marbled" and spotted by subcutaneous ecchymoses. Numerous purplish striae were present over the stretched skin of the lower abdomen and also over shoulders, breasts and hips; and a fine hirsuties was present over the back, hips and around the umbilicus. The skin which everywhere was rough and dry showed considerable pigmentation, particularly around the eyelids, groins, pubes and areolae of the breasts. The peculiar tense and painful adiposity affecting face, neck and trunk was in marked contrast to her comparatively spare extremities.

# Harvey Cushing

## THE PITUITARY BODY

Harvey Cushing (1869-1939), the principal pioneer in neurologic surgery in the United States, believed the surgeon should equip himself in detail with all the disciplines that support his practice, adding the active study of physiology, therapeutics, and pathology to his technical expertise. He was born in Cleveland, graduated from Yale University, received his medical degree from Harvard, and then spent fourteen years at the Johns Hopkins Hospital, where he worked under Halsted in surgery and Osler in medicine. Many years later, after the latter's death, Cushing wrote *The Life of Sir William Osler*, for which he won the 1926 Pulitzer Prize. He returned to Harvard University in 1912 as professor of surgery and also became surgeon-in-chief at the then-new Peter Bent Brigham Hospital. Forced to retire from Harvard at the age of sixty-three, he joined the faculty at Yale, where he spent the rest of his career.

This monograph on the pituitary displays his comprehensive scientific approach. It begins with a brief account of the anatomy, physiology, pathology, and chemistry of the hypophysis. The main text, on clinical manifestations of disordered function, is a detailed discussion of forty-seven cases. The last part of the book is a survey of the incidence, symptomatology, and treatment of pituitary disorders, including his new operative methods. The work on the pituitary was followed by his *Papers Relating to the Pituitary Body* (1932), which reported more of his research in that field.

By the time he wrote his first major monograph, Cushing was already an internationally famous surgeon with a long record of successful research in anesthesia, bacteriology, hypertension, and the control of hemorrhage. He had also performed experimental thoracic surgery on dogs (anticipating lung surgery in man, which he lived to see) and heart surgery (which began soon after his death in 1939 at the age of seventy). Cushing continuously extended his knowledge and treatment of intracranial tumors and published five books on aspects of this research between 1917 and 1938. In addition to his surgical practice and investigations, Cushing was a scholar, historian, and biographer, with an expert's knowledge of the medical books of the Renaissance.

Cushing's writing on what he called "dyspituitarism" stimulated interest in the wide-ranging effects of the ductless glands and helped establish endocrinology as a separate medical specialty. Of course, he is eponymically immortalized by the syndrome that bears his name. His personality and energy had a profound influence on a generation of surgical teachers.

Harvey Cushing. *The Pituitary Body and its Disorders. Clinical States Produced by Disorders of the Hypophysis Cerebri.* Philadelphia, 1912.

The report of Case No. 1 of pituitary basophilism (Cushing's syndrome), originally reported in Cushing's 1912 book, is shown here as it appeared in 1932 in his historic definitive description of the disease.

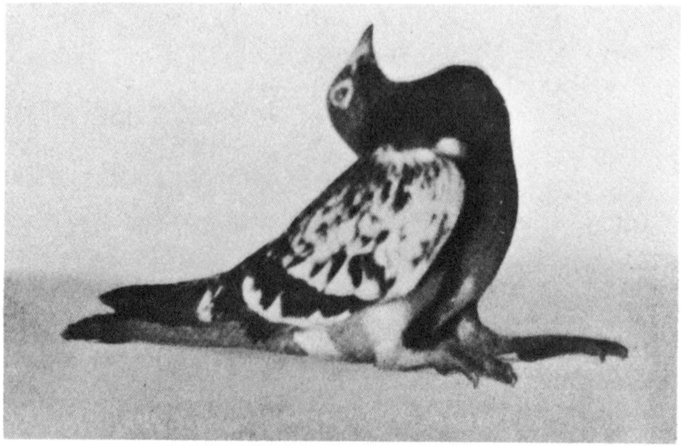

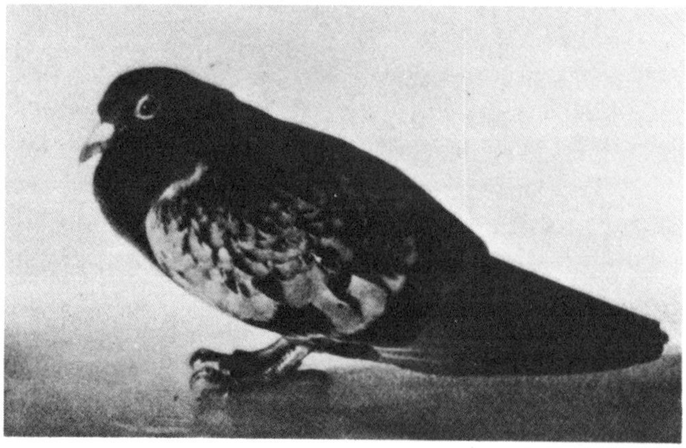

# Casimir Funk

## THE VITAMINS

The biochemist Casimir Funk (1884-1967), born in Poland and educated in Switzerland, Germany, and France, undertook to find the cause of beriberi while working at the Lister Institute in London. It had been recognized that a diet of polished rice would cause beriberi in humans and polyneuritis in pigeons. Using this animal model and starting with the assumption that a deficiency of amino acids was responsible for beriberi, Funk succeeded in isolating the protein factors in polished rice and rice polishings, only to discover that they had no curative effect on the birds. He persisted, pursuing the line that some other nitrogenous substance must be the antiberiberi factor he sought. Finally, he succeeded in isolating and crystallizing a potent compound that cured the neuritic birds and, it was later established, could prevent or cure human beriberi. This substance is now known as thiamine, or vitamin $B_1$.

After further investigation, Funk was able to differentiate the pellagra-preventing factor, niacin. For a paper published in the *Journal of Physiology* in 1912, he coined the term "vitamine-fraction," later shortened to "vitamin."

Funk's book on vitamins was published in Germany when he was thirty. Prophetically calling his work "a first step in a new direction for physiology and pathology," he dealt in turn with several diseases and showed them to be caused by a lack of essential foodstuffs. He described nutritional defects in infants and deficiency diseases in cattle and discussed the chemistry of growth and the role of the vitamins in growth and metabolism. His book opened the way for many advances in preventive and therapeutic medicine.

During World War I, Funk emigrated to the United States and worked in the laboratories of various hospitals in New York, including Cornell Medical College. He went back to Europe after the war and there carried on biochemical research in the pharmaceutical industry. In a pharmaceutical laboratory in Paris, he began a study of sex hormones and was the first to detect and measure appreciable quantities of male hormone in the urine of men. This proved to be one of the basic developments in the isolation of sex hormones.

After returning to the United States again in 1927, he remained in industry for the rest of his professional career, filling part-time or full-time positions with various chemical and pharmaceutical companies.

Casimir Funk. *Die Vitamine: ihre Bedeutung für die Physiologie und Pathologie. . . .* Wiesbaden, 1914.

Funk's pigeon before and after treatment with yeast vitamins. The dramatic change occurred within eight hours after the bird had received the complex of B vitamins found in yeast.

It stimulates osteogenesis; whereas the metal, when used, furnishes only temporary fixation and inhibits osteogenesis in its immediate vicinity, exposes the parts to infection, and in certain instances contributes to the necessity of a subsequent operation for amputation or the removal of the offending metal.

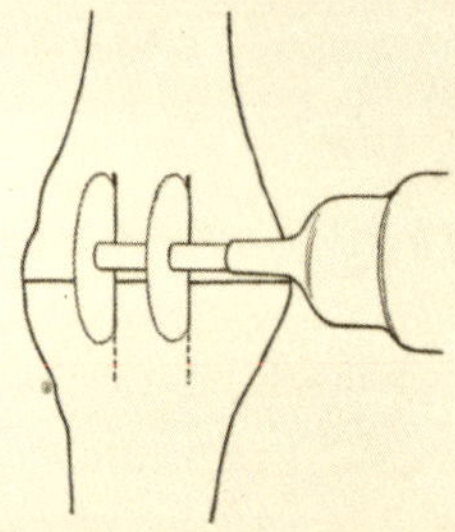

Fig. 214.—Twin saw-cuts to form gutter for inlay graft after wedge has been removed as shown in Fig. 213.

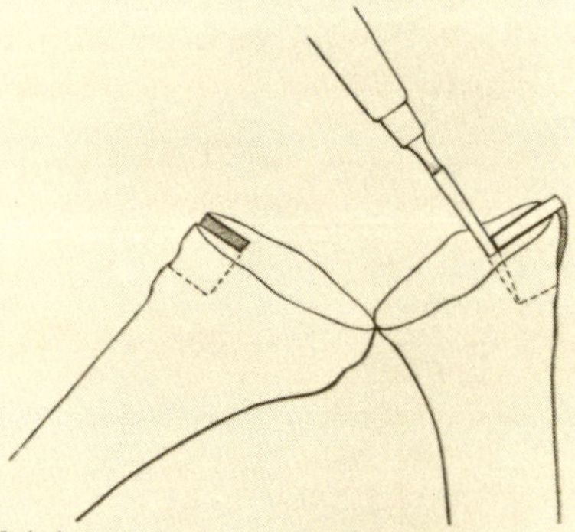

Fig. 215.—Method of removing strips of bone between twin saw-cuts to form gutter for inlay graft.

## THE USE OF THE BONE GRAFT FOR STIFFENING THE KNEE-JOINT IN INFANTILE PARALYSIS

Extensive or partial paralysis of the muscles controlling the knee-joint often causes instability to such a degree that the

# Fred Houdlett Albee

## BONE-GRAFT SURGERY

Fred Albee (1876-1945), professor of orthopedic surgery at the New York Postgraduate Medical School, was a pioneer in introducing living bone-graft surgery. As a boy, he had helped his grandfather graft fruit trees; from him Albee acquired a knowledge of the remarkable restorative capacity of a graft as well as the talent for exactitude and precision that characterized the brilliant work of his professional career. Another boyhood fascination was machinery, especially sawmills. At the age of nine, he improvised a water-driven rotary saw that was not refined enough to cut wood but did an excellent job on rutabagas. Eventually, this ingenious device formed the basis for the electrically powered Albee bone mill, which permitted rapid and accurate bone cuts under sterile conditions in the operating room.

Albee's bone-grafting technique was a striking improvement over the earlier methods for stabilizing fractures and encouraging osteosynthesis that had been introduced by Sir William Arbuthnot Lane in London between 1894 and 1907. Albee's work was developed on a large scale in the United States, Austria, and England only after World War I.

His clinical achievement was founded on extensive experiments on animals (chiefly dogs and sheep) and careful study of his predecessors' work and records. He began to apply his results in surgical practice in 1911, when he transplanted a piece of tibia into the spine of a patient with Pott's disease.

*Bone-Graft Surgery* outlines his principles and techniques and describes his cutting machines and special saws. It deals in detail with bone grafts for repairing lesions of the spine and in fractures, remodeling or ankylosing the hip joint, fixation by inlay of tuberculous joints, infantile paralysis, and osteoarthropathy. Albee also described his wedge graft for habitual dislocation of the patella and the use of grafts in diseases and deformities of the foot and leg, with an addendum of "miscellaneous uses." Twenty-five years later, he surveyed his experiences in a revised edition of this book.

Fred Houdlett Albee. *Bone-Graft Surgery*. Philadelphia, 1915.

Albee's innovative bone-grafting techniques were simply and clearly explained by text and diagrams. Specially designed tools were of his own invention.

To Mr. Lilly.
Compliments
of
F. G. Banting.

LES PRIX NOBEL

EN 1924—1925

# DIABETES AND INSULIN

Nobel Lecture delivered at Stockholm on
September 15th 1925

By

FREDERICK G. BANTING

STOCKHOLM 1925
IMPRIMERIE ROYALE. P. A. NORSTEDT & FILS

# J. J. R. Macleod and F. G. Banting

## THE ANTIDIABETIC FUNCTIONS OF THE PANCREAS...AND INSULIN

Banting and Best's discovery in 1922 of insulin, the antidiabetic pancreatic hormone, was the dramatic climax to a long search. Frederick Grant Banting (1891-1941) conceived an idea for achieving pancreatic control of diabetes almost by chance while working at London, Ontario, in 1920. J. J. R. Macleod (1876-1935), professor of physiology at the University of Toronto, an authority on carbohydrate metabolism, thought the problem intractable, because he knew of the unsuccessful research of workers in previous decades. Nevertheless, in May, 1921, he gave Banting financial support and laboratory space at the university and appointed Charles H. Best, a graduate student, to assist him. By August, they had produced a pancreatic extract that controlled the diabetes of a depancreatized dog; by January, 1922, they had made a crude extract from beef pancreas, and clinical trials had begun in human subjects.

Macleod called in J. B. Collip, who contributed his biochemical expertise to purifying the new extract. Production of insulin in quantities suitable for clinical use was begun by American scientists in the laboratories of Eli Lilly and Company, and the practical treatment of diabetes was at hand.

The first report on insulin research appeared in an article by Banting and Best in the February, 1922, issue of the *Journal of Laboratory and Clinical Medicine,* and other journal articles followed. In January, 1923, Macleod and Banting recounted the history of the discovery in the Beaumont lectures given before the Wayne County Medical Society in Detroit, and these were published as a small book the next year. The first, delivered by Professor Macleod, was a historical review. It traced the development of knowledge about the pancreas from 1682 to the current time. The second lecture, also by Macleod, reviewed the Toronto laboratory experiments that led to the trial of insulin in man. The third and final lecture was given by Dr. Banting. After detailing aspects of the animal studies, he reported on the first clinical use of insulin in diabetic patients.

Banting and Macleod were awarded a Nobel Prize in 1923. Banting shared his portion of the prize with Dr. Best, and Macleod divided his with Collip.

The Lilly Library at Indiana University contains an outstanding collection assembled by J. K. Lilly, Jr., of early papers concerning this successful research.

J. J. R. Macleod and F. G. Banting. *The Antidiabetic Functions of the Pancreas and the Successful Isolation of the Antidiabetic Hormone—Insulin.* London, 1923.

This copy of Banting's Nobel Lecture of 1925, with its inscription, is a prized item in the Lilly Library's fine collection of historical documents relating to the discovery and development of insulin.

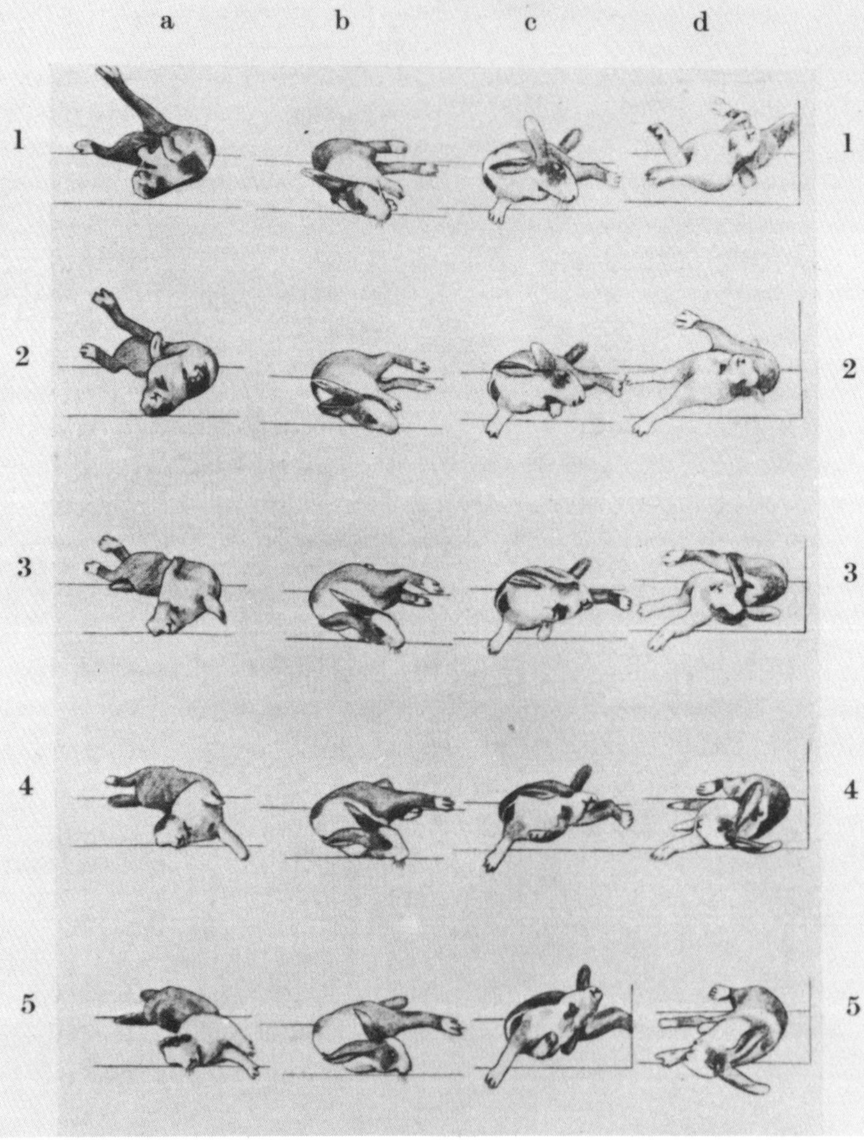

# Rudolf Magnus

## BODY POSITION

Magnus (1873-1927), who was born in Brunswick, Germany, became professor at Utrecht in the Netherlands in 1908 at the age of thirty-five and founded the Institute of Pharmacology there. His work on the neurophysiologic effects of toxic drugs led him to study the nervous control of posture. Inspired by Sir Charles Sherrington, he concentrated his research on the maintenance of balance in the animal and human body and on reaction to movements, such as rotation.

In the 1820's, Flourens had demonstrated the role of the semicircular canals in maintaining equilibrium. A dual function of the inner ear, with its different receptors for hearing and for balancing, had been suggested by earlier workers. Magnus, however, firmly established that the entire control of balance is situated in the middle ear.

*Körperstellung* ("Body Position") was a result of some fifteen years of research in Magnus's laboratory. Many of his approximately one hundred and fifty papers had been published in *Pfleuger Archiv,* and he also summarized his work in several distinguished lectures.

This notable monograph on body posture consists of twelve fully illustrated chapters. It reported on the extensive experiments by which Magnus gathered comparative and human neurologic evidence for his conclusions. After a survey of the problems, he discussed posture, balance, compensatory eye movements, postural reflexes, conditions after extirpation of the labyrinth on one side, conditions after double labyrinth extirpation, labyrinth reflexes in progressive movements, the functions of the otoliths, centers of balance, effect of poisons, and postural reflexes in newborn animals. Magnus's observations and conclusions proved to be of the greatest importance for understanding how ever-faster movement, particularly flight, can disturb balance. He laid a foundation for studying weightlessness in extra-atmospheric exploration.

Magnus's intellectual versatility found expression in a series of outstanding lectures on Goethe as a scientist. During World War I, he served in German army hospitals and after the war coordinated research on the treatment of victims of chemical warfare. He enlarged the Institute of Pharmacology at Utrecht with financial assistance from the Rockefeller Foundation in the United States. Numerous honors were bestowed on him by scientific societies and institutions in six countries.

Rudolf Magnus. *Körperstellung, experimentell-physiologische Untersuchungen über die einzelnen bei der Körperstellung in Tätigkeit tretenden Reflexe, über ihr Zusammenwirken und ihre Störungen.* Berlin, 1924.

The rolling movements of experimental animals that had been subjected to middle-ear surgery. The drawings show disturbances in equilibrium, righting, and balance.

content of crude brew at Oxford with the medium and strain of fungus then in use was about 1 to 2 units per ml. Sixty per cent. of this might be lost during extraction and purification, so that on the evidence then available every case of severe sepsis might need the brewing and processing of as much as 2,000 litres of medium. It appeared therefore that the cost would be high and the number of cases that could be treated by parenteral injection would be few. Dr. Richards deserves great credit for his courage in deciding to recommend the expenditure of large sums of government money on the project of producing penicillin, for his decision rested in the first instance on the experimental results and the few clinical trials from Oxford, and on the opinion of the Oxford workers that synthesis of penicillin in the near future did not appear to be likely. In October and December 1941 initial meetings were held under the chairmanship of Dr. Vannevar Bush at which, amongst others, representatives of manufacturing companies were present. At these meetings plans were made for the distribution of work on penicillin in its various aspects. Penicillin became available to the Committee on Medical Research in March 1942 and during the rest of that year a total of 122 million units was supplied. At the time of Florey's and Heatley's visit it had been expected that some of the first penicillin supplies from American manufacturers would be made available in Oxford. However, only half a million units arrived, the reasons being, in the first place, manufacturing difficulties, and in the second, with the entry of America into the war in December 1941, the appropriation by the Committee on Medical Research of all supplies for clinical trial. Although this caused much disappointment in Oxford, where arrangements had been made for further clinical trials, too high a tribute cannot be paid to the enterprise and energy with which the American manufacturing firms tackled the large-scale production of the drug. Had it not been for their efforts there would certainly not have been sufficient penicillin by D-day in Normandy in 1944 to treat all severe casualties, both British and American.

### Early production in England

In England by the beginning of 1942 small-scale production was being carried out by Imperial Chemical Industries Ltd., who supplied material for some of the clinical investigations. But the fact that so little penicillin was available from outside sources spurred the Oxford workers to further efforts. Brewing was increased and Sanders designed and, with the help of Kent, constructed a second type of extraction apparatus. This depended on mixing acidified brew with amyl acetate and breaking the emulsion so formed with a Sharples centrifuge (Figs. 95 to 98).

In September 1942 Kemball, Bishop & Co. Ltd. began to take part in production. They brewed the material in London and brought the crude brew in 150 to 200 gallon lots in milk churns to Oxford, where it was put through the extraction plant. To preserve the penicillin from destruction by bacteria in transit a small amount of formalin was added to the brew. The output of Imperial Chemical Industries Ltd. increased too, though by present-day standards the amount produced was minute.

### Second series of clinical trials in England

By the beginning of January 1942 enough material had been collected to

# Sir Howard Florey
## and associates
## ANTIBIOTICS

The introduction of penicillin was the most dramatic advance in the treatment of infectious disease since Jenner's cowpox vaccine. In 1921, Alexander Fleming identified lysozyme, a valuable antibacterial enzyme that is present in many animal tissues. He made a second and even more historic discovery eight years later, when he observed the inhibiting effect of the mold *Penicillium* on bacterial growth. Unfortunately, he failed to stabilize its extracts sufficiently for any practical application beyond laboratory use.

Howard Florey, professor of pathology at Oxford, selected Fleming's penicillin for special study in 1938 when, with the help of the biochemist Ernst B. Chain, he began an intensive search for antibacterial agents. They purified penicillin and found it so promising that they devoted their whole laboratory to the production of material for clinical trials. These succeeded dramatically in 1941. In the urgency of war demands, Florey turned to his American friends for large-scale development. The next thirty months saw an unprecedented coalition of the industrial, academic, and governmental research facilities of two countries (see facing page). By 1944, penicillin was being produced in quantities sufficient for treating the casualties of World War II, and soon after this it was available for nonmilitary clinical use.

Florey, Chain, and Fleming were awarded the Nobel Prize in 1945 for their significant contribution to medicine. It is interesting that, during the 1950's, at Florey's suggestion, the Oxford laboratories pioneered in the discovery and development of the cephalosporin family of antibiotics.

In this great two-volume survey, *Antibiotics,* Florey and his team reviewed the first decade of their achievement. There is a historical review by Florey himself and an account of the team's methods. Other chapters describe the many antibiotics derived from natural sources and discuss their modes of action on bacteria. Eighty-four pages of bibliographic citations of journal articles on antibiotics are included. More than half of volume two is devoted to penicillin.

As a sequel, Florey edited a four-volume *Clinical Application of Antibiotics,* published from 1952 to 1961, on other antibacterials.

The multiauthored text of *Antibiotics* marks a significant change in medical literature. The rapid proliferation of scientific data and specialized journals in addition to technical advances leading to prompt printing and dissemination has revolutionized the spread of information. Journal articles have become the medium by which discoveries are announced, and now it must be said that the days of the great single "notable medical books" have almost come to an end.

H. W. Florey, E. Chain, N. G. Heatley, M. A. Jennings, A. G. Sanders, E. P. Abraham, and M. E. Florey. *Antibiotics. A Survey of Penicillin, Streptomycin, and Other Antimicrobial Substances from Fungi, Actinomycetes, Bacteria, and Plants.* 2 vols. London, 1949.

On this page of the monumental *Antibiotics,* tribute was paid to the pharmaceutical industry for its role in supplying penicillin to the wounded of World War II.

# Index of Authors

Acknowledgments

Mr. LeFanu and the editors wish to acknowledge their indebtedness for help in the preparation of this book to a number of individuals, institutions, graphic print services, and published resource materials.

In Mr. LeFanu's words, "I owe a debt of gratitude to my old friend Mr. John Carter who invited me many years ago on behalf of Mr. J. K. Lilly, Jr., to compile the list of two hundred key books in medical literature; to the late Mr. David Randall, the Lilly Librarian, for very kindly suggesting a collaboration with him in a study of Mr. Lilly's medical books; to Mr. Randall's notable catalog published by the Lilly Library, *Medicine, An Exhibition of Books Relating to Medicine and Surgery from the Collection Formed by J. K. Lilly*; and to the authorities and librarians of several libraries in London, in particular the British Museum, the Royal Society of Medicine, the Wellcome Institute for the History of Medicine, and most of all the Royal College of Surgeons of England."

Many of the illustrations have been reproduced directly from the original books in the Lilly Library. Other sources of illustrations include the following:

The Bettmann Archive, Inc., New York—illustrations for Auenbrugger, Boerhaave, Boyle, Cadogan, Drake, von Liebig, Lind, Mesmer, Nightingale, Osler, Röntgen, Semmelweis, Simpson, Stokes, Underwood, and Wenckebach.

Indiana University Art Museum—illustration for Freud.

The National Library of Medicine, Washington, D. C., with the assistance of Ms. Lucinda Keister—illustrations for Avicenna, Bichat, Cesalpino, Corvisart, Dioscorides, Fracastoro, von Graefe, von Haller, Holt, Kircher, Pott, Ramazzini, Ricord, Rokitansky, and Virchow.

Professor Laignel-Larastine, Editor: *Histoire générale de la médecine, de la pharmacie, de l'art dentaire et de l'art vétérinaire*, 3 vols. Paris: Albin Michel Editeur, 1949—illustration for Hahnemann.

The Rockefeller University Archives, courtesy of the New York Academy of Medicine—illustration for Noguchi.

In preparation of the biographical essays, the following books have been helpful:

J. F. Fulton: *Selected Readings in the History of Physiology*, Ed. 2 (completed by L. G. Wilson). Springfield, Ill.: Charles C Thomas, Publisher, 1966.

Fielding H. Garrison: *An Introduction to the History of Medicine*, Ed. 4. Philadelphia: W. B. Saunders Company, 1929.

C. C. Gillispie, Editor: *Dictionary of Scientific Biography*. New York: Charles Scribner's Sons, 1970.

Leslie T. Morton: *Garrison and Morton's Medical Bibliography*, Ed. 2. London: Grafton and Co., 1954.

John H. Talbott: *A Biographical History of Medicine*. New York: Grune & Stratton, Inc., 1970.

John L. Thornton: *Medical Books, Libraries and Collectors*, Ed. 2. London: André Deutsch, 1966.